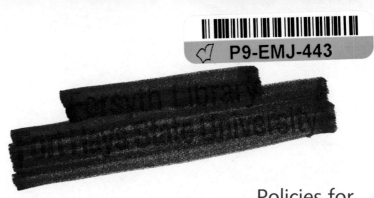
Policies for

an Aging Society

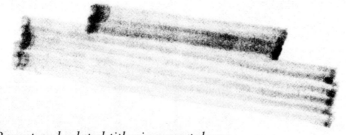

Recent and related titles in gerontology:

Robert H. Binstock, Leighton E. Cluff, and Otto von Mering, eds. *The Future of Long-Term Care: Social and Policy Issues*

Robert H. Binstock, Stephen G. Post, and Peter J. Whitehouse, eds. *Dementia and Aging: Ethics, Values, and Policy Choices*

Leighton E. Cluff and Robert H. Binstock, eds. *The Lost Art of Caring: A Challenge to Health Professionals, Families, Communities, and Society*

Tom Hickey, Marjorie A. Speers, and Thomas R. Prohaska, eds. *Public Health and Aging*

Robert B. Hudson, ed. *The Future of Age-Based Public Policy*

Leslie C. Walker, Elizabeth H. Bradley, and Terrie Wetle, eds. *Public and Private Responsibilities in Long-Term Care: Finding the Balance*

Joseph White. *False Alarm: Why the Greatest Threat to Social Security and Medicare Is the Campaign to "Save" Them*

ROBERT H. BINSTOCK, *Consulting Editor in Gerontology*

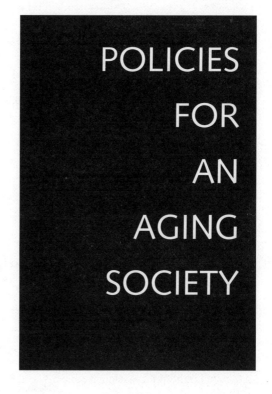

POLICIES FOR AN AGING SOCIETY

Edited by

Stuart H. Altman & David I. Shactman

THE JOHNS HOPKINS UNIVERSITY PRESS
Baltimore & London

© 2002 The Johns Hopkins University Press
All rights reserved. Published 2002
Printed in the United States of America on acid-free paper
9 8 7 6 5 4 3 2 1

The Johns Hopkins University Press
2715 North Charles Street
Baltimore, Maryland 21218-4363
www.press.jhu.edu

Library of Congress Cataloging-in-Publication Data

Policies for an aging society / edited by Stuart H. Altman and
David I. Shactman.
    p. ; cm.
Includes bibliographic references and index.
  ISBN 0-8018-6907-2 (pbk. : alk. paper)
    1. Aged—Government policy—United States 2. Aged—Services for—United
States. 3. Aged—Medical care—United States. 4. Health care reform—United
States. 5. Health policy—United States. 6. United States—Social policy.
7. United States—Economic policy.
    [DNLM: 1. Health Services for the Aged—economics—United States—
Congresses. 2. Health Care Reform—United States—Congresses. 3. Health
Policy—United States—Congresses. 4. Social Responsibility—United States—
Congresses. WT 31 P766 2002] I. Altman, Stuart H. II. Shactman, David.
  HQ1064.U5 P62 2002
  362.6'0973—dc21   2001004975

A catalog record for this book is available from the British Library.

Copyright in this book excludes the work of Paul N. Van de Water, which he
performed as an employee of the U.S. government.

Contents

Preface

This book addresses the challenges of providing health and income security to the aging U.S. population. It focuses on economic and budget challenges as well as policy options and political constraints. Changes in some of these areas raise the question of the value and accuracy of this material over time.

Those of us attuned to the policy debates in Washington tend to focus on the short term. Indeed, short-term economic forecasts are frequently revised according to changes in economic growth or the passage of legislation, such as the tax bill of 2001. But such changes, unless they are unusually large or particularly long in duration, seldom have a substantial effect on long-term projections.

This volume goes to press shortly after the tragic events of September 11, 2001. In the short term, the impact of those events will result in a slower rate of economic growth than was previously projected and a shift in resource allocation toward increased expenditures for defense and homeland security. But although the short-term economic outlook is less rosy than it was when these chapters were written, the long-term outlook has changed to a much lesser extent. The economic challenges of providing for an aging society are chiefly dominated by demographic trends and by the future trajectory of health expenditures.

The full consequences of the terrorist attack in September 2001 will still not be known when this collection is published, but it could affect the long-run budget outlook in several ways. First, terrorism is imposing new costs on the private economy that could reduce productivity and increase inflation. Second, the additional costs of national defense and homeland security could leave less revenue that might otherwise be "saved" for elderly entitlements by reducing the national debt. Steuerle and Van DeWater examine the sensitivity of budget projections to such increased expenditures in Chapter 4.

Whether the economic capacity to fund elderly entitlements remains approximately the same or becomes somewhat diminished in the light of the events in 2001, the policy options remain unchanged. Questions about defined benefit, defined contribution, private accounts, and the like will be at the very heart of the policy debate. In fact, if fewer resources are available to fund elderly entitlements, it will make consideration of these issues and options all the more critical.

Acknowledgments

This volume reflects the efforts of many individuals. As editors, we were most fortunate to work with an extraordinarily accomplished group of authors, many of whom are recognized internationally for leadership in their disciplines. They brought to this collection a wide variety of ideas and perspectives about how America and Americans can begin to address the challenges of an aging society.

We are particularly appreciative of the Robert Wood Johnson Foundation for both the generous funding and the inspiration for the conference that became the genesis for this book. Steven Schroeder, the president of the foundation, suggested at a meeting in the spring of 1998 that we might try to replicate the Sun Valley conference series that was held in the 1970s. The concept of the Sun Valley series was to bring together a small, multidisciplinary group of experts in a retreat setting to focus on one overriding issue of public policy.

The issue we decided on will touch the lives of each of us and our families: in an environment of constrained resources, what policies should America pursue to provide health and income security to an aging population? The Council on the Economic Impact of Health System Change, an RWJ-sponsored research group, undertook the planning for the conference. Housed at the Schneider Institute for Health Policy at the Heller School, Brandeis University, the council is a nonpartisan, educative organization that focuses on national health care policy.

The conference was held at the Lansdowne Resort and Conference Center in Lansdowne, Virginia, in October 1999. In addition to the contributing authors, this book has been enriched by the ideas and discussions raised at the conference by the following individuals: Nancy Barrand, Karen Davis, Jack Ebeler, John Hoff, Madge Kaplan, Julie Kosterlitz, Dwight McNeill, Marilyn Moon, Joseph Neel, June O'Neill, John Palmer, Martha Phillips, Uwe Reinhardt, Brian Rosman, John Rother, Dallas Salisbury, Richard Saltman, Thomas Saving, Robert Solow, Larry Thompson, Kenneth Thorpe, Stanley Wallack, Michael Weinstein, and Janet Yellen.

A special debt of gratitude is owed to the council staff members who helped plan the conference and assisted with the manuscript. In particular, Brian Rosman and Patricia Aloise were instrumental in helping to formulate this publication. Our gratitude is also extended to Ann Cummings and Mary Flynn.

Finally, but certainly not least important, the people at the Johns Hopkins University Press helped bring this project to fruition. The efforts of Wendy Harris were indispensable, and her ideas and suggestions are pervasive in this manuscript. Lois Crum performed a meticulous job of copyediting. Special thanks are also owed to Robert Binstock for his suggestions during the process of organizing this edited volume from a complex body of work.

Contributors

Henry J. Aaron, Ph.D., is Bruce and Virginia MacLaury Senior Fellow in the Economic Studies Program at the Brookings Institution, Washington, D.C. Dr. Aaron has served as Assistant Secretary for Planning and Evaluation at the Department of Health, Education, and Welfare and has chaired an Advisory Council on Social Security. He is a member of the Institute of Medicine, the American Academy of Arts and Sciences, and the advisory committee of the Stanford Institute for Economic Policy. He is currently Chairman of the Board of the National Academy of Social Insurance and is a member of the Board of Directors of Abt Associates and the Center on Budget and Policy Priorities. He is the author or coauthor of sixteen books and the editor or coeditor of fourteen others.

Stuart H. Altman, Ph.D., Sol C. Chaikin Professor of National Health Policy at the Heller School for Social Policy and Management, Brandeis University, is an economist whose research interests are primarily in the area of federal and state health policy. He has been Deputy Assistant Secretary for Planning and Evaluation/Health at the Department of Health, Education, and Welfare. He is currently Co-Chair of the Governor/Legislative Health Care Task Force for the Commonwealth of Massachusetts. Professor Altman is a member of the Institute of Medicine of the National Academy of Sciences; a member of the Board of Overseers of the Beth Israel Deaconess Medical Center, Boston; and Co-Chairman of the Board of the Schneider Institute for Health Policy at the Heller Graduate School, Brandeis University. He is the Chair of the Robert Wood Johnson Foundation–sponsored Council on the Economic Impact of Health System Change.

Robert H. Binstock, Ph.D., is Professor of Aging, Health, and Society at Case Western Reserve University. A former president of the Gerontological Society of America, he has served as director of a White House Task Force on Older Americans and as chair and member of a number of advisory panels to federal, state, and local governments and foundations. Professor Binstock is the author of more than two hundred publications on politics and policies affecting aging.

Lynn Etheredge is an independent consultant specializing in health policy and retirement issues who works with the Health Insurance Reform Project at George Washington University. Mr. Etheredge has worked extensively for the Office of Management and Budget and also in many capacities in the public and private sectors. He has participated in government, academic, and policy think tanks. Mr. Etheredge is author of more than seventy publications.

Victor R. Fuchs, Ph.D., is the Henry J. Kaiser, Jr., Professor Emeritus at Stanford University and is a Research Associate of the National Bureau of Economic Research. Dr. Fuchs's published work covers a wide spectrum of subjects ranging from health and medical care to issues of family, gender, and children. He is the author of nine books, the editor of six others, and has published more than one hundred articles.

John Geanakoplos, Ph.D., is Director of the Cowles Foundation for Research in Economics at Yale University and is an external professor in the economics program at the Santa Fe Institute. He is a fellow of the Econometric Society and of the American Academy of Arts and Sciences and is a partner in Ellington Capital Management.

Jonathan Gruber, Ph.D., is a Professor of Economics at the Massachusetts Institute of Technology. He is also the Director of the Program on Children at the National Bureau of Economic Research, a coeditor of the *Journal of Health Economics,* and an Associate Editor of the *Journal of Public Economics.* Professor Gruber has served as Deputy Assistant Secretary for Economic Policy at the Treasury Department. His research focuses on the areas of public finance and health economics. He is the author of numerous articles in journals and books.

Richard D. Lamm is Director of the Center for Public Policy and Contemporary Issues at the University of Denver. He served as the Governor of Colorado from 1975 to 1987. He was Chairman of the Pew Health Professions Commission and a public member of the Accreditation Council for Graduate Medical Education. Governor Lamm is a frequent guest on nationally televised public affairs programs and has published extensively in newspapers, magazines, and journals throughout the United States. He has written or coauthored six books.

Theodore R. Marmor, Ph.D., is a Professor of Public Policy and Management at the Yale School of Management and Professor of Political Science, Yale University. Professor Marmor is the author of numerous publications and is frequently engaged in television and radio debates and commentaries.

Jerry L. Mashaw, Ph.D., is the Sterling Professor of Law at the Yale School of Law and Professor in the Institute for Social and Policy Studies, Yale University. He is a board member of the National Academy of Social Insurance. Professor Mashaw is the author of various books and writes frequently on social welfare issues.

Olivia S. Mitchell, Ph.D., is the International Foundation of Employee Benefit Plans Professor of Insurance and Risk Management at the Wharton School of the University of Pennsylvania, where she also directs the Pension Research Council, a research center on pensions. She is a member of the National Bureau of Economic Research and is a coprincipal investigator of the Health and Retirement Study at the University of Michigan.

Alicia H. Munnell, Ph.D., is the Peter F. Drucker Professor in Management Sciences at Boston College's Carroll School of Management. She is also the Director of the Center for Retirement Research at Boston College. Professor Munnell was a member of the President's Council of Economic Advisers and served as Assistant Secretary of the U.S. Treasury for Economic Policy. Currently she serves on the boards of the National Bureau of Economic Research and the Pension Rights Center. Professor Munnell has written extensively on tax policy, Social Security, public and private pensions, and productivity.

Norman J. Ornstein, Ph.D., is a Resident Scholar at the American Enterprise Institute for Public Policy Research, Washington, D.C. He also serves as an election analyst for CBS News. Dr. Ornstein writes regularly for *USA Today* as a member of its Board of Contributors and writes a column called "Congress Inside Out" for *Roll Call* newspaper. He is a member of the Board of Directors of the Public Broadcasting System and of the Board of Trustees of the U.S. Capitol Historical Society. He has authored or coauthored several books.

Mark V. Pauly, Ph.D., holds the positions of Bendheim Professor and Chair of the Department of Health Care Systems at the Wharton School, University of Pennsylvania. He has appointments in three departments, Health Care Management, Insurance and Risk Management, and Business and Public Policy. In addition, Professor Pauly is an Associate Editor of the *Journal of Health Economics* and of the *Journal of Risk and Uncertainty*. He is an active member of the Institute of Medicine. Professor Pauly has made significant contributions to the fields of medical economics and health insurance.

Rudolph G. Penner, Ph.D., is a Senior Fellow at the Urban Institute and holds the Arjay and Frances Miller chair in public policy. Previous posts in government include Director of the Congressional Budget Office, Assistant Director for Economic Policy at the Office of Management and Budget, and Deputy Assistant Secretary for Economic Affairs at the Department of Housing and Urban Development. He is the author of numerous books, pamphlets, and articles on tax and spending policy and has authored columns for various newspapers.

Wendell E. Primus, Ph.D., is the Director of Income Security at the Center on Budget and Policy Priorities. Previously, he served as the Deputy Assistant Secretary for Human Services Policy in the Office of the Assistant Secretary for Planning and Evaluation. He was chief economist for the Committee on Ways and Means and Staff Director of the Subcommittee on Human Resources of the U.S. House of Representatives. Dr. Primus has had an extensive and varied career in the fields of government, academia, and research.

Joseph F. Quinn, Ph.D., is the Dean of the College of Arts and Sciences and Professor of Economics at Boston College. He is a founding member of the National Academy of Social Insurance and serves on the Board of Governors of the Foundation for International Studies on Social Security and on the Editorial Board of the *Review of Income and Wealth*.

David I. Shactman, M.P.A., M.B.A., is a Senior Research Associate at the Schneider Institute for Health Policy at Brandeis University and the Project Director of the Council on the Economic Impact of Health System Change. In his capacity as Director, he has been the author of numerous reports and publications. His primary research has been in the areas of hospital mergers and consolidation, access to health insurance coverage, and health policy issues for aging populations.

C. Eugene Steuerle, Ph.D., is a Senior Fellow at the Urban Institute, Washington, D.C. Among his various positions in the Treasury Department, Dr. Steuerle has served as the Deputy Assistant Secretary of the Treasury for Tax Analysis. Dr. Steuerle has published more than five hundred columns in two series: "Straight Talk on Social Security and Retirement Policy" for the Urban Institute and "Economic Perspective" for *Tax Notes Magazine*. He recently began the column "After Tax" for *Financial Times*. He is also the author, coauthor, or editor of 9 books, more than 150 reports and articles, and 45 congressional testimonies or reports.

Paul N. Van de Water, Ph.D., is Assistant Deputy Commissioner for Policy at the Social Security Administration. Previously he served as Associate Commissioner for Research, Evaluation, and Statistics at Social Security and as Assistant Director for Budget Analysis at the Congressional Budget Office. He has written extensively on Social Security, Medicare, and governmental finance and has testified before several congressional committees. Dr. Van de Water is a Woodrow Wilson Fellow and a founding member of the National Academy of Social Insurance.

Joseph White, Ph.D., is Professor of Political Science, Luxenberg Family Professor of Public Policy, and Director of the Center for Policy Studies at Case Western Reserve University. Professor White's research interests and publications have focused on federal budgeting policy and politics, Congress, health care finance, Social Security, and Medicare. He has written and coauthored numerous books and publications.

David A. Wise, Ph.D., is the Stambaugh Professor of Political Economy at the John F. Kennedy School of Government at Harvard University. He is also the Area Director of Health and Retirement Programs and Director of the Program on the Economics of Aging at the National Bureau of Economic Research and a Senior Fellow at the Hoover Institution at Stanford University. He has written extensively on the retirement incentives of defined benefit pension programs in the United States and on retirement incentives in public social security programs around the world. More recently, he has addressed the economic implications of personal retirement programs in the United States as well as other programs relating to the aging of the U.S. population.

Stephen P. Zeldes, Ph.D., is the Benjamin Rosen Professor of Economics and Finance at Columbia University's Graduate School of Business. He is a Research Associate with the National Bureau of Economic Research and a member of the board of the Pension Research Council. Professor Zeldes has served as a member of the Technical Panel on Trends and Issues in Retirement Saving, which reported to the 1994–96 Advisory Council on Social Security. He was also a member of the National Academy of Social Insurance Panel on Social Security Privatization. His research has been published in leading academic journals.

I
INTRODUCTION

Overview

Issues and Options for an Aging Population

David I. Shactman, M.P.A., M.B.A., and Stuart H. Altman, Ph.D.

The United States has entered the twenty-first century with a balanced budget and an unprecedented period of continuous economic prosperity. But like many other developed countries across the globe, it will face a difficult challenge in the future providing income and health security to an aging population. As recently as 1970, the three major programs for elderly persons (Social Security, Medicare, and Medicaid) accounted for roughly 20 percent of the total federal budget. By 1999 those programs accounted for 45 percent, and the Congressional Budget Office (1999, 2000) predicts that they will account for 68 percent by the year 2030. If Social Security, Medicare, and Medicaid consume more than two-thirds of the federal budget, where will the money come from to pay for everything else? Even with a steadily growing economy and a larger federal budget, the country will have great difficulty sustaining this kind of expenditure growth in one economic sector unless taxes are raised or spending in other areas is severely reduced.

The United States is a wealthy country. Most other developed nations have older populations and are less affluent. Yet most of them have been able to fund elderly entitlement programs that are relatively more generous than those in the United States. This raises several questions that we address in this chapter: How did the problem of funding elderly entitlements arise? Why is it difficult to get elected officials to do anything about it? And if they were to act, what kind of policy options might they consider?

HOW DID THE PROBLEM OF FUNDING ELDERLY ENTITLEMENTS COME ABOUT?

How did a wealthy country like the United States reach a point where it must apparently make painful decisions to sustain its relatively modest elderly entitlement programs? The answer chiefly lies in a combination of three factors: the nature of its entitlement programs, demographic change, and the rate of increase in health care costs.

The Nature of Entitlement Programs: Pay-as-You-Go versus Prefunding

In the case of both Social Security and Medicare, the United States has adopted pay-as-you-go social insurance systems. In such systems the working generation pays for the costs of the retired generation. The alternative is a prefunded system in which each generation sets aside sufficient money to pay for its own estimated future benefits. In a prefunded system, a large population bubble, such as the baby boomers, would set aside a sufficient amount of funds in their working years so that in their retired years there would be no shortfall for any other generation to pay. In contrast, for a pay-as-you-go system to cover the expenses of larger and larger retiring generations, increased amounts of money are required from the working generations. The situation in the United States can be compared to a private company that has promised pension benefits to retired workers but has not set aside funds to pay the benefits. That company would have an unfunded liability equal to the present value of those promised benefits. Over the life of the Social Security system, the United States has built up an unfunded liability of nearly $10 trillion (Geanakoplos, Mitchell, and Zeldes 1998). As the baby boom population retires, the working generation will have to pay for the unfunded amounts in addition to any contribution they may make toward their own retirement. The same is largely true of the Medicare program, in which the taxes of the working generation fund the Medicare costs of the retired generation.

Demographic Change

The second factor that will make it difficult for the United States to fund elderly retirement programs is the well-heralded demographic challenge arising out of the pending retirement of 76 million baby boomers. Today, one of eight Americans is over 65 years old. It is estimated that by 2060 the proportion of the population over 65 will increase by 50 percent and the proportion over 85 will triple (U.S. Bureau of the Census 1999, 25). However, estimates of demographic change and its impact on future spending are based on a number of uncertain factors, such as birthrate, average life expectancy, age-specific health status, and immigration policy.

The U.S. birthrate peaked around 1960 at 25 births per thousand population, but it fell sharply afterward before leveling out at slightly more than 14 per thousand (U.S. Bureau of the Census 1999, 75). The Congressional Budget Office (CBO) uses low-, medium-, and high-cost estimates of future population growth. The medium estimates project an approximate continuation of the current birthrate. However, if the rate was to change again at anything approaching the magnitude of change since 1960, the demographic impact would be radically different. The high-cost estimates by CBO would result in roughly a doubling of the projected budget shortfall, whereas the low-cost estimates would eliminate the projected deficit entirely. A change in the birthrate would not have an impact on the amount spent on elderly persons until late in the century, since those retiring before 2065 have already been born. But it would have a significant impact on the number of workers available to support the growing elderly population.

Life expectancy also influences demographic projections. In the United States it has been increasing steadily, having risen from 70.8 years in 1970 to an estimated 76.4 in 2000 (U.S. Bureau of the Census 1999, 93). The increase in life expectancy is projected to continue at a rate of roughly one month every two years. Together, the birthrate, life expectancy, and immigration determine what is known as the *dependency ratio:* the ratio of the number of working-age people (age 20–64) to the number of retirees (people over age 65). In 1960 there were 5.1 workers to each beneficiary, but today there are 3.4 workers to each beneficiary, and that number is expected to fall to 2.1 by the year

2040 (see chapter 4). The dependency ratio is a useful measure because it indicates the potential burden on the younger generation to support the elderly.

A number of researchers believe that longevity might increase considerably faster in the years ahead because of revolutionary progress in biotechnology and genomics. The impact of greater longevity on the cost of retirement programs is somewhat uncertain, depending on another important factor—age-specific health status. In the past, increases in longevity meant longer retirement periods and increased Social Security payments, along with declining health status and increased medical costs. This is still the case, but two factors may be changing, partly as a result of improved age-specific health status. First, the long-term trend toward earlier retirement appears to have reversed itself. Research by Joseph Quinn (1999) shows that the average retirement age declined steadily in the United States from age 70 in 1950 to age 62 in 1985, but since 1985 the average retirement age has actually increased. Recent changes in the Social Security program to remove any implicit penalties for working past retirement age could strengthen this apparent trend. It is too early to state definitively whether this is a one-time change or a reversal in the long-term trend, but later retirement would reduce the shortfall in the Social Security trust fund.

The second factor affecting the economic impact of improved health status is the long-term decline in age-specific disability. Research by Kenneth Manton has indicated that age-specific disability rates for elderly Americans declined by approximately 1.5 percent per year between 1982 and 1994 (Singer and Manton 1998). Manton contends that this rate of decline will continue over the next seventy years as the capabilities of medicine continue to expand. A healthier elderly population would likely lead to longer work lives and later retirement ages, consistent with the findings by Quinn. It could also lead to what is called a *compression of morbidity*, in which individuals experience good health throughout their elderly years until nearly the time of death. Such a change would have significant implications for elderly medical costs, since chronic disease and disability now account for a large portion of total health costs. All of this is somewhat speculative, because most advances in medical technology are still "cost-increasing," and medical spending still increases significantly as individuals age.

In total, many uncertainties affect demographic projections and their impact on elderly expenditures. These uncertainties affect the extent but not the overall direction of future spending caused by demographic change. What is certain is that one of the chief reasons why a wealthy country such as the United States confronts challenges in funding its elderly security programs is the steep rate of aging of the population that will begin after the year 2010.

The Rate of Increase in Health Care Inflation

In addition to program structure and demographics, a third factor influencing the difficulty of providing for an aging society is the rate of increase in health care spending. The United States saw medical expenditures, as a proportion of gross domestic product (GDP), rise steadily throughout the second half of the twentieth century. Total health expenditures as a proportion of GDP rose from 5.1 percent in 1960 to approximately 14 percent today (Levit et al. 1998, 100). During the same time, the government share of health care spending nearly doubled, from 25 percent to almost 50 percent (107). Although some of the increase can be attributed to the organization and financing mechanisms that make up the U.S. health care system, most analysts now agree that technology is the most important driver of health care costs. Newhouse (1993) estimates that advances in health care technology account for up to 50 percent of health care inflation. A disproportionate amount of health expenditures occurs near or at the end of life, so an older population has a large impact on health expenditures. Fuchs (1998) projects that if medical spending on elderly persons continues to increase at past rates, it could reach 10 percent of GDP by the year 2020—more than double what it was in 1995. Not all analysts agree with Fuchs's conclusion. Those who support the compression-of-morbidity theory believe that some of the future technological advances in medicine will be cost-reducing. They contend that some of the "halfway technologies" of today that treat symptoms (e.g., chemotherapy, insulin) will be replaced by "full technologies" that fully cure or even prevent particular diseases. As a result, they argue, the long-range growth rate in health care costs will be reduced. Although some are optimistic that these predictions will eventually become reality, there is little evidence that technological advances will reduce cost any time soon. Hence, the historical rate of health care inflation is likely to continue, and the Medicare program will be more difficult to finance in the long term than Social Security.

As a result of these three forces, even a wealthy country such as the United States faces a challenge in funding its future elderly entitlement programs. Long-term projections by CBO indicate that if the United States follows current policies, spending will eventually outpace revenue. If no corrective action is taken, annual deficits will ultimately balloon and wreak havoc on the economy.

WHY IS IT DIFFICULT FOR ELECTED OFFICIALS TO ACT?

With ample time to prepare, one might expect that legislators would seek to restructure the financing or the spending on future elderly entitlements. However, a number of factors make political action difficult. Perhaps the most significant is the degree of uncertainty inherent in long-term projections. It is difficult to bring individuals with a wide array of perspectives to consensus under normal circumstances, but it is all the more difficult when they do not agree on the underlying data. Since economic projections can differ substantially, political factions can use different projections either to support their particular ideological position or to oppose those of the other party.

Policy change becomes even more difficult when the problem under consideration is far away. This is clearly relevant in the case of Medicare and Social Security, both of which are now accumulating surpluses in their trust funds. Current projections show that the Medicare and Social Security trust funds will not be depleted until approximately 2028 and 2038, respectively. Given those projections, it is hard for elected officials to resist spending some of the surplus funds on politically popular spending programs or tax reductions, actions that will exacerbate the long-term problem. Asking legislators who are up for reelection in two years to make short-term sacrifices now for benefits that will not accrue for thirty to forty years is a very difficult proposition. Given the political dangers inherent in reforming these popular entitlement programs, it is no wonder that legislators have thus far largely avoided taking action on these issues.

The existing political alignment also augurs strongly against change. We currently see a president who was narrowly elected despite losing the popular vote, an evenly divided Senate, a slim Republican majority in the House, high congressional turnover, weak leadership, and sharp ideological divisions between the two major parties. The collective impact of these factors makes any legislative action difficult, particularly if it requires a large degree of consensus building and cooperation.

To make matters more difficult, policymakers, depending on their ideological beliefs, recommend a wide variety of potential solutions. Those on the liberal end primarily want to avoid cutting the budgets of entitlement programs. Hence, they argue that "demography is not destiny" and seize on the uncertainty issue. They oppose taking actions that may not be necessary if economic best-case scenarios play out. Many in this camp advocate the use of budget surpluses to increase access to entitlements. Political factions on the center-left are also concerned about program cuts, but they worry that if changes are not enacted now to ease the budget shortfall, the adjustment will eventually be so steep that adequate funding will be impossible to secure. Many in these groups would support gradual tax increases to prolong the solvency of the trust funds. Those on the center-right also frequently support the need for current action. However, their concern is focused on avoiding deficits or eventual tax increases. Organizations such as the Concord Coalition or the Committee for a Responsible Federal Budget would fall into this category. They tend to support spending curbs or program restructuring that would result in lower spending. Also on the right, especially among those who are more conservative, are proponents of tax cuts. They believe that the government should return surplus taxes to the taxpayers and that sufficient money will remain to fund entitlement programs, particularly if those programs are reformed to become more efficient. Many conservatives, as well as others across the political spectrum, would comprehensively restructure entitlement programs for reasons ranging from economic efficiency to political ideology.

Given these widespread differences among policymakers along with the uncertainty of economic projections and the long-term nature of the problem, it is a difficult climate in which elected officials must act. Nonetheless, as the financing problem gets closer at hand and the public becomes better informed of the issues, there will be increasing pressure on elected officials to set forth what Lynn Etheredge calls a "national retirement policy." In so doing, a wide variety of policy options might be considered.

WHAT ARE THE POLICY OPTIONS TO CONSIDER?

In the most general sense, the potential policy options are quite straightforward. To fund our current entitlement programs over the long term, we must eventually choose one or more of the following options:

1. Take no action and depend on the growth of the economy to generate sufficient revenues to fund future needs.
2. Increase spending on elderly persons without a proportional tax increase and allow budget deficits.
3. Raise taxes and increase spending for elderly entitlement programs.
4. Raise elderly spending and reduce spending in other government-supported areas, such as defense, environment, housing, and education.
5. Restructure current elderly entitlement programs, reducing their size and scope or increasing their efficiency, or both.

The first four options are basically political decisions based on economic and budget projections and on national spending priorities. They are inherently dependent on projected revenue flows (taxes), projected spending on elderly entitlements, economic growth, and the economic impact of increased budget deficits or decreased levels of national debt. Although economic projections are subject to much uncertainty, they stake out the parameters of the long-term budget problem. They provide the context for the political debate and policy decisions that must follow.

We devote the first part of this volume to an overview of the issues related to providing health and income security to an aging population. Entitlement spending in the United States is examined and is then compared with that of other industrialized countries. Part 2 examines and analyzes current U.S. economic and budget projections. We address basic questions such as, What is the likelihood that the economy will grow fast enough to pay for future elderly entitlement programs? How large is the estimated budget shortfall? How large a tax increase would be necessary to avoid the shortfall, and what impact would such a tax increase have on the economy? What would be the likely impact of paying for increased entitlements with deficit spending? What would be the impact on discretionary spending if entitlements continue to grow as expected?

Much of the current debate concerns programmatic alternatives. Neither raising taxes nor cutting elderly entitlement programs is a popular course of action. Hence, policymakers seek to find more attractive options. Reforming or restructuring entitlement programs to make them more cost-effective is a win-win alternative. But reforming universal social programs such as Social Security and Medicare has economic, philosophical, and political repercussions. An analysis of the major programmatic alternatives is presented in part 3. We consider universal versus means-tested programs, defined benefit versus defined contribution, private individual accounts versus public trust funds, and prefunding versus pay-as-you-go; we look at diversifying investments to include equities, providing incentives for longer work lives, and aligning incentives across entitlement programs.

In the final part, we view the potential policy options in the context of the current political environment. What political elements must ordinarily be present for elected officials to undertake major program reform? Given the current political climate, what is the likely potential for significant reform in the near term?

The purpose of this volume is to set forth the issues that must be considered as the United States confronts the challenges of providing for an aging population. Although economics provides much of the context, it is also important to focus on the programmatic and the political. In so doing, political science and social philosophy are fundamental. We refrain from recommending any particular set of policies or supporting any political philosophy. Because this book is primarily organized to be used as a textbook, we have attempted to present a balanced and wide range of perspectives from experts of various political persuasions. Hence, many of the chapters are consecutively paired with opposing viewpoints and can be assigned together to provide a comprehensive understanding of different issues. Our intention is to offer an objective source of knowledge, so that students, policymakers, public affairs professionals, and ordinary citizens will be able to better assess the challenges we face as we determine how to provide for an older population.

A SYNOPSIS OF THE CHAPTERS

"The single most important long-run fiscal issue facing the developed world is the aging of its populations." Beginning with that provocative statement, Jonathan Gruber and David Wise provide us with an international perspective on policies for an aging society. They point out that all developed countries provide guaranteed income support and health insurance coverage to their elderly citizens. As populations have aged in these countries, the response of their governments has been simply to increase spending on elderly persons. For example, between 1980 and 1995, when the percentage of the population over age 65 in OECD countries increased by 20 percent, those countries raised their spending on elderly persons by 25 percent. The authors estimate that if current trends hold in these countries, average elderly spending (excluding health services) as a proportion of GDP will rise from 8.2 percent today to 11.4 percent by 2050, an increase of nearly 40 percent. Funding such increases will be a significant economic challenge.

Gruber and Wise compare U.S. spending on elderly persons with spending in other selected OECD countries. In terms of income replacement, the U.S. Social Security program is rather modest. At early retirement age, which is 62 in the United States but 60 in the other sample countries, the U.S. program replaces 41 percent of income. That is the lowest percentage replaced by any OECD country except for Canada and far less than is replaced by France and the Netherlands, where it is 91 percent. In terms of its national income, spending on elderly programs is fairly modest compared to that of other developed nations. Of the thirteen OECD countries examined by Gruber and Wise, the United States ranks in the lower third, spending about 8.4 percent of GDP on elderly persons, compared to an average of 10.9 percent among the thirteen countries (including health care).

Given that other countries in the developed world are spending a greater proportion of their wealth on elderly persons and that this proportion is expected to rise, the authors next ask what they are getting for their money. They draw the following conclusions. First, those countries that provide a strong monetary incentive to retire early find that their workers do retire earlier and, hence, they displace private earnings with public dollars. Second, they conclude that overall there is little relation between the wealth of elderly persons and the amount of spending on elderly entitlements. However, the overall impact of social spending on wealth masks important differences across income classes. Public benefits to wealthier people have simply replaced private funds they otherwise would have provided themselves. But public benefits to poorer recipients have helped significantly in keeping them out of poverty. Third, they find that OECD countries did not increase total spending as their population aged but simply reduced spending on the younger generations. On average, they reduced spending on the nonelderly 0.33 percent for every 1 percent increase in the elderly population. Concluding as provocatively as they began, the authors state that "if current trends continue, the brunt of the burden of an aging society will be borne through reduced spending elsewhere, including spending on the nonelderly."

With the benefit of an international perspective, we turn to part 2 of the book, on the U.S. economic and budget framework. Henry Aaron provides an overall context warning about the uncertainties inherent in long-term projections and the limitations of using them to formulate policy. According to Aaron, long-range budget projections are valuable because they restrain legislators from spending money in the future, when both the legislators and the money may no longer be around. The projections may also be effective in "goading" lawmakers to enact otherwise unpopular or unpleasant reforms. But in regard to policies affecting the major entitlement programs, Aaron is clear about their limitations, contending that projections of long-term deficits tell us only a little of value in reforming the structure of these programs.

Aaron formulates two major questions about long-term budget projections: What do we know that is reliably certain, in the face of uncertainty? and How should long-term projections be employed to influence policy? Economic and political conditions fluctuate considerably over time, he warns, and the consequence of policy changes can be deleterious and long lasting because, once effected, they are difficult to undo. He suggests that we often know the direction but not the magnitude of change. For example, if productivity increases by 0.5 percent annually, incomes will be 29 percent higher by the year 2050. A larger but plausible increase in productivity of 1.5 percent annually, however, would increase incomes by 114 percent by 2050, engendering an entirely different set of budget projections and policy responses.

How should we act in the face of such uncertainty? Citing work by Auerbach and Hassett, Aaron concludes that uncertainty should not justify procrastinating with regard to financing policies such as actions to close a projected deficit. However, he contends, most of the policy debate is not about financing but about structure.

According to Aaron, most potential structural changes in Social Security and Medicare have little or nothing to do with budget projections. In the case of Social Security, he identifies four major structural issues: private accounts versus a public trust fund; defined benefit versus defined contribution; investment in equities as well as government bonds; and prefunding versus pay-as-you-go. He argues that the advantages and disadvantages of the first three do not depend on budget projections and can be debated independently of long-term projections. Only the decision whether or not, or how much, to prefund, is closely tied to budget estimates.

Aaron sums up by reiterating the usefulness of long-term budget and economic projections and the importance of fiscal policy as part of the larger domain of public policy. But "fiscal policy," he concludes, "is not health policy and . . . is not pension policy."

Having been forewarned about the limitations of long-term projections, we examine the details of how they are formulated. Eugene Steuerle and Paul Van de Water provide a comprehensive explanation of current economic and budget estimates and their sensitivity to changes in underlying factors. Steuerle and Van de Water begin by summarizing the current budget outlook. Under the October 2000 baseline assumptions (with no new tax cuts or spending programs), the U.S. economy will yield large surpluses over the next twenty years. However, as entitlement expenses for the baby boomers kick in, the budget will go into deficit by 2028 and use up all of the accrued surpluses by

2037. Following that, debt will begin to accumulate, and with projected interest rates higher than the growth rate of the economy, debt will theoretically balloon to 100 percent of GDP by 2062—a rosy picture for the near future, but sobering over the long-run.

The authors explain, as we mentioned earlier, the high degree of uncertainty involved in these estimates. For example, the Social Security Administration makes high-, middle-, and low-cost demographic projections. Summed over the next sixty years, the difference between the high and low projections amounts to an astonishingly large number—4 percent of GDP, or more than $4 trillion. Other sources of uncertainty arise from such factors as growth in wages, interest rate levels, and policy assumptions for taxes and spending. Although the degree of uncertainty means that long-run projections are not likely to be accurate, the authors believe that these projections will "indicate the extent to which future policymakers may have to alter old promises to fit new circumstances."

The next part of the chapter deals with the crowd-out issue in the United States. Just as Gruber and Wise portrayed elderly entitlement costs reducing spending on nonelderly persons in other countries, Steuerle and Van de Water exhibit similar findings for the United States. Whereas total health and retirement costs consumed just 10 percent of the U.S. federal budget in 1950, they now consume more than half. Fortunately, in the United States, this increase was somewhat painlessly absorbed by cuts in the relative proportion of the budget spent on defense. Defense spending fell from 14 percent of GDP just after the Korean War to 3 percent today. Clearly, as the authors point out, such reductions cannot continue. Hence, further increases in health and retirement costs will have to come out of nondefense spending (or increased taxes), which is apt to engender considerably more political opposition. This has already begun to happen: Steuerle and Van de Water show that nearly every budget category is expected to decline as a proportion of GDP between 1993 and 2004. Nevertheless, one must be aware that the economy as a whole is growing, so some expenditures are growing in absolute terms even as they are shrinking as relative proportions of the budget.

In the final section of the chapter, Steuerle and Van de Water discuss potential policy alternatives in terms of their impact on budget projections. They consider three kinds of policy options: increasing savings, controlling health care costs, and increasing the supply of labor. Among these, the most predictable benefit is derived from increasing the supply of labor by encouraging longer work lives.

This chapter by Steuerle and Van de Water clarifies some of the complexities of the budget process and focuses on the value, importance, and sensitivities of long-range projections. It provides a context from which readers can consider the economic impact of general changes in tax and spending policies and specific changes in entitlement programs.

The next two chapters provide differing perspectives on the long-term budget projections and their implications for policy. Wendell Primus is relatively optimistic about funding future elderly entitlements, provided that the political debate does not become too polarized. Primus does not think the economy would have a major problem adjusting to a rise in spending on the order of a few percentage points over a number of years. He gives examples of previous adjustments of that magnitude, including a 3 percent rise in government spending as a proportion of GDP between 1965 and 1968.

Primus supports prefunding future deficits by accumulating surpluses and "paying for" any new spending or tax reductions by reducing existing spending or adding new revenue. Using the Social Security surpluses to reduce government debt, he explains, will result in increased savings and investment and produce a larger economy and lower interest rates over time. The additional revenues generated can help alleviate the future entitlement deficit.

The converse is also true. If some of the surplus is used for tax cuts or increased spending, some of the surplus dollars will be spent on consumption rather than investment. Government debt and the interest paid on it will be larger than if the surplus was "saved." Deficits will occur earlier, debt will rise sooner, and there will be fewer resources to support aging entitlement programs. Nevertheless, the large surplus makes it difficult for legislators to ignore politically popular tax cuts or spending programs for a problem that might not arise for many years.

Rudolph Penner is more pessimistic than Primus about our funding for elderly entitlements. Penner explains that a debt explosion and economic collapse will eventually occur if policies remain unchanged. It will take some time for that to happen, but he is not sanguine that the corrective actions needed to prevent it will be undertaken. His primary concerns are twofold: first, that policy is moving in exactly the wrong direction. Instead of talking about policies to reduce the projected deficit, most discussions have been about how much to cut taxes and how much to increase spending. Second, the longer we wait to enact corrective policies, the more difficult it will be to close the budget gap. For example, if no action is taken until the year 2020, the size of the required correction doubles relative to GDP. Although current estimates of the fiscal gap have now been reduced to 0.5 percent, that still represents an immediate correction of more than $40 billion. Since any reductions in entitlements would have to be gradually phased in, total spending cuts would be larger—even if they began today. Delaying action, or, worse, enacting tax cuts or new spending programs, would make the necessary corrections that much more difficult.

Having warned about the consequences of not funding future entitlements, Penner asks what happens to the welfare of the nation if elderly entitlements are funded but they assume a growing proportion of GDP? Here the answers are less clear. In general, Penner explains, higher taxes distort individual behavior and lower economic efficiency. But the impact of raising taxes to pay for increased Social Security and health benefits depends on behavioral issues and is quite unclear. If elderly individuals substitute public benefits for private savings they would otherwise have accumulated themselves (crowd-out), the economic impact would be quite negative. However, if public benefits mostly substitute for private transfers from younger generations, the economic impact would be slight. Economists do not agree which of these scenarios better reflects reality. And it may be, at least at the present time, that people prefer more entitlement spending and are willing to bear the cost.

Penner observes that the cost to nonelderly persons will become more apparent after the baby boomers begin to retire. The annual growth in GDP for uses other than Social Security and Medicare will fall from 1.6 percent between 2010 and 2020 to 1.3 percent between 2020 and 2030 and to 0.9 percent between 2040 and 2050. At the same time, there will be a major reduction in per capita growth of GDP for nonelderly individuals. When nonelderly individuals begin to feel the impact of these restraints, they may then demand changes in elderly entitlement programs.

Joseph White provides a thoughtful conclusion to this section. Although he recognizes the need for advance budget planning and incremental reform, he states emphatically that a budget crisis never existed. White contends that there is no economic basis for either radical structural change or for drastic cuts in elderly entitlement programs. Extending Aaron's arguments, he points out the weakness of forecasts that project that current policies will continue, without correction, up to the point of economic disaster. Long-term budget estimates became relevant to policy debates, he argues, only when government agencies "began extrapolating current law to the point of total irresponsibility and then modeling the results." Too much about future economic projections is unknown, he reasons, and "ignorance is not a good basis for policy choice."

White argues that economics does not have a large influence on whether the budget becomes unmanageable. The major impact of economics is after the budget becomes unmanageable, when budget deficits begin to rise, interest payments increase, and significant economic feedbacks occur. Analyzing the numbers, he determines that if nothing were done until 2020, an increase in revenues from 2020 to 2040 of 5 percent of GDP (from 19.2% to 24.2%) would likely pay for current entitlement programs. He concludes that the decision to pay for these programs twenty years from now is well within our economic capabilities and hence is a value decision, not a matter of economic facts. Furthermore, he argues, we should question the wisdom of making policy decisions far in the future for other people who will have to live with them.

White believes it is politically unlikely that the government will accumulate huge surpluses. However, he recommends that we continue to reduce debt and interest and, perhaps, to establish private Social Security accounts with some of the surplus. He also advocates restraint in Medicare and Medicaid spending, moderation in the amount of tax cuts, and avoidance of large discretionary spending programs. He believes that incremental reform of Medicare and Social Security could be helpful and that some structural reforms could be tried. Furthermore, the issue of how to fund longer life expectancies should be addressed.

All of these recommendations together would not come close to eliminating the eventual deficit. However, he argues, they would produce a less difficult baseline and make policy decisions easier and more manageable for future generations. White concludes by stating that long-term budget forecasts, interpreted correctly, show the value of cautious budget policies and incremental program reform but do not indicate an economic crisis or even a severe difficulty.

The next section of the book explores the policy alternatives. We begin with two opposing views about universal social insurance. Theodore Marmor and Jerry Mashaw believe that universal social insurance systems are preferable on grounds of both equity and efficiency. Richard Lamm believes that in a world of limited resources, the universal elderly entitlements we now have cannot be sustained, and unless we limit and prioritize them we will end up rationing in an amoral fashion.

Universal social insurance allows us to "manage the risks of economic [or health] misfortune that will befall some of us at any one time and threaten all of us over the course of our lifetimes." "This social ideal . . . produces an us-us rather than a we-them political dynamic," guaranteeing that everyone is entitled to basic income and health security in a dignified and deserving manner, and not as a handout from the more fortunate. Thus begins a quite elegant defense of our universal social insurance programs by Marmor and Mashaw.

The authors point out that since most Americans hold universal social insurance programs in high regard, most of the political opposition has focused on issues of affordability rather than social equity. They contend that the potential budget shortfall arising from the retirement of the baby boomers is now being used by long-time opponents of Social Security and Medicare to derail the social insurance programs that serve both the middle class and the poor.

After making a strong case for social equity, Marmor and Mashaw make the case for affordability. In the case of Social Security, they argue that demographic projections are overstated. Although the ratio of working people to elderly persons will fall, the impact will be partially offset by a decrease in the number of children. They contend that the budget shortfall in Social Security is relatively small and that a payroll tax increase of just 0.8 percent (0.4% employer and 0.4% employee) would immediately put the program in long-term balance. Even without such a tax increase, the authors believe the program could be brought into balance by enacting the "Ball plan." The Ball plan contains several relatively small adjustments in payments and benefits and invests 40 percent of the trust fund into equities. They contrast the Ball plan to numerous privatization proposals favored by economic conservatives. Privatization, they argue, would shift risk from the government to individuals, remove the redistributive nature of the program, and fail to protect poor or disabled persons and those who happen to invest their savings poorly.

In the case of Medicare, they claim that the program can be expanded to include long-term care and pharmaceutical benefits and that its financing can still be adjusted to deliver benefits at a cost similar to such programs in other countries. The authors claim that cost could be controlled in three areas: provide less needed services, provide less unneeded services, and pay less for service providers. They favor reducing payments to "medical providers of all sorts," as well as considering increases in payroll tax rates. Marmor and Mashaw argue that the public strongly supports the Medicare program and would be willing to pay increased taxes but should not have to tolerate the pattern of health expenditures that now exists. "Our problem," they conclude, "is not that we have attempted too much but that we have completed so little."

Richard Lamm, in contrast, would argue that we cannot afford what we have already promised, to say nothing of adding new entitlements. Lamm believes that when limited funds meet unlimited demands, they must be budgeted and prioritized. In fact, he states that it is unethical not to have a system of priorities, for those in government have an ethical duty to maximize the health of the entire population. Under the current system, Lamm contends, "it is likely that we deny more people more health care than any other industrial country."

Lamm states that "the price of modern medicine is to honestly admit that all health care systems ration." The technological advances driving the capabilities of medicine mean that we can no longer pay for everything that is beneficial to everyone. That is hard for us to accept, he explains, because admitting that our present health care system is not sustainable requires us to give up the dream of a total universal and egalitarian health care system.

He argues that physicians are not the best individuals to judge resource allocation; they must be focused on the individual doctor-patient relationship, whereas the equitable allocation of resources for a society requires a larger view. Medical ethics controls the behavior of the provider but cannot control macroallocation decisions. To maximize the health of the group, he asserts, one must occasionally suboptimize what is available to individuals. In our country, he continues, we should limit what is available, but instead we limit access. That is to say, we ration the "who" instead of the "what," and as a result we have over 40 million uninsured people who do not have equitable access to health care.

Lamm makes the case for both intergenerational and distributive equity. He points out that we spend three times as much taxpayer money on the elderly as we do on our children, leaving our children a burden of unpaid debt. He argues that even though our entitlement programs are popular, they have become unjust to our children. "It is not a nation-building strategy," he points out, "to spend significantly more on the last generation than we do on the next generation."

Lamm contends that Americans must take a wider view than maximizing the health of each individual in order to maximize the total health and well-being of the society at large. He urges us to extend "the health care floor" rather than "raising the research ceiling," so that we confront the problem of the uninsured and guarantee all citizens decent access to basic health care services.

Mark Pauly takes it as a given that if tax rates are to remain within levels that will not cause significant economic distortions in the future, the design features of our major social insurance programs must be modified. Thus, he contends, we have a better chance of preserving the advantages of our current social insurance programs if those programs are converted to a means-tested form using defined contributions.

Pauly begins by postulating a continuum in which universal social insurance programs are on one end and means-tested benefits are on the other. Classical social insurance programs have open-ended, broad eligibility and tightly defined benefits that are prescribed by the state. As one moves along the continuum, eligibility becomes less open-ended and the way benefits can be used becomes more flexible.

Means-tested, defined contribution programs are not only more affordable than universal defined benefit programs, Pauly states, but they also are more equitable. Why should the working generation, with many low-income wage earners who are paying regressive payroll taxes, pay for the retired generation, who, on average, are financially better off? He also recommends defined contribution programs on grounds of economic efficiency because individuals can match their contributions to their personal preferences. This is particularly relevant in the case of health care, where wealthier people, who are less risk averse, might be forced by a defined benefit to purchase more insurance than they would otherwise prefer.

Pauly suggests that one might want to phase in the defined contribution nature of programs according to income. For example, in regard to health care, he suggests that a universal benefit floor be established for low-income individuals with benefits comparable to today's Medicare program. If one believes that lower-income people have less capacity to bear risk or less knowledge to make investment decisions, one could restrict the use of funds at lower incomes as in a defined benefit program. Then, as income and the capacity to bear risk increase, individuals could be given more of a defined contribution plan and more freedom of choice in the way they use their benefit. Similarly, in the case of Social Security, as individuals get wealthier they could have more choice as to how to invest retirement funds and how to choose a pattern of future payouts.

Alicia Munnell expresses an almost totally opposite point of view, concluding that a change in entitlement programs from defined benefit to defined contribution would have a profoundly negative effect on society. Munnell opposes such a change on both economic and philosophical grounds. The whole point of having a Social Security system, she explains, is to provide workers with a predictable and dependable retirement benefit. Retirement income that depends on one's skills as an investor or on market returns is inconsistent with the goals of the program. Similarly, a medical care contribution that may not keep pace with the cost of health care fails to ensure elderly health security.

Munnell cites a number of disadvantages of a defined contribution Social Security system. These include considerably higher administrative costs, the danger that individuals would make early withdrawals, the lack of automatic annuitization (without a fixed schedule of annual payments, individuals could exhaust their retirement money too quickly), and the likelihood that the income redistribution in today's system would be reduced or eliminated. It is not clear, she states, whether a defined contribution system is any more efficient or whether it will result in increased or decreased total savings. She supports the arguments put forth by Geanakoplos, Mitchell, and Zeldes in chapter 12 that a shift to defined contributions would not in itself raise the return on contributions. The only advantages, she contends, are greater freedom for individuals to control their savings and less involvement of government. Munnell does not believe that these advantages outweigh the loss of social risk pooling or the increased administrative costs.

She is less definitive on the net benefit of a defined contribution health system. The Medicare system, she explains, is complex and often criticized for being inefficient in its payment policies. It is possible that a change to defined contribution would enable more competition as individuals shopped for value, although such an occurrence is by no means certain. A shift to defined contribution could also bring about a number of negative consequences. If contributions did not keep pace with the cost of medicine, the risk for payment would shift from the government to individuals. In addition, the insurance pool could be broken up as both wealthier and healthier people might choose high deductible or catastrophic plans, leaving those with high expected health costs in traditional full-service plans where the premiums would escalate. These factors combined could negatively impact the poorest and least healthy individuals, exacerbating the uneven distribution of wealth that traditional social insurance programs attempt to alleviate. Munnell concludes that the disadvantages of a change to defined contribution outweigh the uncertain prospects of reduced health costs.

Munnell also opposes a change to defined contribution on more philosophical grounds. The history of social insurance programs, she explains, began hundreds of years ago when people bound together to help each other. The concept was one of social solidarity, in which all would be contributors to a fund that anyone could use if needed. This is a very different concept from public assistance, she points out, which is paternalistic and often condescending and stigmatizing to those who avail themselves of its benefits. Our social insurance systems, she contends, are stable, predictable, supported by the middle class, and insulated from the changing whims of politicians. Changing them to defined contribution systems would end that stability and put the most vulnerable of our population at risk.

Many advocates of Social Security reform claim that a privatized social security system would pay a higher rate of return to recipients. Geanakoplos, Mitchell, and Zeldes argue that such claims are untrue, and although there may be some valid reasons to support privatization, a higher rate of return is not one of them.

The reason people become confused about privatization proposals, these authors explain, is that three different elements are often mixed together: privatization, diversification, and prefunding. Privatization means replacing the government's trust fund and obligations to pay Social Security benefits with individual accounts. Diversification means investing funds (either personal accounts or trust funds) into a range of assets, possibly including shares of stock. Prefunding means replacing the current pay-as-you-go system with one in which each generation sets money aside for its own retirement. Any one of these elements can exist without the other two. Geanakoplos, Mitchell, and Zeldes explain them one at a time.

The authors identify a common misperception that occurs because individuals receive benefits that represent a seemingly low rate of return (about 2.2%) on the taxes they pay in to Social Security. On the surface, it seems to many people that if they had private accounts, they could earn a higher return by investing in stocks, corporate bonds, or even risk-free government bonds. What they fail to take into account is that in our pay-as-you-go Social Security system, the working generations pay the benefits for the retiring generations. In return, the next younger working generations will pay the benefits for them. The present working generations have to pay about $9 trillion in benefits to those who will retire before them. Even if Social Security accounts are privatized, the country is not going to default on the benefits owed to older Americans who have already paid their Social Security taxes. Hence, that $9 trillion still has to be paid by the younger generations.

Geanakoplos, Mitchell, and Zeldes contend that the net rate of return current workers will derive from Social Security, after properly accounting for the $9 trillion that they must collectively pay, will not be raised by simply changing the system to private accounts.

The authors contend that neither diversifying investments nor prefunding will raise the overall rate of return for Social Security. Nevertheless, there may be other valid reasons to diversify investments or to prefund. For example, a transition to a prefunded system would increase returns for future generations. However, that increase would come at the expense of current generations, who would have to support both the prefunding and the existing pay-as-you-go obligations during the transition.

In conclusion, Geanakoplos, Mitchell, and Zeldes suggest that the Social Security reform debate should focus on the trade-off between returns among different generations; the benefits of offering all households a diversified portfolio; and, if funds are diversified, whether diversification should be accomplished via private accounts or trust fund investments. It is important to note that general agreement does not exist on all of these issues. Nevertheless, Geanakoplos, Mitchell, and Zeldes argue forcefully that privatization of Social Security will not yield higher rates of return.

In addition to major structural reforms of our current entitlement programs, there are a number of less dramatic policy alternatives that could help to alleviate the long-term budget shortfall. One such alternative is to provide incentives for longer work lives. Joseph Quinn has performed seminal research on the retirement trends and work patterns of older Americans.

Quinn states his major findings early in the chapter. He tells us that a century-old trend of earlier and earlier retirement is now over, and has been for at least fifteen years. Quinn explains that the labor force participation of older Americans began falling in the late 1800s and fell precipitously after World War II. For example, in 1950 more than 70 percent of 65-year-old men were in the labor force, but that fell to 30 percent by 1985. Since 1985, however, the retirement trends of both men and women have reversed.

Quinn hypothesizes that the reasons for the change in trend could be permanent changes in the work environment or the temporary strength of the economy, or both. He finds support for both reasons. However, the strength of the economy explains only a part of the diverging trend. Most of the change, he argues, is permanent. It is likely the result of a combination of factors such as the elimination of mandatory retirement, the reduction of Social Security work disincentives, the increased proportion of defined contribution pensions, increased longevity, and improved age-specific health status.

Quinn's research has far-reaching implications, because longer work lives have a powerful effect on the potential budget shortfall. If public policies and private employment incentives are structured to encourage older Americans to work longer, it can satisfy the changing preferences of workers and the increased labor demand of employers as well as ameliorating the long-term budget problem. In fact, Toder and Solanki estimated that if the number of years of retirement could be kept constant as longevity increases, the ratio of labor supply to (needs-weighted) population would remain approximately constant through the year 2040.

Another policy area that holds promise is aligning consistent incentives across separate retirement programs. Lynn Etheredge identifies the need for a national retirement policy. Today, our three major retirement income streams (Social Security, Medicare, and private pensions) are not coordinated and often work at cross-purposes. A national retirement policy would provide consistent incentives for people to work longer and give them more flexibility to allocate various sources of retirement funds to best suit their individual needs.

Etheredge identifies four specific areas in which a coordinated policy could help finance the future retirement needs of the baby boom generation. The first is providing incentives for people to extend their work lives. Etheredge explains the need to structure programs so that individuals do not have to sacrifice benefits by working longer. He also points out current disparities in the age people are eligible to receive benefits under different programs. Medicare age eligibility is 65, but Social Security is 65 (gradually changing to 67) with an option for early eligibility at age 62. Lump-sum private pensions are available without penalty at age 59.5. If age eligibility was aligned across programs, individuals would be able to have consistent incentives to work longer. For example, one can now work past age 65 without sacrificing

Social Security payments, but the individual or his or her employer would have to sacrifice Medicare benefits. Etheredge also recommends a retirement bonus to encourage more work years. He proposes a ten-thousand-dollar lump sum bonus, paid when the individual retires, for each year of work beyond age 65. He contends that the amount government would save by not paying Medicare and Social Security benefits during that period, and in interest and additional tax revenue, could be used to pay for the bonus.

The second area in which Etheredge recommends change is the expansion of pension coverage. More than half of American workers do not receive private pension benefits. He recommends that individuals who do not have access to employer-sponsored pensions be allowed to use additional Social Security withholding to invest in private pensions.

Etheredge also advises that use of the separate tax advantaged savings streams be made more flexible, allowing people to choose how they spend their retirement accounts. For example, he advocates that private pensions be required to include a rollover option for beneficiaries to purchase long-term care insurance. He suggests combining public and private funds to encourage the purchase of long-term care insurance. This could be accomplished by the government's guaranteeing payment for all long-term care after two years for individuals who privately insure the first two years of long-term care services.

Taxing private pensions is Etheredge's fourth recommendation. He compares the benefits of public health and income security programs against the tax favored treatment of private pensions. He concludes that support for public programs should be given a relatively higher priority. Etheredge contends that before cuts are made to the universal social insurance programs, closer scrutiny should be given to the $9.5 trillion in private pension accounts. He warns against jeopardizing the largely successful private pension system but argues that a small tax would be equitable given the tax advantages conferred on these accounts. A 0.25 percent tax on tax qualified pension balances would raise about $24 billion annually. Etheredge concludes that closer coordination among Medicare, Social Security, and private pensions could help alleviate the challenge America faces in financing future retirement.

Moving from potential policy options to political feasibility, the final section of the book examines the political context for the reform of elderly entitlement programs. Does the political landscape of today favor efforts for comprehensive reform? Norman Ornstein examines the political landscape as of March 2001, about one month after the beginning of the Bush presidency. Although Ornstein speaks about individual and party politics particular to this time period, there are many general policy implications that can be drawn from his specific examples.

"The 2000 elections were the most consequential in the modern era," Ornstein contends, because both houses of the Congress and the presidency were "up for grabs," as well as the political balance in a large number of state legislatures. Rarely, if ever, in recent U.S. history has so much power been so closely contended in a national election.

The results of the election have left the country divided as evenly as possible in partisan political terms, and Ornstein draws the following conclusions that will bear on future policy initiatives. First, the evenly divided nature of the House and Senate will mean that comprehensive or controversial legislation will be difficult to enact. Second, the fact that the leadership of both houses of Congress could be altered in the next election augurs against bold or risky action from either party. The close party balance in Congress is likely to continue, furthermore, and may similarly impact the next several election cycles. Third, the typical normal ideological distribution that we have had in the post–World War II era no longer exists. Using a football metaphor, Ornstein explains that most elected officials used to be clustered ideologically between the 35- and 40-yard lines on both sides of the midfield stripe. Now, he observes, the 107th Congress is bimodal, especially in the House, with many elected officials between the 10- and 20-yard lines and a good number behind the goalposts. As a result, there is a large difference between the majority and minority leaders in each committee, and there is a great deal more animosity and mistrust. Fourth, there is weak leadership and a lack of loyal followers because three-quarters of congressional members are new since 1990 and 45 of 100 senators are presently serving their first term.

Given these facts, neither party is likely to be a majority force or exhibit strong national leadership. Hence, the parties will scramble for voter blocs and "traction" issues from which they can mobilize their ideological base, attack their opponents, draw some support from the center, and avoid issues that could be damaging with swing voters.

This is particularly true in the case of Social Security and Medicare reform, where neither party wants to be labeled by the other as insensitive or nonsupportive. In such an atmosphere, legislators are more likely to give in to spending increases than to make tough budget decisions. They are unlikely to attempt the kind of reforms that would require trust and cooperation between the two major parties.

What is likely to change that will make the environment more open to comprehensive reforms? Ornstein believes that financing elderly entitlements will eventually be perceived as a zero-sum game, pitting increased spending for elderly programs against funds for all other discretionary programs. Such a perception might bring about the impetus for significant reform, but entitlement spending is not yet being seen in that context. A restoration of trust and respect between the major parties would also be conducive to substantive change, but, again, the prospect of such a change in attitude is not on the immediate horizon. Ornstein observes that a major national crisis could bring about such an attitude change. In the meantime, the prospect of turning politicians away from the party positioning and budget politics of today does not appear very promising.

Robert Binstock considers the factors that must be present in the political context to improve the prospect for significant change that Ornstein finds so bleak. Binstock observes that only under rare circumstances do we tend to consider sweeping or comprehensive policy initiatives. Such circumstances generally arise out of major social, economic, or political developments or a confluence of political leadership. In our society, he contends, there are many barriers to comprehensive change. Among these are the constitutional separation and fragmentation of power, a historical tendency toward incremental change, and the difficulty of implementing change in a pluralistic environment. Binstock explains that there is a retirement industry replete with stakeholders who benefit from the status quo and who will strongly resist change. Furthermore, the lack of an immediate crisis militates against mobilizing the resources for change, particularly in regard to elected politicians who are not apt to support short-term sacrifices for distant long-term goals.

Binstock explores the circumstances that might enhance the potential consideration of entitlement policies involving comprehensive change. He observes that the combination of advance planning, distant startup, and gradual implementation can be used as a strategy to phase in large-scale change. As an example, he cites the Social Security Reform Act of 1983. That legislation extended the eligibility age for Social Security from 65 to 67. But the changes did not begin to take place until twenty years after the legislation was enacted (2003). They were then phased in at the rate of one month per year so that the two-year extension will not be fully implemented until the year 2027.

Binstock also identifies the importance of framing the issue in the proper context. He explains that for any issue to be salient with the public, it must compete with all other issues and crises as a form of media entertainment. Framing the issue as a crisis about government programs simply does not elicit the kind of crisis response necessary to attract significant attention. Hence, Binstock recommends that the issues be framed in terms of people and not programs. Focusing on the potential impact on families would be most effective, he argues, because nearly everyone is personally affected by the aging of family members.

Binstock concludes by warning of the dangers of policy inaction. If we postpone action now, our economy may not be as prosperous in the future, and the challenge of meeting the obligations of our elderly entitlement programs might be "economically and politically overwhelming." Although major reform is difficult, Binstock holds out the hope that it can be accomplished by using strategies that have worked in the past.

A fitting and final perspective is provided by Victor Fuchs. One must assume a holistic view, Fuchs reasons, in order to understand the financial implications of our aging population. In Fuchs's definition, a holistic view includes the financing of all goods and services for the elderly, not only what elderly persons spend on themselves but also the transfers they expend that come from younger generations. A holistic view requires that the totality of programs for elderly persons be considered as opposed to evaluating reforms one program at a time.

Fuchs explains that as death rates in the United States decline and life expectancy rises, elderly persons face a number of problems associated with aging. Among these are two financial problems: low income and high medical expenditures. In assessing the financial security of elderly persons, Fuchs points out, one used to be able to consider income and health expenditures separately, because the capabilities of medicine were less and expenditures were not ordinarily large. That is no longer the case, and since money is fungible, it no longer makes sense to separately consider spending on health and income security programs. Hence, Fuchs defines the concept of "full income" as the sum of personal income plus health care expenditures not paid from personal income. The concept of full income, he contends, is a necessary element in a holistic framework.

He raises two questions about the full income of elderly Americans: how much of their full income is devoted to health care, and how much of it is provided by the young (citizens less than 65 years of age)? Fuchs estimates that elderly persons spent 35 percent of their full income on health care in 1997 and that 56 percent of total elderly expenditures was provided by the young. He further estimates that if health care grows 3 percent faster than other expenditures, 52 percent of elderly persons' full income will be devoted to health care by the year 2020 and 62 percent of their total expenditures will be paid by the young. Fuchs's computations are per capita, so they do not even include the fact that the ratio of elderly to nonelderly persons will increase.

Given these estimates of spending, Fuchs contends that many elderly persons will be "health care poor." That is, they will spend large portions of their resources on health but will not be able to afford other necessities of life. Furthermore, the increased spending by young persons to support these expenditures will compete with and crowd out other important expenditures until the burden on young persons will eventually become unbearable. This will occur, Fuchs argues, even acknowledging that a growing elderly component of the population will require increases in taxes.

There are two possible escapes, he posits, from this bleak scenario. The first is to reduce the growth in health care expenditures, and the second is to require elderly persons to assume more of the financial burden. Reducing the rate of growth in health care expenditures, he reasons, may not be feasible; and even if it is, it may not be desirable. The chief driver of health care spending is technology, and improved medical technology contributes to longer and better-quality lives. Present evidence suggests little political will or public support to slow the pace of technological advances in medicine.

Hence, Fuchs reasons, elderly persons themselves must eventually assume more of the financial burden. To do so, he argues, elderly persons need more income from savings and more income from earnings. Addressing savings, he recognizes that the ability to save varies directly with income and that poor persons cannot be expected to increase savings. However, he observes wide variability in the amount people save within the same income groups, and he concludes that as long as savings are voluntary, many people will not save. Hence, without being specific, he recommends that the United States consider a program of compulsory savings.

Addressing income, he observes that the number of work years has not kept pace with increases in life expectancy. He calculates that the number of years not working for 65-year-olds has increased during the period from 1975 to 1995 from 11.7 years to 13.7 years in the case of men and from 17.3 to 17.8 years in the case of women. Fuchs recommends policies that encourage longer work lives. He advocates reexamining all policies that create high marginal tax rates for elderly workers and all laws that make it more costly for employers to hire and retain elderly workers.

CONCLUSIONS

What conclusions can be drawn from this collection of ideas that traverses the political and ideological landscape? In broad economic terms, there is substantial agreement that an aging population that is living longer and spending increasing amounts on health care will present a formidable economic challenge. The extent of the challenge is uncertain, and although wide differences of opinion exist, most would concur that current policy should at least include economic precautions about the future needs of our aging population.

We think this collection reflects the thinking that major program reforms are at least as much a matter of values as they are of economics. But opinions vary, and whereas some argue that comprehensive, structural changes in income and health security programs are required, others recommend no more than incremental reform combined with informed economic preparedness.

Regardless of what position one assumes on these issues, there is little question that it is necessary to assess the total requirements of our aging society. Whether or not we should assume Victor Fuchs's holistic view or accept Lynn Etheredge's call for a national retirement policy, the magnitude of our economic challenge should not go unheeded. Today's policies should be evaluated not only for their current value but also against the backdrop of the future needs of an aging population.

Large tax cuts or huge new social spending programs are not consonant with many of the economic projections contained in this volume. And a comprehensive aging policy seems unlikely in today's fractured political arena. Yet the politics of budget surpluses and divided party leadership have moved us toward policies that ignore future social and economic exigencies. Honest differences about the nature and scope of policy reform are prevalent in this volume, but the need to consider the implications of present policies on the future needs of an aging population is clear.

REFERENCES

Congressional Budget Office (CBO). 1999. *The Long-Term Budget Outlook.* Washington, D.C.: U.S. Government Printing Office, December 14.

———. 2000. *The Budget and Economic Outlook: Fiscal Years 2001–2010.* Washington, D.C.: U.S. Government Printing Office, January.

Fuchs, V. 1998. Provide, Provide: The Economics of Aging. NBER Working Paper no. 6642, National Bureau of Economic Research, Cambridge, Mass.

Geanakoplos, J., O. S. Mitchell, and S. P. Zeldes. 1998. Would a Privatized Social Security System Really Pay a Higher Rate of Return? NBER Working Paper no. 6713, National Bureau of Economic Research, Cambridge, Mass.

Levit, K., C. Cowan, B. Braden, J. Stiller, A. Sensenig, and H. Lazenby. 1998. National Health Expenditures in 1997: More Slow Growth. *Health Affairs* 17:6.

Newhouse, J. P. 1993. An Iconoclastic View of Health Cost Containment. *Health Affairs* 12 (suppl.): 152–71.

Quinn, J. 1999. Retirement Trends and Patterns among Older American Workers. Paper presented to the Council on the Economic Impact of Health System Change, Lansdowne, Virginia, October 21–23.

Singer, B. H., and K. G. Manton. 1998. The Effects of Health Changes on Projections of Health Service Needs for the Elderly Population of the United States. *Proceedings of the National Academy of Sciences* 95 (December): 15618–22.

U.S. Bureau of the Census. 1999. *Statistical Abstract of the United States, 1999.* Washington, D.C.: U.S. Government Printing Office.

2

An International Perspective on Policies for an Aging Society

Jonathan Gruber, Ph.D., and David A. Wise, Ph.D.

The single most important long-run fiscal issue facing the developed world is the aging of its populations. In virtually every developed country, there will be a steep increase in the ratio of elderly persons to the working-age population over the first half of the twenty-first century. Figure 2.1 shows the ratio of the number of persons aged 65 or older to the number aged 20–64 for a sample of ten countries. In six of the countries, this ratio will exceed 0.5 by 2050; in Spain it will exceed 0.6, so for every working-age person there will be 0.6 retirement-age persons. As is immediately apparent, the developed world is moving into uncharted territory during this period.

Moreover, this population aging is happening in environments that are unprecedentedly generous to the elderly citizens of developed nations. In every nation, elderly persons retire into a world of guaranteed income support and health insurance coverage. And thus far, the reaction of the developed world to population aging has been simply to increase spending on elderly persons. From 1980 to 1995, as the percentage of the population over age 65 in OECD nations rose by almost one-fifth, the percentage of GDP transferred to elderly persons rose by almost one-quarter.

But it should be immediately apparent from Figure 2.1 that such a reaction to population aging is not sustainable. Simple projections,

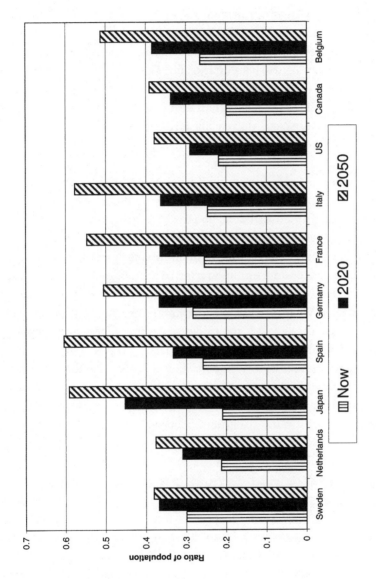

Fig. 2.1. Ratio of the population aged 65+ to the population aged 20–64. *Source: Gruber and Wise 1999b.*

described in more detail below, suggest that if the current relationship between population aging and social spending on elderly persons continues, the share of GDP that developed nations transfer to elderly persons will rise by almost 40 percent between now and 2050, reaching more than 11 percent of GDP by the midpoint of the century. This would require either enormous increases in the tax burdens on the relatively small group of workers or enormous reductions in spending on other age groups. Moreover, this is not a medium-run phenomenon that will disappear in the second half of the twenty-first century; due to decreasing mortality and decreasing fertility, we are seeing a secular shift in population composition that will persist for the foreseeable future.

This chapter considers both the institutions through which elderly persons are supported by the public sector and the implications for elderly persons and government budgets. We focus on the OECD nations for which data are most readily available. We very briefly review the panoply of public programs targeted to elderly persons and document the size of spending on them, relative to both national economies and government budgets, and how this varies across the relatively similar OECD nations. We review what this increased spending is buying elderly persons by providing some evidence on the relationship between social insurance program incentives and labor supply, between public spending and average elderly incomes, and between public spending and poverty rates. Then we ask what the demographic transition bodes for the future: if countries do not change their behavior, what is the likely path for their fiscal situations? And where is the burden of paying these high fiscal bills likely to fall?

WHAT DO PUBLIC PROGRAMS IN DEVELOPED COUNTRIES DO FOR ELDERLY PERSONS?

Each developed nation has a unique set of programs to support elderly persons, and it is difficult and potentially misleading to attempt to categorize the nature of elderly support simply. Nevertheless, we attempt to do so, providing enough flexibility to discuss the major types of programs and the kinds of deviations from the norm that one observes.

Income Support Programs

Every developed nation (and indeed the vast majority of less-developed countries as well) has some form of universal income support program for its elderly population. Table 2.1 illustrates the structure of these social security programs for the sample of countries reviewed in Gruber and Wise 1999b. It first shows the early and normal entitlement ages for these programs. The early entitlement age is the age at which benefits can first be claimed, whereas the normal retirement age is a benchmark measure against which benefits are sometimes (but not always) adjusted. For example, in the United States, individuals claiming their Social Security benefits early (between ages 62 and 65) are subject to an actuarial reduction of those benefits. In fact, in most countries in the Gruber and Wise study, the modal age of entitlement was the early entitlement age; the "normal" age of entitlement in fact is no longer normal.

The next column shows the typical replacement rates available to a married male worker (with a nonworking spouse) at the age of early entitlement. Two things are notable about this figure. First, in some countries it is quite high; in France, for example, the typical worker who retires at age 60 replaces 91 percent of the earnings on his or her preretirement job. Second, it is quite variable across countries, with retirees in the United States replacing only 41 percent of their earnings if they retire early.

This table obscures important differences in the structure of income support programs. In the United States, the primary support program is Social Security, which is not means tested but is conditioned on modest labor force attachment. In Canada, in contrast, there are three types of programs: a universal demogrant (conditional only on citizenship) at age 65, an earnings-related pension available at age 60, and means-tested transfers available at age 60. In Germany, although the official age of early entitlement for Social Security is age 60, workers can entitle themselves to their full benefits by becoming unemployed at age 57. In Italy, until recent reforms were put in place, entitlement was conditional only on thirty-five years of labor market experience, so that individuals who started work at age 20 could retire at age 55 with full benefits.

Table 2.1. Institutional Features of Social Security Programs

Country	Early Retirement Age	Normal Retirement Age	Replacement Rate at Early Retirement Age
Belgium	60	65	77
Canada	60	65	20
France	60	65	91
Germany	60	65	62
Italy	55	60	75
Japan	60	65	54
The Netherlands	60	65	91
Spain	60	65	63
Sweden	60	65	54
United Kingdom	60	70	48
United States	62	65	41

Source: Gruber and Wise 1999a.

An important complement to income transfer programs is disability programs, such as Disability Insurance in the United States. There is significant variation across developed countries in the extent to which these programs truly screen applicants on the basis of disability, as opposed to acting as backdoor routes to early retirement. In the United States, disability screening is severe, with only about one-third of applicants initially approved; as a result, fewer than one-seventh of older (age 60–64) men are on disability. In Sweden, disability screening is much more lax, and as a result one-third of 64-year-old men are on disability. Similarly, a large fraction of employees in Germany "retire" through the disability program. Indeed, a much larger fraction of employees retire through the disability and unemployment programs than through the social security program (Borsch-Supan and Schnabel 1999).

Health Insurance

In most developed countries, elderly persons do not receive particularly special care under the health care system; health care (or health insurance) is a universal entitlement to which elderly persons benefit as do the remainder of the population. The United States is exceptional in having largely private insurance for the nonelderly population and a public entitlement for elderly persons through the Medicare program. The only other major industrialized nation with a separate system of health care for elderly persons is Japan. Elderly persons are differentiated in many other countries, in that health care is financed by payroll taxation so that retirees bear no funding burden. But the fundamental structure of care and insurance is similar for the elderly and the nonelderly. This linkage heightens even further the dependence of elderly persons on nonelderly portions of public budgets.

Developed countries also use a variety of mechanisms to attempt to control medical costs. In the United States, public insurance costs through Medicare are primarily controlled through cost sharing on the patient side and restrictive provider reimbursement, although for many services cost sharing is limited by either employer-provided or individually purchased supplemental insurance. In many other countries, such as Germany or Italy, there is relatively little cost sharing, but there are stricter controls on provider reimbursement and other rationing mechanisms such as expenditure caps and global budgets (Cutler 1999).

A critical and growing component of health care spending on elderly persons is long-term care. Although in most OECD nations, long-term care is fully publicly funded, there are many differences across developed countries in the public provision of long-term care. In the United States, much of the long-term care is financed by public programs, but the care is provided privately, and wealthy individuals pay their own way. In Italy and Belgium, long-term care is funded through a social insurance scheme. In Canada, there is partial public funding of long-term care, and roughly one-half of the institutions are publicly owned.

Nonhealth in-Kind Transfer Programs

Of the expenditures on nonhealth in-kind programs for elderly persons, the majority goes to residential care, home-help services, and rehabilitation services. Almost every country we study here has at least one program that falls into one of these categories, either specifically for elderly persons or available to elderly persons. The other main expenditure on in-kind programs comes from housing benefits. However, only about two-thirds of the countries that we study have housing benefits. A few countries have other "miscellaneous" in-kind benefits for which elderly persons are eligible, such as food or subsidized public transport. However, the contribution of these programs to the overall social expenditure is quite small.

Facts on Spending

Putting this panoply of programs together, we see a consistent pattern of substantial transfers to elderly persons across developed countries but also substantial heterogeneity in the amount of resources devoted to that group. Figure 2.2 presents the distribution across developed nations of the percentage of GDP that is transferred to elderly persons as cash or (nonhealth) in-kind benefits; these figures capture only current spending, not any future entitlements that are being built up through social security programs. These figures were calculated from the OECD's Social Expenditure Database. For some programs, such as age-targeted social insurance programs, the amount of spending on elderly persons could be assessed straightforwardly. For other programs, such as health care or public housing, it was more difficult. Where possible, we contacted experts from each of the countries to assist us in assessing the distribution of spending through other programs across population groups.

As Figure 2.2 shows, there is wide variation across these fairly similar industrialized nations in their spending on elderly persons. For example, Italy (13.2%) devotes more than four times as much of GDP to elderly persons as does Australia (3.2%). Although the United States is toward the low end, with the government spending only 6.2 percent of GDP on elderly persons, it still spends a larger percentage than Australia, Canada, or Japan and roughly as much, proportionally, as Switzerland. On average, the governments of this sample of developed nations transfer 8.2 percent of GDP to elderly persons through social programs.

This is an understated figure, however, for two reasons. First, for a number of categories of social spending in many countries, we remain unsure about the division of spending between the elderly and the nonelderly. Second, we have not included health care benefits, a large share of which accrue to elderly persons. Figure 2.3 shows the increase

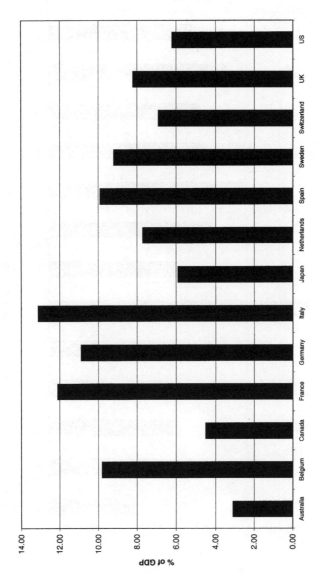

Fig. 2.2. Percentage of GDP spent on elderly persons: No allocation

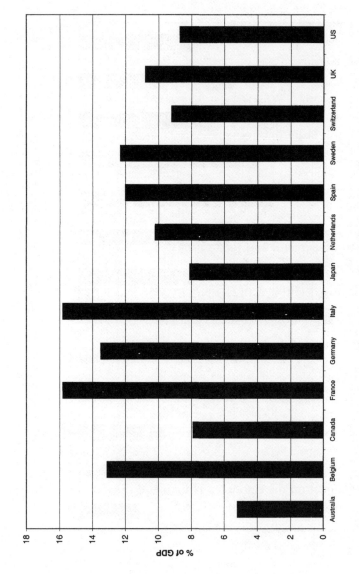

Fig. 2.3. Percentage of GDP spent on elderly persons: Unsure and health allocated by population

to our spending figures if we add spending for health and other catego-ries for which uncertainties remain: for health care, we used the data from OECD 1998 to divide health care spending into the portion spent on the elderly and the portion spent on the nonelderly;[1] for other un-certain categories, we assumed that spending on elderly persons was in proportion to their share of the population. The levels of spending on elderly persons are much higher here, about 2.7 percent higher on av-erage, so across this sample of countries we see 10.9 percent of GDP transferred to elderly persons. For the remainder of the analysis, we use the more conservative estimate, which we can measure accurately.

Part of this variation in spending on elderly persons reflects general preferences for social spending in these nations. Figure 2.4 explores this issue by showing the share of social spending that goes to elderly persons. Italy continues to transfer the largest share of social spending to elderly persons (52%) and Australia the least (less than 20%), but the United States now ranks fifth in share of social spending to elderly persons at 40 percent, and Japan ranks second (44%).

WHAT DOES PUBLIC SPENDING BUY?

This dramatic variation in spending on elderly persons raises the natural question of what increased spending buys for elderly persons. There are two extreme alternatives that one might expect on this ques-tion. This variation could reflect simply variations across countries in the preference for public versus private spending on elderly persons; in that event there would be little net impact on the living standards of elderly persons but rather only a transfer of responsibility for their care. That is, in this extreme alternative, there would be full "crowd-out" of private spending by public spending on elderly persons, with minimal impact on the resources available to them in the long run.

At the other extreme, it is possible that these programs are substan-tially increasing the living standards of elderly persons and that with-out them there would be significantly lower well-being in this popula-tion. In the United States, for example, private health insurance of elderly persons was reported to be quite modest before the publicly provided Medicare program arose in the mid-1960s. At this extreme, crowd-out

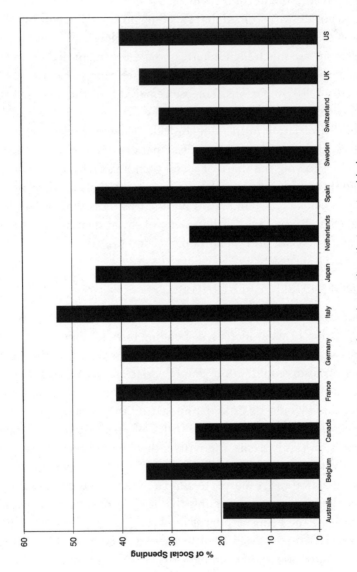

Fig. 2.4. Percentage of social spending that goes to elderly persons

is negligible, and increased transfers to elderly persons bring real benefits to them.

It is difficult with aggregate data to crisply distinguish these extremes and impossible to estimate precisely where, in between, the truth lies. But three important pieces of evidence can be brought to bear that suggest merit to both possibilities. The first, focusing on the labor supply responses to public pension incentives, suggests that there is a substantial crowd-out of work among elderly persons by public pension programs. The second further suggests crowd-out by showing no relationship between the relative incomes of elderly persons and the share of GDP transferred to them. The third, however, demonstrates that the elderly poverty rate is negatively related to transfers to elderly persons, suggesting that at the bottom of the income distribution, these transfers are improving living standards.

Public Pension Incentives and Elderly Labor Supply

One avenue through which the crowd-out noted above can arise is through the labor supply decisions of elderly persons. If larger public programs induce elderly persons to retire earlier, then these programs will simply serve to displace private labor earnings with public pension dollars.

This issue was the topic of a recent study that we directed (Gruber and Wise 1999b). We convened teams of experts from eleven countries to study the relationship between public pension program structures and the retirement decisions of older workers. This study produced three important conclusions. First, as illustrated in Figure 2.5, there is substantial disparity in the labor force participation rates of older workers across developed nations. The countries in this figure are ordered by labor force participation at age 65. At age 50 approximately 90 percent of men are in the labor force in all of the countries. But the decline after age 50 varies greatly among countries. Most men in Belgium are no longer in the labor force at age 65, and only about 25 percent are working at age 60; in Japan, however, 60 percent are working at 65 and 75 percent at age 60.

Second, there is also significant disparity across nations in the incentives for continued work at older ages. Many social security systems,

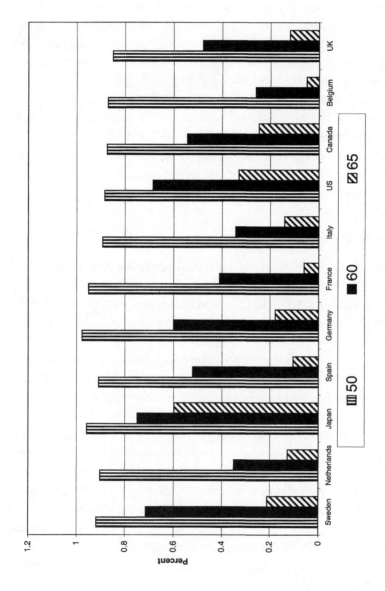

Fig. 2.5. Labor force participation for men by country and age

particularly in Europe, both provide benefits that replace a substantial portion of preretirement earnings and offer no upward adjustment to benefits for work beyond the early entitlement age. As a result, these systems provide substantial "implicit taxes" on work at older ages, since workers can receive virtually their full incomes even if they are retired. This is in contrast to the United States, which has a relatively low replacement rate (41% for the median worker) and provides a significant incentive for work past age 62, by both increasing benefits (6.67 percent for each year worked to age 65) and recomputing benefits to account for higher earnings years at older ages.

Table 2.2 shows the results of detailed calculations of these implicit taxes in the countries in the Gruber and Wise study. These calculations were all made for a hypothetical man born in 1930 who earned the median level of wages throughout his life, with a wife three years younger who never worked. The results are striking. For example, in France, there is an 80 percent tax on work past one's sixtieth birthday, since the replacement rate is so high (91%) and it is not adjusted for additional work. In the Netherlands, the tax rate is 141 percent, since the older person who continues to work not only forgoes benefits equal to 91 percent of his wage but also pays very steep income and payroll taxes on the wages that he earns. In contrast, in the United States, there is actually a small subsidy for continued work at age 62, due to the incentives put in place to continue working at that age.

The third, and perhaps most important, finding of the Gruber and Wise study is that there appears to be a very strong correlation between the retirement incentives put in place by public pension systems and the actual retirement decisions of older workers. We illustrate this point in two ways, using data from our summary paper (Gruber and Wise 1999a). First, we show the "hazard rate," or the conditional exit rate from the labor force, for France, in Figure 2.6. This hazard has a enormous "spike" at age 60, which is the age of entitlement for social security benefits. That is, of the workers still working at age 60, 60 *percent* leave the labor force at that age. This cannot be easily explained by any mechanism other than the public pension structure. Indeed, Gruber and Wise show that fifteen years earlier, when the age of public pension entitlement was 65, there was little labor force exit at age 60

Table 2.2. Retirement Incentives of Social Security Programs

Country	Tax Rate (%) for Working Past Early Retirement Age
Belgium	82
Canada	8
France	80
Germany	35
Italy	81
Japan	47
The Netherlands	141
Spain	−23
Sweden	28
United Kingdom	75
United States	−1

Source: Gruber and Wise 1999a.

and much more at age 65; this spike in the hazard evolved only after the early retirement provision at age 60 was introduced.

Next, we show the relationship between the tax rates documented in Table 2.2 and the extent of early withdrawal from the labor force illustrated by Figure 2.5. Figure 2.7 graphs the total amount of "nonwork" from age 55 to age 65 (the percentage of the male population in that age interval who are not working) against the logarithm of the "tax force" to retire, which is the sum of tax rates on work from age 55 to 69.[2] We see a striking correspondence between these two, with the tax force explaining over 80 percent of the variation in nonwork.

This finding must be interpreted with some caution, of course. There are a host of other factors that differ across nations in a cross section, and these may be correlated with both the tax force and nonwork measures. But this strong relationship suggests that there may be important "crowding out" by large public pension systems along at least one dimension, labor supply. Moreover, work by Richard Johnson (1999) confirms the significant negative impact of retirement incentives on labor supply using within-country changes in retirement incentives for a

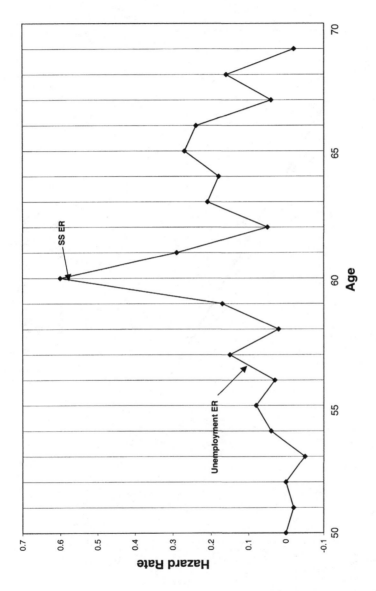

Fig. 2.6. Hazard rates for France

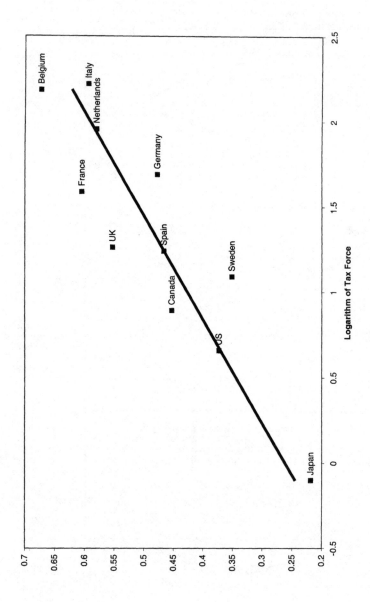

Fig. 2.7. Nonwork versus tax force

sample of countries throughout the twentieth century (see below for a discussion of the advantages of this approach).

Average Incomes of Elderly Persons

Another avenue for understanding the implications of public spending on elderly outcomes is to examine the implications directly for the living standards of elderly persons. We do so by examining the relationship between spending on elderly persons and their relative incomes, from Hauser 1997. The income measure we use is the ratio of the average income of pensioner households (households where there is someone over age 65 who is receiving a pension) to the average income of nonpensioner households.[3] These data are available for only nine of our twelve sample countries.

Figure 2.8 shows the relationship between relative incomes and the percentage of GDP spent on elderly persons. The lack of correspondence between the measures of living standards and the measures of spending on elderly persons is striking, as is the fact that countries that transfer such dramatically differing shares of their incomes to elderly persons show no differences in elderly living circumstances. Canada, which transfers less than 5 percent of GDP to elderly persons, and Germany, which transfers over 10 percent, have essentially the same ratio of elderly to nonelderly incomes; Italy, which transfers over 13 percent, has much lower elderly incomes.

Once again, this result must be interpreted with considerable caution. If countries where there is more underlying structural reason for elderly persons to have lower incomes are the ones that spend more on elderly persons, then that could cause the lack of correlation between spending and elderly living standards. But these findings are nevertheless suggestive of substantial crowd-out of private mechanisms by public mechanisms; where the public sector transfers more to elderly persons, they are no better off on average.[4]

Elderly Poverty Rates

Even if there is no impact on average elderly incomes, it is possible that larger transfers to elderly persons are successful in keeping them

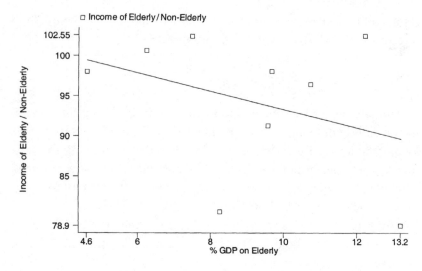

Fig. 2.8. Spending and elderly incomes

out of poverty. A negative impact on poverty rates even while there is
no impact on average incomes could arise either if transfers are tightly
targeted to the poorest elderly or if transfers are raising incomes at the
bottom but lowering them at the top, leading to no impact on average
incomes.

Figure 2.9 therefore compares a measure of the poverty of elderly
persons to our data on transfers to elderly persons as a share of GDP.
This (relative) poverty indicator measures the percentage of individuals aged 65 or older whose incomes are less than 40 percent of the
median disposable income in the nation; these data come from Smeeding
1997. In fact, we do see a striking negative correspondence between
spending and poverty; those nations that spend more on elderly persons do have lower elderly poverty rates. Italy and France, which transfer
more than 12 percent of their GDP to elderly persons, have elderly
poverty rates of less than 5 percent; Australia, Japan, and the United
States, which transfer less than 7 percent, have poverty rates above 18
percent. Although the fit between these two series is not perfect, the
relationship suggests that for every percentage point of GDP transferred to elderly persons, their poverty rates fall by 1.33 percentage
points.

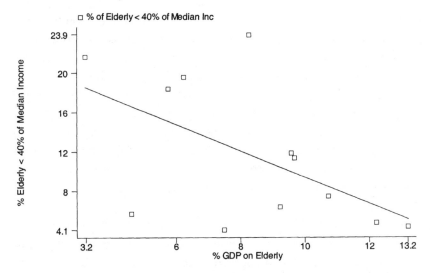

Fig. 2.9. Spending and elderly poverty

Thus, the two different income measures used in the last two subsections paint very different pictures of the impacts of government spending. It is once again important to highlight the suggestive nature of these findings; nonetheless, they do suggest that more spending on elderly persons is successful in removing them from the worst circumstances but that at higher income levels the increased spending is undoing private sources of support.

IMPLICATIONS OF POPULATION AGING FOR PUBLIC SPENDING

Spending on Elderly Persons

A critical question for fiscal policy in developed nations is how public spending on elderly persons will evolve as the demographic transition continues. Making these types of projections based on the past relationship between aging and spending is difficult. But they provide a useful benchmark against which future aging trends can be analyzed.

We make these projections by matching our data on the distribution of spending on elderly persons to data on the aging of populations in

OECD countries. Since we have data on both of these variables over time (since 1980), we can now run panel data regressions, controlling for country-specific dummies to capture time invariant tastes for spending on elderly persons and controlling for year-specific dummies to capture common trends in population and spending around the world for the period 1980 to 1995. That is, for this measure we can consider the more robust method of considering how *within-country changes* in social insurance spending translate into parallel *within-country changes* in health outcomes. This provides a more convincing estimate of the impact of spending than do the simple cross-country comparisons of the previous section.

We in fact find a very strong positive relationship between within-country changes in the share of the population that is elderly and within-country changes in the share of GDP that is devoted to public spending on elderly persons. The first row of Table 2.3 shows the coefficient on the share of the population that is elderly from a regression of elderly spending as a share of GDP on elderly population share, controlling for a full set of country and year fixed effects. There is a precisely estimated coefficient of 0.26; each percentage point increase in the ratio of the elderly population to total population raises spending on elderly persons by 0.26 percentage points of GDP. The elasticity figure at the bottom of the cell, 0.47, shows the elasticity of spending on elderly persons; for each 1 percent rise in the elderly population share, spending on elderly persons rises by 0.47 percent.

Table 2.4 shows the results of using this estimate to extrapolate what will happen to spending on elderly persons over the coming decades if this relationship continues to hold. The first column of this table shows actual spending on elderly persons, as a share of GDP, in 1995. The remaining columns extrapolate spending in future years, based on OECD projections for the elderly share of the population.

The results are striking. We find that, on average, the percent of GDP spent on elderly persons by this projection method would rise almost one-half, from 8.2 percent to 11.4 percent, by 2050. The increase varies substantially across countries, reflecting different patterns of population aging. Australia starts with the lowest spending on elderly persons in our sample but has the highest proportional increase (more than doubling by 2050). Germany, Italy, Japan, and Spain are

Table 2.3. Elderly Population and Social Spending

Dependent Variable	Coefficient on Elderly / Total Population		
Spending on elderly / GDP	0.264	(0.065)	{0.47}
Other nonhealth social spending / GDP	−0.332	(0.129)	{−0.57}
Nonelderly nonhealth spending / GDP	−0.186	(0.104)	{−0.369}
Unsure nonhealth spending / GDP	−0.147	(0.048)	{−2.09}
Health spending / GDP	0.099	(0.069)	{0.22}
Total spending / GDP	0.030	(0.143)	{0.02}
Number of observations	208		

Note: The regressions used control for a full set of country and year fixed effects. Standard errors in parentheses; elasticities in brackets.

projected to see an increase of 4 percentage points or more in spending on elderly persons relative to GDP. Sweden and the United States have relatively modest projected increases of less than 2 percentage points.

Implications for Government Finance

What are the implications of this dramatic increase in spending on elderly persons? Governments can take one of three routes to finance a rising share of elderly persons: reduce spending in other areas, raise taxes, or increase debt. Our evidence suggests that the first of these routes has been chosen more often than the other two.

The second row of Table 2.3 shows a regression of spending on all categories of transfers, excluding health and those transfers we can clearly assign to elderly persons, as a share of GDP, on the elderly population share, once again controlling for a full set of country and year fixed effects. We call this measure "other nonhealth social spending." It is important to highlight that this dependent variable includes our "unsure" categories of spending, some of which may be on elderly persons but which it is impossible to assign cleanly. As a result, in the next two rows of Table 2.3 we divide other nonhealth social spending into categories of spending for which we can clearly assign their impacts to the nonelderly (education, job training), which we label "nonelderly

Table 2.4. Projected Social Spending (as a percentage of GDP) on the Elderly

	1995 (Actual)	2010	2020	2030	2040	2050
Australia	3.1	3.4	4.4	5.3	6.1	6.4
Belgium	9.8	10.1	11.0	12.0	12.4	12.2
Canada	4.6	5.1	6.1	7.3	7.5	7.5
France	12.3	12.7	13.6	14.4	14.9	15.0
Germany	11.1	12.1	12.6	14.0	15.1	15.1
Italy	13.0	14.1	14.9	16.2	17.7	17.8
Japan	6.1	7.8	9.1	9.3	10.1	10.4
The Netherlands	7.3	7.9	9.2	10.5	11.2	10.8
Spain	9.7	10.5	11.2	12.6	14.2	15.0
Sweden	8.8	9.0	9.7	10.0	10.4	10.1
Switzerland	6.8	7.5	8.6	10.0	10.6	10.0
United Kingdom	8.1	8.2	9.3	10.4	10.8	10.8
United States	6.2	6.3	6.8	7.5	8.0	7.8
Sample average	8.2	8.8	9.7	10.7	11.4	11.4

nonhealth spending," and categories for which we cannot clearly do such assignment (disability, housing benefits, rehabilitation services), which we label "unsure nonhealth spending."

These three rows of Table 2.3 deliver a clear message: rising elderly population shares are strongly negatively associated with other nonhealth spending. In fact, the estimated impact of a 1 percent within-country increase in elderly population leads to a reduction in other nonhealth spending/GDP of 0.33 percent. Thus, on net, there is no estimated impact of an increase in the elderly population on transfer spending; the increased transfers to elderly persons are offset by reduced spending in other categories.

As the next two rows show, however, only about 42 percent of this total other nonhealth spending impact is through categories clearly assigned to the nonelderly; more than half is through unsure categories. This makes it somewhat difficult to assess the full welfare implications of the spending reductions that accompany population aging. Even in the limiting case in which all of the "unsure" spending goes to elderly persons, however, we are still seeing a significant negative impact on spending on the nonelderly as the population ages.

Of course, an increase in the elderly population should also increase health spending, and indeed there is a positive relationship with health spending, as the fifth row of Table 2.3 shows, but it is not significant. Adding all three elements (elderly transfers, other transfers, and health), there remains a very small and insignificant relationship between within-country changes in the elderly population and total government transfer plus health spending. This finding suggests that, if current trends continue, the brunt of the burden of an aging society will be borne through reduced spending elsewhere, including spending on the nonelderly.

WHERE DO WE GO FROM HERE?

There is a wide variation in the share of national resources devoted to elderly persons across similar developed nations documented in this study. Part of this variation reflects different shares of the population that is elderly, but this variation explains only about 10 percent of the within-country variance in elderly spending. There are clearly substantial differences across countries in their views on redistribution to the elderly population.

We have explored two dimensions of this redistribution. We first examined the implications for the well-being of elderly persons, for which we found mixed evidence. Across countries, there is very suggestive evidence that more generous retirement income support systems, which generally provide large disincentives to labor supply at older ages, lead to much lower labor supply levels among elderly persons. Perhaps as a reason, there is no correlation between the share of GDP transferred to elderly persons and their income levels. There is evidence, however, that an increase in the level of transfers to elderly persons reduces their poverty rates.

Second, we have shown that increases in the elderly population translate into significant increases in transfers to elderly persons. Indeed, if the trends of the recent past can be extrapolated into the future, population aging over about the next fifty years will result in 11.4 percent of GDP being devoted to spending on elderly persons on average in our sample of developed countries. At the same time, we find that this population aging causes equal reductions in spending elsewhere, so that on net there is no change in transfers as the population ages.

This finding is good news for fiscal balances but potentially bad news for the nonelderly. An important priority for future work is to explore the mechanisms through which population aging affects the spending on the nonelderly. Are the gains that we document in terms of elderly health matched by costly losses in terms of the education, health, or other well-being of the nonelderly? If so, it would appear that national priorities in all of these countries should be to find ways to ease the growing imbalances that aging populations are forcing on us.

NOTES

1. These data show the percentage of total health care spending on elderly persons, not public spending, but for most countries in our sample these are one and the same. For countries for which we did not have these data, we used the sample average percentage of health care spending on elderly persons to assign it. For the United States, we had true data on public spending on elder health, so no allocation was required.

2. We use tax rates after age 65 as well because forward-looking individuals should consider the entire future path of tax rates in making their retirement decisions. As we show in Gruber and Wise (1999a), our conclusions are not sensitive to the formulation of either the nonwork or tax force measures.

3. This is actually a simple average of the series for those aged 65–74 and those aged 75+; these two series are so highly correlated (0.97) that this is a reasonable representation of all those over age 65.

4. It is not obvious whether the correct variable for the analysis here is the share of GDP spent on elderly persons or the share of GDP spent per elderly person (the latter being the former divided by the elderly share of the population). But the results in Figures 2.8 and 2.9 are insensitive to whichever of these definitions is used.

REFERENCES

Borsch-Supan, A., and R. Schnabel. 1999. Social Security and Retirement in Germany. In J. Gruber and D. A. Wise, eds., *Social Security and Retirement around the World*. Chicago: University of Chicago Press.

Cutler, D. 1999. Equality, Efficiency, and Market Fundamentals: The Dynamics of International Medical Care Reform. Harvard University. Mimeographed.

Gruber, J., and D. A. Wise. 1999a. Introduction to J. Gruber and D. A. Wise, eds., *Social Security and Retirement around the World*. Chicago: University of Chicago Press.

————, eds. 1999b. *Social Security and Retirement around the World.* Chicago: University of Chicago Press.

Hauser, R. 1997. Adequacy and Poverty among the Retired. Paper presented at the Joint ILO-OECD Workshop on Development and Reform of Pension Schemes, Paris. December 15–17, 1997.

Johnson, R. 1999. The Effect of Social Security on Male Retirement: Evidence from Historical Cross-Country Data. KC Fed Working Paper, RWP 00-09, December 2000.

OECD. 1998. *Maintaining Prosperity in an Ageing Society.* Paris: OECD.

Smeeding, T. 1997. Financial Poverty in Developed Countries: The Evidence from LIS. LIS Working Paper no. 155, Maxwell School, Syracuse University.

II
THE
ECONOMIC
FRAMEWORK

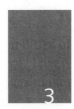

3

Budget Estimates

What We Know, What We Can't Know,

and Why It Matters

Henry J. Aaron, Ph.D.

Conversations about social insurance pensions and health benefits for the elderly revolve around projections or forecasts of the distant future. These projections are valuable in constraining legislators. Projections of deficits may occasionally goad legislators to enact unpleasant reforms. But these projections generally have quite limited value in telling us whether and how to modify the structure of Social Security or Medicare and about the proper way to address problems of long-term care.

Virtually every study or proposal regarding Social Security or Medicare rests on projections of population, economic conditions, and health care costs stretching decades into the future. Indeed, the United States has led the world in using long-term projections of costs to shape debate on its social insurance programs. The use of seventy-five-year projections for Social Security and of twenty-five-year and then seventy-five-year projections for Medicare has resulted in a salutary constraint on legislation. Such projections make it much harder to spend now and pay later, a distressing proclivity of elected officials, who serve *now* and will be retired or dead *later.* Proposing to raise Social Security or Medicare benefits without additional revenue, except when a surplus is projected, is unheard of. By bringing within the current political horizon events that would otherwise remain too distant to matter now, long-term projections can also create a political climate conducive to reforms. Thus, the long-term projections have an almost mystical and largely benign power.

Yet there is a paradox here. We are all justifiably skeptical about forecasts of the prices of stocks next week or of budget surpluses next year. When it comes to health care and pension issues, however, we routinely deal in projections stretching for decades. Even more striking is the apparent willingness of some of us to treat projected deficits as point estimates whose reliability is sufficient to undergird sweeping and immediate changes in program structure.

Of course, the fact that the cone of possibilities widens as one looks further into the future cannot be allowed to paralyze decision making. It is surely better to form one's best guess about the future and act on that judgment than it would be to proceed blithely ignoring projections or to procrastinate until the hazy future becomes the quite certain present. Pensions, after all, represent a roughly seventy-five-year contract with people entering the labor force. If the government is going to take workers' money today and compensate them with benefits much later on, long-term projections are a necessary input into honesty.

If projections were reliable, the road would be clear. Calculate the best policy and the best schedule for phasing it in, and enact it. But we know that projections require frequent and extensive revision. And the range of plausible possibilities widens the further one looks into the future. How, then, should we use them to shape current legislation? There are really three related questions: What do we know with some measure of reliability about the current situation? What will happen if we do not change policy? And how will changes in policy change future events? Each step is marked by uncertainty. The first problem concerns errors in data. The second and third problems concern model uncertainty. The critical and inadequately studied question concerns how data and model uncertainties should shape current policy. I focus on projection or forecast uncertainty as they affect Social Security, Medicare, and long-term care. But all three sources of uncertainty merit more study than they have received.

UNCERTAINTY AND POLICY CHANGES

Imagine a simple and quite fanciful world in which one can choose a given future policy environment with equal ease regardless of the policy environment at any earlier time. In that world, it would be equally possible to have the same defined contribution Medicare plan two decades from now whether or not a defined contribution plan or a defined benefit plan exists, say, ten years from now. It would also be equally possible to have a system of individual accounts instead of part or all of the Social Security system five decades from now whether or not one establishes individual accounts today or in three decades.

That world, of course, is not the one we live in.

- Programs take time to mature. Private accounts will be bigger in 2050 if we start now than if we start in the future.
- Initial conditions matter, and political decision making is costly. It is normally easier to keep a program than to enact it or to repeal it. If we think that private accounts are a bad idea, we must bear in mind that it will probably be harder to kill them once they are established than to prevent their creation.

Note the persuasiveness of uncertainty. We are uncertain not only about the future environment and the direct consequences of legislation but also about the effects of action on the political framework for future decisions. Initial conditions also matter because some imbalances (e.g., surpluses) are easier to respond to than are other imbalances (e.g., deficits), and they produce different outcomes. We could, for example, deal with uncertainty regarding mortality rates in the following three ways: keep a benefit formula that is independent of life expectancy, index benefit amounts to life expectancy, or index the retirement age to life expectancy. If the system is otherwise in balance, the first approach will result in deficits whenever life expectancy rises more than anticipated, creating pressure for some combination of benefit cuts and tax increases. Under the second and third approaches, balance will be maintained through benefit cuts alone, but the cuts will be distributed differently. Congress could legislate anew to produce the same outcome, regardless of initial legislation, but I doubt that any of us would expect the outcomes to be the same.

- The political possibility of change fluctuates. Timing is everything not only in love and war but also in politics. The political environment will be different when the baby boomers are age 60 to 80 from what it is now when they are age 35 to 55.

What this all means is that in deciding what to do, we should weigh the reliability of projections; the time it will take our current actions to take effect; the ease of reversibility; and the ease of future, as compared to current, action. And of course we should recognize the direct and intended economic and political consequences of our current action, which are themselves uncertain.

We typically do not think about policy this way. We normally pretend that we live in the simple world of certain projections and costless and frictionless legislation. We analyze, within certainty models, the effects of well-defined policy changes and evaluate the results. Economists, for example, study the labor supply effects or excess burdens of raising payroll taxes; the effects on financial markets of a change in the assets in which the Social Security Trust Fund are invested; or the rates of return, risks, and administrative costs associated with private accounts. With respect to Medicare, they study the effects on costs of adding coverage of prescription drugs or a stop-loss provision and of converting the program from a defined benefit, fee-for-service program to one with managed care or premium support. Political scientists study political coalitions likely to support or oppose each of these changes. Health policy analysts consider, for example, how the availability of long-term care insurance would influence the willingness of friends and relatives to provide free care and what the costs of such "woodwork" effects would be.

The subject of model uncertainty and its effects on macroeconomic policy received a fair bit of attention a few decades ago, but not much has been heard lately on that subject. One study, by Alan Auerbach and Kevin Hassett (1999), tried in a formal way to come to grips with the extremely difficult issues arising from uncertainty about the future environment and the difficulty of legislating, but no one has addressed all of those issues.

The reason no one has considered all of these questions simultaneously is that the task is laughably beyond our current analytical capacities. We simply cannot simultaneously handle the direct consequences of action (presuming that our point estimates are correct), *and* the direct consequences under alternative properly weighted uncertain contingencies, *and* the direct consequences under plausible models different from the one we have used, *and* the difficulty of modifying policy if current projections are incorrect, *and* the impacts on future legislation of different legislative and political defaults brought about by current actions, *and* whether it would be better to commit now to act at some time in the future than to act now. If we tried to answer those questions all at once, we would rapidly lapse into subjective evaluations for which our analytical training provides no legitimacy. Science does not advance by tackling questions that are too hard to answer. And experts do not retain their reputations by dithering about "maybe's" and "perhaps's" in areas outside their expertise.

Politicians, in contrast, must deal with such questions. They know that forecasts may be absurdly off the mark. They hear from a variety of analysts with models generating diverse and sometimes contradictory prescriptions, and each analyst sincerely believes that his or her model is the best way of looking at an issue. Elected officials, like the rest of us, are loath to admit error. They also fear that if they reverse a decision, voters will punish them at the next election for being weak or indecisive.

As analysts, we pretend that we are simply providing decision makers with information that they must decide how to use. But given the passionate intensity with which many of us push our favored policy options, this pretense is self-serving or self-deluding nonsense. We are wannabe policymakers. But we use analytical frameworks that exclude questions central to political judgment. We exclude those questions because we can't answer them. But our incapacity does not make the questions unimportant or irrelevant. We all hold subjective "priors" about these unanswerable questions (which is a good thing, because they are very important), and these priors may overshadow our analytical judgments (which can also be a good thing, because they may be more important than the analytical conclusions we are trained to reach). Perhaps we should also take seriously the kinds of concerns that trouble decision makers. And perhaps we should not allow theoretical models simplified for analytical tractability to obscure those subjective priors.

WHAT WE KNOW

We often know signs and what is big and what is small, but we seldom have a good fix on values. We know, for example, that the effect of birthrates on the long-run balance of Social Security and Medicare is big and that of divorce rates is comparatively small. We know that birthrates are down from post–World War II highs but are higher than they are in most other developed nations. We have good theories to explain why they probably will not rise much and might fall. This forecast is critical to projections of the long-run financial condition of Social Security and Medicare. It means that the population pyramid will inexorably tend to become a rectangle and that it could even become an inverted pyramid. Should birthrates return to 1950 levels, the projected deficit in Social Security would fall by half and that in Medicare would shrink somewhat less. I think we are on safe ground assuming that little or no financial relief will come from that quarter.

Mortality rates are falling, which is to say that life expectancy is increasing. Furthermore, the ongoing and accelerating revolution in biotechnology could lead to increases in life expectancy considerably larger than are assumed by the Social Security Administration or even by the Bureau of the Census. Such an event, if all else were held constant, would mean financial calamity for Social Security. The effects on Medicare finances would be less certain. In short, how much life expectancy will increase is critically important to our financial projections, but—alas!—that is unknowable.

WHAT WE DON'T KNOW

Signs count, but so do magnitudes. Economic productivity has been rising since the start of the industrial revolution. Growth accelerated sharply in the developed world after World War II, then slowed. More recently, the pace has increased in the United States. We can be confident that productivity will keep on rising, but we cannot be sure how fast. Speed matters. If productivity grows 0.5 percent annually, U.S. residents in 2050 will have 29 percent higher incomes than we do today. At 1.5 percent growth, they will have 114 percent more than we do today. Both growth rates are within the range that responsible forecasters might assume. The difference—nearly equal to income today—will have an important bearing on how future workers feel about paying taxes to support health and pension benefits for the dependent elderly and disabled.

Change in the size and composition of the population depends not only on the fact that birth and mortality rates are falling but also on how much and on net immigration. Together those elements determine population trends. Even if birthrates decline below zero population growth (ZPG) levels, population will continue to rise for some time because younger cohorts are so much larger than older cohorts and because of immigration. But experience in Europe and Japan suggests that we should not rule out population implosion. The only things we do not know are whether that will happen and, if so, when.

Even more troubling is our complete ignorance about the quality of life that people will enjoy as life expectancies increase. We do not know whether the entire process of aging—reduced mental flexibility, deterioration of joints, muscle atrophy, senility, arthritis, decline of libido, and other curses of the aging class—will be delayed. If they are, tomorrow's 75-year-olds may look like today's 50-year-olds. If not, tomorrow's 75-, 85-, and 95-year-olds may just be more numerous than, but not different from, today's.

We do not, therefore, know how long people will choose to work when confronted with any given set of incentives. We know that the twentieth century was marked by a steady decline in the labor force participation rates of men. That trend seems to have come to a halt sometime during the 1980s (Quinn 1998). But experts disagree on whether the halt reflects an unusually strong labor market, in which case the decline will resume when the labor market softens, or whether it is a major shift from a decades-long pattern. If age-specific physical and mental vigor does not increase, the prospects that people will choose to work much longer as their incomes rise cannot be viewed as bright, even if work becomes somewhat less onerous. But if tomorrow's 75-

year-olds physically and mentally resemble today's 50-year-olds, efforts to encourage them to work like today's 50-year-olds are more likely to succeed.

We know that a biological revolution is under way and that the speed of technological advance is inherently unpredictable. I think the evidence is overwhelming that the new technology will tend to push up medical costs in the near future, as it has done for decades. Some claim that technology will lower costs soon. I am skeptical. But my point is that we do not know whether that will happen or when. Meanwhile, we know that changes in human institutions—private organization of the health care system and public Medicare and Medicaid policy—can have first order effects on medical expenditures. Between 1995 and 2000, for example, the Health Care Financing Administration (HCFA) actuaries reduced their projections of the cost of Medicare as a share of GDP by roughly two-fifths (see Table 3.1). Even short-term projections have been subject to massive error (see Figure 3.1). HCFA in 1991 projected that national health care spending in 2000 would claim 16.4 percent of GDP (Sonnenfeld et al. 1991). Two years later, the Congressional Budget Office (CBO) put the share for the year 2000 at 17.5 percent (Lemieux 1993). The current HCFA and CBO projections are 14.3 and 13.9 percent, respectively. Let me be clear. I come not to bury CBO and HCFA analysts, but to praise them. They are top-class professionals—the best we have and as good as we are likely to get—but their projections have not been exactly bang on. The point is that we really do not have a very good fix on where health care spending is going.

We do not know what will happen to the distribution of income—whether inequality will rise or fall or how much. We know that income inequality fell sharply for about three decades following World War II and then rose for the succeeding two decades, restoring the degree of inequality that had prevailed half a century earlier. The Energizer bunny economic expansion that lasted until late 2000 halted the trend to increased inequality, but we do not know what the future holds. Powerful forces are at work—economic globalization, an information revolution, and changes in social norms regarding compensation. Whether inequality widens or narrows will powerfully influence not only the character of the economy of the future but also whether income redis-

**Table 3.1. Projections of Medicare Outlays (as a percentage of GDP)
by HCFA Actuaries**

	Medicare Outlays	
Projection Year	In 2020	In 2040
1995	6.01	8.05
2000	3.50	4.76

Source: Board of Trustees, Federal Hospital Insurance Trust Fund, *Annual Report of the Board of Trustees of the Federal Hospital Insurance Trust Fund* (Washington, D.C.: U.S. Government Printing Office).

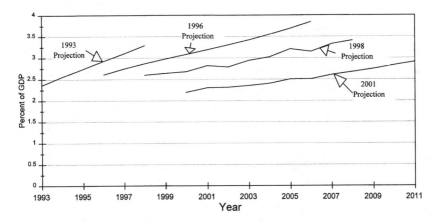

Fig. 3.1. Medicare spending: CBO projections. *Source:* Congressional Budget Office, *The Economic and Budget Outlook* (Washington, D.C.: U.S. Government Printing Office, selected years).

tribution—which is a central element of Social Security, Medicare, and Medicaid—will become more or less important.

WHY IT MATTERS

This list of what we know and what we do not know is short and selective. My point is not just that our long-term projections will not be *exactly* realized but that they may not even be *approximately* correct. I doubt that this observation is controversial, but to drive home the point, I shall sketch two scenarios for life in the latter half of the next century based on projections of key variables that I think are plausible. I freely acknowledge that I am grouping assumptions that are "optimistic" for one scenario and assumptions that are "pessimistic" for the other. Some messy average of the two will probably materialize. But these scenarios are not just a bit different from one another. They portray staggeringly different societies in which economic and social opportunity, the typical life cycle, values, and norms are poles apart. The disparate consequences of less extreme, but more plausible, scenarios should give pause to those of us who currently advocate radical change based on long-term projections.

In "active aging" scenario one, birthrates and net immigration produce essentially ZPG conditions; as a result, population levels off in the next few decades. Mortality rates fall roughly in line with current SSA intermediate projections. But medical science finds ways of forestalling arthritis and senility. Disability rates plunge. Powerful technological advance fuels annual productivity growth averaging 1.5 percent per worker. Educational levels increase, and lifelong learning becomes a reality, not just a slogan. Technological change and improved education cause income inequality to decline. People respond to the liberalized delayed-retirement credit in Social Security, the disappearance of window pension plans, and general cheerleading for lengthened working lives by remaining in the workforce to age 70, on the average, for men and to age 65 for women. The trend to later work partially offsets the tendency of population aging to boost the ratio of retirees to active workers. Around 2020, advances in medical technology become cost-reducing rather than cost-increasing.

In "inactive aging" scenario two, birthrates fall to levels now common in western Europe—1.3–1.6 children per woman. Mortality rates plummet, as medical science first finds effective treatments for, and then ways to prevent, many common cancers and heart disease. Unfortunately, treatments for arthritis and senility do not improve materially. Because age-specific disability rates decline little, the number of disabled elderly explodes and age at retirement does not increase. As a result, the ratio of retirees to active workers skyrockets. Productivity growth slows and the late-twentieth-century increase in inequality continues. Medical technology continues to push up costs, forcing agonizing political and economic choices between dramatically increased health care outlays and rationing.

I want to emphasize once again that these scenarios are extreme. The second, in particular, calls to mind Herb Stein's droll comment that if something cannot possibly continue, it will stop. Scenario two would surely spawn vigorous efforts to counter the rather dire outcomes. In general, how the future unfolds will depend significantly, but not completely, on the policies we adopt now. Even with these qualifications, I hope you will accept my assertion that, for any given set of current policies, plausible scenarios for the United States in 2050 differ so radically from one another that they would elicit entirely different responses today, if we knew for certain which would unfold. But we don't know, and we can't.

IMPLICATIONS

Well, life is uncertain. So what? More specifically, so what for current policymaking regarding pensions and health benefits for the elderly and disabled?

Social Security

The current debate on Social Security revolves around two groups of issues. One concerns how to deal with the projected long-term deficit. The other concerns the best structure for a government-mandated pension system.

To avoid the projected long-term deficit, one must first decide how much to commit to pensions. Then one must pick the best way to pay for them. Although some elected officials have proposed to reduce total pensions to levels that current payroll taxes could support, they have not gotten far. And with good reason. U.S. Social Security benefits are modest compared to benefits in virtually all other developed countries (Gruber and Wise 1999) and provide the average earner a benefit at age 62 barely in excess of the U.S. poverty threshold (Aaron and Reischauer 2001). The drift seems to be toward proposals that would maintain or boost benefits by tapping general revenues in one way or another or by raising the payroll tax base.

So the long-term financial problem becomes a question of fiscal policy—whether to cover benefits at least as large as those currently promised by raising revenues now or later—in the face of uncertainty about future economic conditions. This is the question that Auerbach and Hassett (1999) tackled. They deserve great credit for taking on a formidably difficult problem. To make the problem tractable, however, they simplified heroically in various ways. They set the problem in an overlapping generation model where each generation contained one representative person who lived for two periods. Their only limit to the policy that they analyze—that policy cannot be changed in two successive periods—omits most of the interesting political complexities. Their most important finding is that uncertainty about future economic events is no reason for legislative delay in closing a projected deficit. In fact, uncertainty justifies extra short-term saving because the losses from a worse-than-expected future exceed the gains from a better-than-expected future. Unfortunately, that conclusion collapses if legislation cannot be changed freely whenever new information becomes available. In that event, action should sometimes be deferred. Instead of legislating, the "government may . . . choose not to exercise its valuable option to set policy and, because the impact of its policies on the elderly cannot be reversed in the future, it is more likely to choose inaction when fiscal tightening is called for. Thus, the optimal policy response over time might best be characterized by great caution in general, but punctuated by occasional periods of apparent irresponsibility" (23).

This conclusion is remarkably equivocal, despite the exclusion of many of the politically relevant uncertainties I mentioned before. In addition, with one representative agent per generation, the model omits intragenerational distributional questions, which are matters of central importance to many in the current debate. With each generation living only two periods, economic questions about the effects of when policy is changed on the welfare of various cohorts and the politics of decision making could not be considered. The central insight—that uncertainty about the future should not justify procrastination—is relevant to the current debate on Social Security financing, provided that one treats the current debate as one about financing alone.

Of course, the current debate is not solely, or even mostly, about financing. More than six decades have passed since the Social Security

Act became law. The nation in which Social Security was enacted consisted of one-earner couples, of whom only a small minority were divorced. Few earners had more than a high school education and most had less. Fewer still paid income taxes. Tax sheltered individual savings accounts did not exist—why should they, when almost no one paid income taxes? Even amortized mortgages were uncommon, because the Federal Housing Administration had not yet made them safe for timid bankers. Financial sophistication among the mass of the population was slight to nil.

Well, things have changed. Half of marriages end in divorce. Most women work outside the home. Incomes and educational levels have risen dramatically. Most people pay income taxes and have some form of group or individual tax sheltered retirement saving. It is about time for us to consider whether a social insurance system that suited the United States in 1935 still suits it today. Has financial sophistication increased or financial market risks changed enough to undercut the case for defined benefit social insurance? Are people adequately protected by private pensions and individual saving, so that the risk-spreading characteristics of defined benefit social insurance are no longer needed?

These questions actually break down into four specific issues. Should management of the pension program remain in government hands or be privatized? Should social insurance take the form of defined benefit (DB) or defined contribution (DC) pensions? Should reserve accumulation be increased? And should reserves be invested in assets other than government bonds? Additional issues concern the desirability of sustaining the income redistribution that Social Security now provides and the best way to protect the interests of lesser earners (mostly women) and of surviving spouses (again, mostly women).

If long-term forecasts were reliable, they would bear directly on some of these questions but not on others. The advantages of public versus private management or of DB versus DC pensions do not depend on any long-term projection other than whether the future will be radically different from the past.

- We know that private management is far more costly than public management. Taken in isolation, private management would lower rates of return to pensioners (National Academy of Social Insurance 1998; Zinn 1999; Geanakoplos, Mitchell, and Zeldes 1998; Murphy and Welch 1998).

• We know that DC pensions have been—and are likely to remain— far riskier than DB pensions for individual workers in the U.S. political context.

• We also know that for the past couple of centuries, bonds have yielded less than stocks and that a portfolio consisting only of government bonds would have yielded less than a diversified and somewhat riskier portfolio. We have reason to think that those trends will continue.

• And we know that a central fund managed with a long planning horizon serving all workers is especially well suited to bearing risk because it can spread risk among workers and over time in the way that no DC plan or subnational DB plan can do (Diamond 1997).

We also know that reserve accumulation—that is to say, higher national saving—will increase burdens on the current generation and decrease them for future ones. The decision on how to distribute burdens across generations should be influenced by projections of economic growth.

What this means, I think, is that many of the most important elements of the current debate on the future of Social Security can proceed without much attention to refined long-term financial projections. The question of whether to build sizable reserves is an exception. And one would have to be blind to fail to see the political value of trying to foment discontent and a mood for reform by waving seventy-five-year forecasts in credulous people's faces. But from an analytical standpoint, what we should do about Social Security, other than the question of reserve accumulation, is pretty much independent of whether the actuaries report that the system will have a deficit or a surplus or will be in balance seventy-five years from now.

Medicare

Pretty much the same conclusion holds for Medicare. Whatever our ability may be to forecast pension costs, an impenetrable fog of unknowability shrouds projections of Medicare costs beyond just a few years. Table 3.1 and Figure 3.1 indicate that our past record in projecting the costs of Medicare is quite dreadful. Technological change, by its very nature, is unpredictable, as are its effects on costs. Institutional changes, such as the advent of managed care and legislated reimbursement rates, also have had huge effects on costs. And if you disagree with that assertion, we are really at sea, because we are then left without any explanation for why even short-run projections have been so dreadfully off the mark. Just now, for example, no one knows for sure why growth in the cost of health care slowed in the middle and late 1990s and sped up in 2000 or what will happen in the years ahead.

The projection of a long-term deficit is a goad to legislation. But the structural issues are largely independent of the projected deficit unless a mood develops to force elderly or disabled persons, or both, to shoulder a higher proportion of rising per capita health spending. Once again, the queue of elected officials endorsing such a shift is quite short. Reducing the gaps in coverage—the lack of pharmaceutical benefits, the absence of catastrophic coverage, the spottiness of long-term care coverage—will actually aggravate projected deficits. No serious observer can believe that a cost-conscious army of elderly and disabled health insurance shoppers will drive down costs enough to pay even for these added benefits, much less to eliminate the projected deficits.

Long-Term Care

The discussion of long-term care is instructive precisely because we do not have long-term projections of cost. Instead, we can focus directly on the fundamental policy questions. On these matters, alas, there is little consensus, aside from the view that care in the home or community is nearly always better, and just about as often cheaper, than institutional care. We cannot decide whether long-term care is an insurable event that can be handled by private insurance or whether it must be handled with some form of governmental intervention. If there is to be some form of social insurance, we cannot decide whether it should provide benefits covering the relatively frequent short stays and leave the costly, but relatively uncommon, long stays to be covered by personal budgets or by a means-tested backup, such as Medicaid; or whether social insurance should provide catastrophic coverage that kicks in only after short stays, which would remain an individual responsibility.

Cost projections are certainly relevant to the debate. Different approaches carry different price tags. And demand curves for collective, as well as private, goods slope downward. But I think we understand that there are more important structural issues to be resolved.

Beware of Careless Grouping

My contention that long-term projections have little to do with some of the most important questions in pension and health policy reform has a corollary. It is that the tendency to lump health and pension programs together as "entitlements" and thereby to suggest that they present similar policy challenges is misleading and unhelpful. It would make as much sense—which is to say, no sense at all—to treat pensions, welfare, and the earned income credit as "cash assistance" and to suggest that they pose common problems, or to lump health, education, and scientific research together because they represent "investments and maintenance of human capital," or to lump agricultural subsidies and defense expenditures together because both are financed by personal and corporation income taxes. Although the Social Security Act authorizes both Social Security and Medicare, and the payroll tax finances part of the cost of each program, the quite different policy challenges that arise from each must be solved independently.

Legislative moats do separate some programs that would be best considered jointly. Medicaid for the elderly and disabled and Medicare raise similar problems. Perhaps both of those programs and social service grants for the elderly should be treated as a unit. Some of us who, for our sins, follow tax policy are appalled at the drawer full of tax sheltered accounts that avid savers accumulate because of piecemeal legislation. Coordination in these and other areas could simplify life and improve the effectiveness of federal policy.

CONCLUSION

What this all adds up to is that long-term projections provide an admirable political discipline forcing elected officials to adopt a longer-than-customary perspective. Accordingly, they may stimulate action earlier than it would otherwise occur. It is quite important, I believe, that legislators continue to work within these constraints. The long-term projections reinforce the case for fiscal policy to boost national saving, a case that is pretty strong even without the projected deficits in Social Security and Medicare. But major proposals for reform of Social Security, Medicare, or long-term care should address the structure of pensions and of noncash benefits. Fiscal policy—which is to say, the determination of how much government revenues and expenditures should contribute to or subtract from national saving—is an important aspect of public policy. It is worth careful attention of policy analysts as well as elected officials. But it is not health policy and it is not pension policy.

ACKNOWLEDGMENTS

I want to thank Peter Diamond and William Gale for helpful comments on an earlier draft and Ben Harris for research assistance. I incorporated elements of this chapter in my presidential address to the Association for Public Policy Analysis and Management, "Seeing through the Fog: Policymaking with Uncertain Forecasts," *Journal of Policy Analysis and Management* 19, no. 2 (spring 2000): 193–206.

REFERENCES

Aaron, H. J., and R. D. Reischauer. 2001. *Countdown to Reform: The Great Social Security Debate.* 2nd ed. New York: Century Foundation.

Auerbach, A. J., and K. A. Hassett. 1999. Uncertainty and the Design of Long-Run Fiscal Policy. NBER Working Paper no. 7036, National Bureau of Economic Research, Cambridge, Mass.

Diamond, P. 1997. Macroeconomic Aspects of Social Security Reform. *Brookings Papers on Economic Activity* (fall): 1–66.

Geanakoplos, J., O. S. Mitchell, and S. P. Zeldes. 1998. Would a Privatized Social Security System Really Pay a Higher Rate of Return? In R. D. Arnold, M. J. Graetz, and A. H. Munnell, *Framing the Social Security Debate: Values, Politics, and Economics.* Washington, D.C.: National Academy of Social Insurance.

Gruber, J., and D. A. Wise, eds. 1999. *Social Security and Retirement around the World.* Chicago: University of Chicago Press.

Lemieux, J. 1993. Projections of National Health Expenditures: 1993 Update. Congressional Budget Office. Washington, D.C.: U.S. Government Printing Office.

Murphy, K. M., and F. Welch. 1998. Perspectives on the Social Security Crisis and Proposed Solutions. *American Economic Review* 88, no. 2 (May): 142–50.

National Academy of Social Insurance. 1998. *Report of the Panel on Privatization of Social Security National Academy of Social Insurance.* Washington, D.C.: National Academy of Social Insurance.

Quinn, J. F. 1998. The Labour Market, Retirement, and Disability. Paper presented at a conference on Income Support, Labor Markets, and Behavior, Australian National University, Canberra, November 24–25.

Sonnenfeld, S. T., D. R. Waldo, J. Lemieux, and D. R. McKusick. 1991. Projections of National Health Expenditures through the Year 2000. *Health Care Financing Review* 13, no. 1 (fall): 1–27.

Zinn, H.-W. 1999. Why a Funded System Is Needed and Why It Is Not Needed. Paper presented to the 55th IIPF Congress, Moscow, August 23–26.

4

Long-Run Budget Projections and Their Implications for Funding Elderly Entitlements

C. Eugene Steuerle, Ph.D., and Paul N. Van de Water, Ph.D.

Policy for the long term is driven by far more than numbers, particularly numbers about costs. Nonetheless, numbers help clarify the nature of budgetary trade-offs, and the production of long-term projections is a growth industry. Members of Congress and administration officials are clamoring for numbers, and staff members are striving to meet the demand. Long-run modeling efforts are under way at the Social Security Administration, the Congressional Budget Office, the Employee Benefit Research Institute, the Urban Institute, the Heritage Foundation, Cornell University, and numerous other sites.

Since long-term budget projections are not going to disappear but are likely to become more common, policymakers need to understand their underlying concepts, assumptions, and limitations. This chapter provides a primer or user's guide on long-term budget projections. It summarizes the long-run budget outlook, the sensitivity of long-run budget projections to changes in assumptions, the issues of resource allocation raised by the projections, and the budgetary and economic effects of major policy proposals.

In the course of this survey, it will become clear that the demand for long-run projections is fueled not simply by improvements in computational technology but also by the extent to which current law makes promises for the future. Indeed, current commitments for health and retirement benefits will absorb most or all of the projected growth in federal revenues for the foreseeable future (Steuerle et al. 1998, chap. 4).

THE NUMBERS: LONG-RUN BUDGET PROJECTIONS

Social Security, Medicare, and Medicaid are the largest but not the only federal programs that provide benefits to people age 65 or older. Together, they account for 86 percent of estimated federal spending on elderly persons (see Table 4.1). Retirement benefits for federal civilian and military retirees and benefits for veterans make up most of the rest. But not all spending for Social Security, Medicare, and Medicaid is devoted to elderly persons. One-eighth of Medicare benefits are provided to long-term disabled workers; one-quarter of Social Security benefits are received by disabled workers, young survivors, and retirees under age 65; and two-thirds of Medicaid assistance goes to low-income persons with disabilities or families with young children. All in all, however, spending for these three programs provides a reasonable approximation of federal spending on elderly persons.

Federal spending on people age 65 or older now represents about 35 percent of the federal budget and 6.4 percent of gross domestic product (GDP). Thirty years ago, spending on elderly persons represented only 22 percent of the budget and 4.2 percent of GDP. If current laws and policies continue, the Congressional Budget Office (CBO) estimates that 43 percent of the budget and 7.1 percent of GDP will be devoted to elderly persons after ten years—the period covered by the president's budget submission and the congressional budget resolution.

To analyze the fiscal situation beyond the usual ten-year budgetary horizon, CBO also produces long-run projections of federal receipts and expenditures. In contrast to CBO's ten-year baseline budget projections, the long-run projections of taxing and spending are often based on simple rules using historical patterns rather than current law. Also, because the long-run projections are designed to focus on macroeconomic relationships, they use the categories of the national income and product accounts rather than those of the federal budget (CBO 2000).

Making budget projections even a few years ahead is fraught with difficulty. When the Balanced Budget Act of 1997 was passed, for example, CBO projected that the federal budget would run a *deficit* in

Table 4.1. Estimated Federal Spending for Elderly Persons under Selected
Programs, 1971–2010 (by fiscal year, in billions of dollars)

	1971	1980	1990	2000	Projected 2010
Mandatory Programs					
Social Security[a]	29	85	196	307	471
Federal civilian retirement	2	8	21	33	50
Military retirement	1	2	7	14	21
Annuitant's health benefits	*	1	2	4	9
Special benefits for coal miners and black lung	*	1	1	1	1
Supplemental Security Income	1	2	4	6	10
Veterans' compensation and pensions	1	4	7	9	14
Medicare	8	29	96	189	377
Medicaid	2	5	14	33	73
Food stamps[b]	*	1	1	1	1
Total	44	137	349	597	1,026
Discretionary Programs					
Housing	*	2	4	7	10
Veterans' medical care	1	3	6	9	13
Administration on aging programs	*	1	1	1	1
Low-income home energy assistance program	n.a.	*	*	*	1
Total	1	6	11	18	24
Total					
All federal spending on people 65 or older	46	144	360	615	1,050
Memorandum: Federal spending on people 65 or older					
As a percentage of the budget	22	24	29	35	43
As a percentage of GDP	4.2	5.3	6.3	6.4	7.1
Per elderly person (in 2000 dollars)	8,896	11,839	15,192	17,688	21,122

Source: Based on data in CBO 2001.
Notes: * = less than $500 million; n.a. = not applicable.
[a]Includes Tier 1 of Railroad Retirement.
[b]Includes the federal share of states' administrative costs and nutrition assistance to Puerto Rico.

fiscal year 2000 of $48 billion, or 0.5 percent of GDP (CBO 1997). In fact the budget recorded a *surplus* of $236 billion, or 2.4 percent of GDP. If the estimated fiscal balance can shift by 3 percent of GDP in just three years, then the range of uncertainty fifty or seventy-five years from now is clearly vast.

Although CBO typically updates its ten-year budget projections twice a year, its long-run projections are calculated less frequently. The most recent long-run projections date from October 2000 and do not reflect two major developments. In January 2001 CBO upped its projections of surpluses by increasing the assumed rate of growth of real GDP by 0.3 percent a year. Then in May 2001 the president and Congress dipped into the surpluses by enacting a large reduction in taxes. On balance, the October 2000 projections overstate the near-term surpluses, but the numbers are still in the right ballpark.

Although the federal budget could remain in surplus for several decades, it faces mounting pressures in the very long run. Under the October 2000 projections, the surplus grows from over 2 percent of GDP in 2000 to 4 percent of GDP in 2010. After 2010, however, the retirement of the baby boom generation and continued growth in the cost and use of medical care will cause the surplus to shrink. The surplus will disappear by 2040, and deficits could reach 12 percent of GDP by 2060 (see Table 4.2). These projections indicate a very high probability that government budgetary policy is on an unsustainable path due to growth in benefit payments that cannot be met by the projected growth in revenues.

As the projected deficits grow, the federal government will have less fiscal flexibility, because the three large entitlement programs will absorb an increasing share of the budget. Together, Social Security, Medicare, and Medicaid now account for about 45 percent of noninterest spending. Their share of the noninterest budget is projected to rise to roughly 55 percent in 2010, 65 percent in 2020, and 70 percent in 2030. Over the same period, they will nearly double as a share of GDP— from 7.5 percent today to 15 percent in 2030.

Social Security and Medicare operate through trust funds. Earmarked revenues (including payroll taxes and interest on trust fund balances) are credited to the funds, and the programs' obligations (both benefits and administrative expenses) are paid from the trust funds. Social Se-

Table 4.2. Federal Receipts and Expenditures (by calendar year, as a percentage of GDP)

	Actual					Projected					
	1960	1970	1980	1990	2000	2010	2020	2030	2040	2050	2060
NIPA receipts	18	19	20	20	21	20	20	20	20	20	20
NIPA expenditures											
Social Security	2	3	4	4	4	4	5	6	6	6	7
Medicare	0	1	1	2	2	3	4	6	7	7	9
Medicaid	0	[a]	1	1	1	2	2	3	4	4	5
Subtotal	2	4	7	7	7	9	12	15	16	18	20
Other noninterest	14	15	14	12	8	7	7	7	7	7	7
Net interest	1	1	2	3	3	[a]	−2	−3	−3	[a]	6
Total	17	20	22	22	18	16	16	18	20	24	32
NIPA deficit (−) or surplus	1	−1	−2	−3	2	4	4	2	[a]	−4	−12
Primary deficit (−) or surplus	3	[a]	[a]	[a]	5	4	2	−1	−3	−5	−7
Debt held by the public	46	28	26	42	34	−8	−41	−49	−37	−5	67
Memorandum:											
GDP (trillions of dollars)	1	1	3	6	10	16	24	36	55	81	115

Source: Office of Management and Budget, Bureau of Economic Analysis, CBO 2000.

Note: NIPA = national income and product accounts.

[a] Less than 0.5 percent.

curity currently receives hardly any general revenues; income taxes on Social Security benefits represent less than 2 percent of the program's income. Medicare's Supplementary Medical Insurance Trust Fund, however, gets three-quarters of its income from general revenues.

Including interest and general revenues, the Social Security and Medicare trust funds are currently taking in more than they are spending, but they face insolvency in the longer run. Medicare's Hospital Insurance (HI) trust fund will start running deficits in 2021 and will be depleted in 2029 (Board of Trustees, HI Trust Fund 2001). The two Social Security trust funds (Old-Age and Survivors Insurance and Disability Insurance, or OASDI) will start running deficits in 2025 and will exhaust their assets in 2038. Outgo will begin to exceed noninterest income in 2016 (Board of Trustees, OASDI Trust Funds 2001).

In the past, the projected depletion of trust fund balances has often provided the impetus for taking painful steps to increase taxes or scale back scheduled benefits. The imminent exhaustion of the Social Security trust funds spurred action in 1983, and shortfalls in the Hospital Insurance trust fund served a similar function in 1997. Although such deadlines are artificial from an economic point of view, they can have real-world consequences.

Federal Debt and the Economy

What to do with the near-term surpluses has become a contentious political issue. In its budget for fiscal year 2002, the Bush administration proposes to pay down all of the federal debt that can easily be redeemed over the next ten years. The administration would not attempt to redeem nonmarketable debt, such as savings bonds, or long-term bonds that would not mature until after 2011. The administration opposes federal investment in the private sector and argues that funds not needed for debt reduction should be returned to the public through lower taxes in the future (U.S. Office of Management and Budget 2001, 227–28).

In contrast, CBO's long-run budget projections assume that the government will invest its surpluses in nonfederal assets after debt held by the public is eliminated. When deficits return, those assets are drawn down. Eventually, the government must resume issuing debt to the public. That result stems from some simple budgetary arithmetic and straightforward economic analysis.

The arithmetic involves a concept known as the primary deficit or surplus—the deficit or surplus excluding interest payments to (or from) the public. If the primary deficit is zero and the interest rate on the debt equals the rate of growth of the economy, both debt and GDP will grow at the same rate, and the debt-to-GDP ratio will remain constant. If the primary deficit is greater than zero (as is projected to occur some time after 2020), however, the debt-to-GDP ratio will rise. If the interest rate also exceeds the growth rate, the debt-to-GDP ratio will grow even faster (CBO 1985, 88–93).

CBO's long-run analysis is designed to account for the effect of deficits on the economy, and those economic feedbacks greatly accelerate the accumulation of debt. When publicly held debt grows faster than the economy, the federal government places increasing demands on credit markets. The growth of debt drives up interest rates and reduces the share of economic output that is available for private capital formation. As a result, the growth of productivity slows and may eventually cease. The rise in interest rates increases the numerator of the debt-to-GDP ratio, and the slowdown in productivity decreases its denominator. Together, these two factors make the accumulation of debt more explosive.

Because even a small primary deficit can lead to an explosion of debt if continued for many years, a projection that the debt will eventually explode provides no information about the size of the policy actions that must eventually be taken to put the budget on a sustainable path. The "fiscal gap" provides a convenient summary of the size of the fiscal problem. That gap is the amount by which spending must be cut or taxes increased, starting immediately, to keep the debt-to-GDP ratio from exceeding its current level over the next seventy-five years. In CBO's October 2000 projections, the fiscal gap is 0.8 percent of GDP, or about $74 billion in today's terms.

Sources of Growth in Spending

The projected growth of Social Security, Medicare, and Medicaid—and the resulting pressure on the federal budget—stems from the interaction between the demographic and economic projections, on the one hand, and the features of the three programs, on the other.

Demographic Factors

Because most of the people who will be working or drawing benefits during the next twenty or thirty years have already been born, the primary demographic factor affecting the budget projections in the near term is the recent pattern of births. The post–World War II baby boom of 1946 to 1964 was followed by a baby bust during the late 1960s and the 1970s. Although the number of births rebounded after 1973, it has never regained the peak established in 1961. The large cohort of baby boomers will start to reach age 62—the age of initial eligibility for Social Security retirement benefits—in 2008. At the same time, the smaller cohorts of Generation X and Generation Y will be reaching their years of peak earnings and entering the labor force, respectively. This demographic shift will strain the federal budget by causing spending for elderly persons to increase more rapidly than taxes paid by workers.

Improvements in longevity add to the budgetary pressures. As life spans increase, more people survive to age 65, and those who live to become eligible for retirement benefits draw Social Security and Medicare benefits for more years. In 1940 the average cohort life expectancy at age 65 was 12.7 years for men and 14.7 years for women. Today, life expectancy at age 65 has risen to 16.2 years for men and 19.6 years for women. The Social Security actuaries estimate that life expectancy at age 65 will increase by about one year by 2020 and two years by 2040, although many demographers believe that improvements in longevity will be even greater (Board of Trustees, OASDI Trust Funds 2001, 78).

These projected demographic changes are summarized in the aged dependency ratio, which compares the number of aged people to those of working age. For Social Security, the comparable concept is the ratio of beneficiaries to covered workers. That ratio has been roughly constant for the past twenty-five years at about 30 beneficiaries per 100 covered workers. It will begin to rise toward the end of this decade, when the leading age of the baby boom becomes eligible for Social

Security retirement benefits, and it will really take off in the following two decades. The Social Security actuaries project that there will be 32 beneficiaries per 100 covered workers in 2010, 40 in 2020, and 47 in 2030 (Board of Trustees, OASDI Trust Funds 2001, 48).

To some extent, improvements in health status will blunt the effects of greater longevity on the federal budget. Health could potentially improve so much that the use of medical care over a lifetime would decrease as life spans increased. Although that extreme outcome is unlikely, it does appear that as people live longer, their additional years of life are generally marked by health and vigor rather than by disease and disability. Thus, an increase in the number of people age 65 or older is likely to lead to a less than proportional increase in spending on Medicare and Medicaid. Improvements in longevity and health status could also lead to a lower rate of receipt of benefits from Social Security Disability Insurance (DI), but the data so far show no signs of such a reduction. To the contrary, the rate of receipt of DI benefits is increasing, and the Social Security actuaries project that this trend will continue.

Although people are living longer, the age at which people begin to draw Social Security retirement benefits has declined sharply over the years. For men, the average age at which benefits are claimed dropped from 68.7 in 1950 to 66.8 in 1960. After early retirement benefits for men were introduced in 1962, the average age of initial receipt dropped further—to 64.4 in 1970 and 63.9 in 1980. Since 1980 the average age at which benefits are awarded has remained roughly stable, suggesting that the trend toward earlier retirement may have abated. Nonetheless, two-thirds of men claim Social Security benefits before age 65 (Social Security Administration 2000, table 6.B5). In 2000 Congress repealed the Social Security earnings test for people above the normal retirement age, but the effect of this change has yet to appear in the data.

Even though Social Security benefits are actuarially reduced if they are claimed before the normal retirement age, early retirements still impose costs on Social Security and the economy. First, they reduce economic output and cut tax revenues. Second, to the extent that policymakers seek to achieve adequate levels of benefits for early retirees, they require overall benefit levels to be higher. If people worked longer, not only would they have more private resources to support themselves in retirement, but also Social Security would be able to provide better benefits to people at older ages (Steuerle and Bakija 1994, 44).

Programmatic Factors

In addition to demographic factors, the structure of the Social Security, Medicare, and Medicaid programs themselves is a critical element in their projected growth. If benefits per recipient were lower, for example, or if they grew more slowly, an increase in the number of recipients would have less effect on the budgetary totals.

For Social Security, there are several ways of looking at the level of benefits. As currently structured, the program is designed to provide a stable replacement rate—the ratio of a person's real benefit to his or her earnings just before retirement. For a hypothetical unmarried 65-year-old who always earned the economy-wide average wage and retires at the normal retirement age, the annual benefit is currently about $12,000, and the replacement rate is about 42 percent. The lifetime value of this benefit is roughly $160,000 for a man and $225,000 for a woman (based on figures in Steuerle and Bakija 1994, 103). The replacement rate will remain constant in the future for workers who retire at the normal retirement age, and the real benefit will grow at the same rate as real earnings. By 2030 the hypothetical average earner is projected to receive a benefit of about $17,300 a year in today's dollars—about 45 percent above the current level (Board of Trustees, OASDI Trust Funds 2000, table III.B5). Because many workers have years with little or no earnings, however, the typical retiree has earnings and benefits below those of this hypothetical worker.

In Medicare, average outlays per enrollee total nearly $5,500 a year. The lifetime value of these benefits is about $105,000 for a 65-year-old man and $135,000 for a woman of the same age. Federal Medicaid spending per aged enrollee is about $6,300, of which $1,700 is for acute care and $4,600 is for long-term care. Unlike Social Security, however, Medicare and Medicaid are open-ended programs. Benefits are specified not as a dollar amount but as a bundle of services for which beneficiaries are eligible. Thus, spending for Medicare and Medicaid grows not only on account of increases in real earnings and in the number of beneficiaries, as with Social Security, but also with increases in the cost and use of medical care. In Medicaid this tendency has been held in check to some extent by requiring recipients to enroll in managed care plans. But in Medicare enrollment in managed care plans (now part of Medicare+Choice) is optional and saves little or nothing for the taxpayer in any event.

Driven by the development of new drugs, procedures, and technologies, the growth in health care spending has generally outpaced the growth of the economy. Between 1970 and 1993, national health expenditures rose from 7.1 percent to 13.7 percent of GDP. Although that ratio has not changed much in the past few years, signs of more rapid increases in health costs have begun to emerge, and most analysts believe that the recent experience is just a temporary lull. Projections from the Centers for Medicare and Medicaid Services (formerly the Health Care Financing Administration) assume that national health expenditures will reach 16.2 percent of GDP by 2008 (Smith et al. 1999). The projections team cites, as factors contributing to the projected acceleration in spending, slower growth in enrollment in managed care plans, a movement toward less restrictive forms of managed care, increased state and federal regulation of health plans, and an upturn in the underwriting cycle for private health insurance.

Clearly, health care spending cannot continue to absorb an ever increasing share of our economic output. Determining when an unsustainable process will stop, however, is not an easy matter. Until recently, both CBO and the Medicare actuaries assumed that after twenty-five years, medical costs per person would rise no faster than compensation per hour. But in their most recent reports, both agencies assume that growth in health care spending per capita will continue to exceed the growth in per capita GDP by about one percentage point a year for seventy-five years (Board of Trustees, HI Trust Fund 2001, 9–10).

The Sensitivity of the Projections

Although the upcoming demographic pressures on the budget are a virtual certainty, long-term budget projections must be used with caution. Just a few years ago, in May 1996, CBO estimated that the long-run fiscal gap was 5.4 percent of GDP. That figure dropped to 4.1 percent in March 1997, 1.6 percent in May 1998, and 0.8 percent in October 2000.

This large change in the numbers vividly illustrates the sensitivity of long-run budget projections to the assumptions that underlie them. These assumptions can be divided into three categories—demographic assumptions (such as birthrates, longevity, and health status), economic assumptions (such as the rate of real wage growth or the real interest rate), and policy assumptions (such as the rate of taxation and the amount of discretionary spending).

Demographic Assumptions

Projected fertility and birthrates have little effect on the projections for the next twenty-five years, because people under age 25 pay few taxes and collect relatively few federal benefits. In the longer run, however, fertility rates are an important determinant of the size of the labor force, the amount of the tax base, and (ultimately) the spending for health and retirement benefits. Increases in longevity can have a more immediate impact on the costs of the retirement system, and their effect also grows with time.

To assess the effects of alternative assumptions, the Social Security and Medicare actuaries develop low-cost and high-cost scenarios in addition to their best-guess case. The low-cost demographic path assumes a smaller increase in longevity and higher fertility rates than the intermediate case. (It also assumes a slightly higher rate of immigration.) As a result, there would be fewer Social Security and Medicare beneficiaries and more taxpayers to foot the bill. The high-cost path assumes a greater increase in longevity and lower fertility rates, and its effect on the budget projections is just the opposite.

CBO has estimated the impact on the long-run budget projections of using the Social Security actuaries' low-cost and high-cost population paths. Over the next 20 or 30 years, their effects are relatively modest. Over 75 years, however, they swing the fiscal gap by more than 1 percent of GDP (see Table 4.3).

Table 4.3. Change in the Fiscal Gap under Alternative Economic and Demographic Assumptions (as a percentage of GDP)

	Change in Fiscal Gap
Population	
Optimistic assumption	−1.2
Pessimistic assumption	1.4
Productivity	
Optimistic assumption	−1.3
Pessimistic assumption	1.1
Health Costs	
Optimistic assumption	−1.5
Pessimistic assumption	2.8

Source: CBO 2000, 16.

Economic Assumptions

On the economic side, a critical assumption is the rate of growth of real wages—that is, the excess of wage growth over inflation. Unlike changes in the aged dependency ratio, changes in real wage growth move both federal receipts and expenditures in the same direction.

As indicated earlier, Social Security is designed to provide a retirement benefit that bears a specified relationship to a beneficiary's earnings before retirement. Thus, an increase in a worker's real wages increases both taxes paid and benefits that will ultimately be received. Once a worker is on the benefit rolls, however, his or her benefits are indexed to keep pace with inflation, but they are not adjusted for increases in the real income of those in the labor force. As a result, an increase or decrease in the rate of growth of real wages affects tax payments immediately but affects Social Security benefits only with a lag. This lag reduces or increases the cost of Social Security benefits relative to taxable payroll or gross domestic product.

The effect of real wage growth on the cost of Medicare and Medicaid is more complicated. Medicare and Medicaid both guarantee a package of medical care services, and the provision of those services is very labor intensive. Thus, if a change in the growth of real wages was mirrored by a change in the cost of medical services as well as in payroll taxes, Medicare's financial balance would be little affected. CBO makes precisely that assumption after the first ten years (although not before). The Medicare actuaries assume that only 60 percent of Hospital Insurance benefits are affected by wages. Under CBO's assumption, an increase or decrease of 0.5 percentage point in productivity growth (and, hence, the growth in real wages) will reduce or increase the fiscal gap by a little more than 1 percent of GDP.

The assumed rate of growth of health care costs has an even more powerful effect on the long-run budget projections. In its intermediate projections, CBO assumes that the annual cost growth per enrollee in Medicare in excess of wage growth (that is, excess growth in health costs) will slow from 2.1 percent to 1.1 percent between 2010 and 2025 and will remain the same thereafter. If excess cost growth slowed to zero, the fiscal gap would shrink by 1.5 percent of GDP. If no slowdown occurred, the fiscal gap would grow by 2.8 percent of GDP (see Table 4.3).

Policy Assumptions

Extrapolating current budgetary policies for seventy-five years involves making many judgments, and those judgments can have big effects on the results. The projected level of discretionary spending and the rate of taxation are two such key assumptions.

Discretionary spending is that controlled by the annual appropriations process. It includes almost all spending on national defense and the day-to-day operations of the federal government. CBO's ten-year baseline budget projections assume that discretionary spending will grow with the rate of inflation. Because the economy is projected to grow faster than the rate of inflation, discretionary outlays drop as a percentage of GDP from 6.2 percent in 2001 to 5.1 percent in 2011. After ten years, CBO assumes that part of the future growth in real incomes will be devoted to discretionary spending and that it will grow at the same rate as GDP. If discretionary spending grew forever at the rate of inflation, it would continue to shrink as a share of GDP, and it would be 2.7 percent of GDP lower by 2060. Alternatively, if discretionary spending was held constant as a share of GDP from the start (and not allowed to drop for the first ten years), it would be higher by 1.1 percent of GDP from 2010 on.

Changes in tax policy can also have a significant effect on the long-run projections. For example, in June 2001 President Bush signed Public Law 107-16, the Economic Growth and Tax Relief Reconciliation Act. If the provisions of that bill are made a permanent part of law (many of them sunset at the end of 2010), they will reduce revenues and increase the primary deficit by 2 percent of GDP in the long run (based on data in Friedman, Kogan, and Greenstein 2001).

THE ISSUE: HEALTH AND RETIREMENT VERSUS EVERYTHING ELSE

A rich economy can afford many things. At the beginning of the twenty-first century, the average individual living in the United States is five times richer than one living at the beginning of the last century. At the beginning of the next century, she or he may be five times richer again. Whatever the ultimate multiplier, we will assuredly be much better off in terms of more output, better health care, and longer lives. In many ways, therefore, it is wrong to say that the nation cannot afford much more in the way of retirement leisure and continually higher shares of national income spent on health and retirement. But what we *can afford* is a different issue from what we *should spend*.

Over most of the last half of the twentieth century, the drop in defense spending allowed spending for elderly persons to grow without substantial changes in average tax rates. Yet defense, which declined from 8 percent of GDP in 1970 to 3 percent at the end of the century, is not going to decline by another 5 percentage points. Over the past few years, not only defense has provided an offset to rising spending for retirement and health. Nondefense discretionary spending slipped from 3.7 percent of GDP in 1995 to 3.3 percent of GDP in 2000. Under President Bush's budget, it is projected to fall to 2.7 percent of GDP by 2011 (CBO 2001).

Several questions arise in considering the best course for the future. First, to what extent should the fiscal gap be closed through tax increases? Taxes raise revenues, but they also inhibit saving and work effort. In general, economists theorize that the next one percentage point addition to tax rates would cause more distortion than the previous percentage point increase did. Second, even if tax rate increases are possible, what is the best use of the additional money? A typical couple retiring today is promised nearly $0.5 million in Social Security and Medicare benefits; for higher-income couples retiring in three decades, the total is closer to $1 million. Individuals now retire for about one-third of their adult lives. Are additional years of retirement a higher priority for the nation than doing something about poverty, illiteracy, or urban blight?

Finally, within budget groupings, are moneys being allocated in the fairest and most efficient way? Should the public money available to the retired increasingly go toward health insurance instead of cash benefits, which give elderly persons more freedom and flexibility to spend money according to the priorities that they set? Would some of the funds currently scheduled for Medicare be better spent to help the nonelderly meet their medical bills? Should additional steps be taken to reduce poverty among the oldest old?

We cannot answer these questions here. But they center the issue of retirement and health on issues of relative, rather than absolute, valuation. More health care or freedom to retire is better than less; however, it is not necessarily better than alternative uses of the same societal resources, whether by individuals acting privately or through their government.

THE POSSIBILITIES: ASSESSING THE EFFECTS OF REFORMS

Various options are available to deal with projected shortfalls in retirement and health programs, and many of them are intended to affect the economy as well as the budget. Some aim to increase society's resources by increasing saving or lengthening the work life. Others would control the growth of health care costs by regulating prices, quantities, or technology or by moving toward a defined contribution or capitated-payments system.

In May 2001 President Bush appointed the President's Commission to Strengthen Social Security. The president has asked the commission to make recommendations for modernizing and restoring fiscal soundness to Social Security using six guiding principles. The commission will issue its final report by the end of 2001.

The ten-year baseline budget projections currently used in the congressional and executive budget processes assume that taxes and spending will follow current laws and policies. Also, a single set of economic assumptions is used to evaluate all budgetary proposals. Over a relatively short time horizon, this approach poses few problems. Most proposed policy changes would not have a significant effect on aggregate economic activity during such a brief period. Moreover, if there is general agreement on a proposed change in course (in recent years, for example, deficit reduction), its effects can be included in the economic assumptions underlying the baseline budget projections (CBO 1995).

The approach used for ten-year estimates is less satisfactory in comparing alternative budgetary policies over the very long run. First of all, the very concept of current policy is not well defined over such a lengthy period. Is it really current policy that increasing numbers of taxpayers should become subject to the alternative minimum tax, as a mechanical extrapolation of current law would assume? Is it really current policy that discretionary spending should shrink forever as a share of GDP, as current budget rules provide? Not likely. Moreover, over a seventy-five-year period, the choice of budgetary policies can have very significant macroeconomic feedbacks. Often, however, there is no professional consensus on their magnitude.

For these reasons and more, no government agency has yet produced consistent long-run estimates of the economic and budgetary effects of specific policy proposals. CBO has so far avoided this morass by using its long-run model for descriptive and analytical purposes but not to evaluate proposed legislation. The Social Security and Medicare actuaries face the baseline problem to a lesser extent in their cost estimates, since they are not required to prepare projections for the entire federal budget. In comparing the consequences of alternative plans to ensure solvency for Social Security and Medicare, however, current law does not provide a realistic benchmark because it is not sustainable. The 1994–96 Advisory Council on Social Security compared its proposals to what it called present-law pay-as-you-go—a construct in which payroll taxes would be increased to finance current-law benefits on a pay-as-you-go basis. The President's Commission to Strengthen Social Security is wrestling with the same issue.

Increasing Saving

A variety of Social Security proposals, for example, attempt to go beyond simple benefit and tax changes and to increase saving in other ways. President Bush has charged the President's Commission to Strengthen Social Security with developing a system of voluntary personal retirement accounts that would augment traditional Social Security. Others have recommended transferring a portion of general revenues to Social Security as a way of warding off future tax cuts. If such efforts succeeded in increasing saving in the trust funds or in individual accounts, two questions would then arise: Would that additional saving increase government saving as a whole? And would national saving also increase?

The Effect of Policy Changes on Saving

To determine the net impact on government saving of a policy that increased saving in one area, one must know how much other government expenditures and taxes would change if that policy were adopted. Putting Social Security payroll taxes into private accounts could be treated as an immediate expenditure of government, for example, whereas promises made under traditional Social Security are not treated as an outlay until funds are spent as benefit payments. Thus, conversion to individual accounts recognizes liabilities up front and tends to raise the current deficit. One then has to make some assumption about how government will react. If Congress targeted a balanced total budget, then conversion to individual accounts would imply reducing expenditures or increasing taxes by an amount roughly equal to the conversion. If the target was a balanced non–Social Security budget, no offsetting changes would be required.

The attempt to save the Social Security surpluses raises the same types of issues. The Social Security trust funds have been classified as off-budget since 1985; and at least through most of the 1990s, it was thought that this label had no effect on congressional action. By the end of the 1990s, however, Congress and the president were making a significant effort to run total surpluses at least as large as the Social Security surpluses—suggesting that the off-budget designation was having some effect after all. What will happen when those off-budget items start running deficits rather than surpluses? At that point, if Congress aims for a non–Social Security (and possibly non-Medicare) deficit of zero, then the fact that Social Security trust funds are off-budget could decrease, rather than increase, government saving.

Equally thorny is the issue of how much private saving would adjust to a change in Social Security or Medicare. One theory asserts that private saving tends to react directly, almost immediately, and in the opposite direction to changes in government saving, offsetting it dollar for dollar. It is as if citizens made a calculation of what was in their own accounts and government accounts simultaneously and always kept the two on some target line. But one need not go so far as this rational expectations theory to note that increases in government saving tend to increase the supply of loanable funds to the private sector, which in turn uses some or much of those loanable funds to finance additional consumption. In effect, new sources of loanable funds lead to borrowing not just for investment but for consumption as well (Steuerle 1990).

If people are forced to save in individual accounts, many analysts believe that they would react by reducing their contributions to 401(k) plans, defined contribution pension plans, and other vehicles for saving. Those least likely to be able to make such offsets are those who are not saving in the first place. Note that each individual does not have to offset pension saving directly. The individual might simply maintain more mortgage or credit card debt.

Reductions in promised benefits will induce more private saving, although the amount is uncertain. Suppose a person had a target benefit of $25,000 to replace a final wage of $40,000. If Social Security benefits are reduced, say, from $16,000 (a 40% replacement rate) to $14,000 (a 35 percent replacement rate), then the individual has an inducement to make up all or part of the $2,000 annual loss through other pensions or savings to restore retirement goals.

The Effect of Saving on Economic Growth

The next question to be raised is how much additional saving adds to growth in the economy. Some economists attribute to each dollar of additional saving the expected marginal return that they believe can be captured by the next additional dollar spend on business investment—usually 8 to 10 percentage points in real rate of return. For several reasons, however, this figure may be too high. First, additional saving may end up adding to nonbusiness investment, such as education, homes, cars, durable goods, or some form of public investment. The rate of return on these investments, unless they are carefully chosen, tends to be below the rate on physical capital employed by the corporate sector. Second, the marginal return to capital falls as capital investment rises (diminishing returns to capital). Some believe it falls significantly—that the best opportunities for investment have already been seized. Finally, the earnings-to-price ratio of the current stock market implies a real return of about 4 percent. It is possible, therefore, that at least temporarily the returns to capital—if reflected accurately in the earnings-to-price ratio—are below historical averages. Of course, if the market fell back toward normal, then higher returns would be available for later investments.

Even if one assumes that the real rate of return on additional saving is high, it would take a long time for additional saving to have a big effect on the economy. The physical capital stock is about $35 trillion, and the stock of human capital is probably three to four times as much. Thus, increasing saving by as much as 1 percent of GDP would increase the stock of physical capital by only about one-fourth of 1 percent, and the stock of physical and human capital by maybe one-sixteenth of 1 percent. Accordingly, it would still take many years to increase GDP by even a few percent when the saving rate is permanently increased by 1 percent of GDP. For example, CBO estimated in October 2000 that saving total surpluses would require that the government save about 1.5 percent of GDP more each year than saving only the off-budget surpluses, yet it would add only 3 percent to GDP (and even less to consumption) by 2030 (CBO 2000).

The Effect of Economic Growth on the Budget

It might at first be thought that if more saving is generated, then the returns to that saving would accrue to the benefit of those who own the assets. Under most economic theories, however, much of the return would inure to the benefit of workers. Indeed, most economic models posit that labor and capital keep a relatively constant share of the total income in the economy. For example, more capital leads to a greater demand for labor as either a substitute (it is now relatively cheaper) or a complement (it is now needed more to run the machines). More demand for labor means higher wages for workers.

Growth is important because it produces higher incomes, which, in turn, increase tax collections. In terms of total revenues, it makes little difference whether the additional income is attributed to labor or to capital. Typically, workers pay Social Security and personal income taxes at an average marginal rate in excess of 30 percent. Capital owners typically pay the corporate income tax rate of 35 percent and a few cents in individual income tax (most capital income is not recognized at the individual level). Of course, payroll taxes on earnings from labor go directly to the Social Security and Medicare trust funds; income taxes on capital do not. Therefore, any reform that increases taxes on labor under current law would include some attribution of increased funds (and higher future benefits) to Social Security, whereas any additional taxes raised on capital would almost all go into general revenues.

Many reformers like to argue that they can somehow take all of the additional growth they have generated and distribute it to meet their objective, whatever it is. Thus, some would impose a higher tax *rate* but argue that, with higher incomes in the future, no one will be worse off in the sense of having a lower after-tax *level* of income. Others want to impose a lower replacement *rate* but argue that with higher income no one will be worse off if they can be prevented from having a lower benefit *level*.

Such analyses tend to ignore the impact of growth on programs as they are currently designed. As explained earlier, more growth in the economy leads directly to higher wages and higher Social Security and Medicare benefits for future retirees. The gains to the Social Security and Medicare trust funds therefore tend to be modest.

Increasing the Supply of Labor

Although the effect of proposed reforms on saving is extraordinarily difficult to quantify, the effect of one reform on labor supply is estimated to be quite strong. That reform is an increase in the initial age of eligibility for benefits—now age 62 for Social Security and age 65 for Medicare. Since most people at those ages have insufficient assets to support their retirement and health insurance costs, the age of eligibility for benefits has a significant impact on the decision to retire and on labor force participation (Gruber and Wise 1999). Although other features of Social Security and Medicare also affect labor force participation, empirical studies have generally found those effects to be small (Burtless 1984).

The economic consequences of changes in labor supply are significant. One interesting statistic is the nonemployment rates of males and females over the past few decades. The nonemployment rate, a measure of the percentage of all adults who are not employed, includes both unemployment and retirement but is dominated in recent years by retirement decisions, including those due to the aging of the population. Over the post–World War II period from 1948 to 1997, the nonemployment rate for men rose from 14.2 percent to 26.3 percent. However, that increase was more than offset by the decline in the nonemployment rate for women. As a result, despite the extraordinary growth in nonemployment of men, the nonemployment rate has fallen almost continually throughout the past half century (see Table 4.4).

Since World War II, the nonemployment rate has risen only in years around a recession. In contrast, the actuaries' current projections assume an increase in the nonemployment rate of about 0.4 percentage points every year for about twenty to thirty years running once the baby boomers start retiring. The annual change is not far from what is experienced in a mild recession, but unlike a recession, this situation involves compounding of the increase year after year. The total change is on the order of the decline in the labor force during the Depression, but this time it would be permanent.

At the same time, the history of female labor force participation suggests that labor demand and other societal influences can operate as very powerful forces to encourage work. Thus, if private and public

Table 4.4. Nonemployment Rate of People Age 20 or Older (by calendar year)

Year	Males	Females	Total
1948	14.2%	69.3%	42.6%
1997	26.3	42.2	34.5
2030	33.6	49.2	41.7

Source: Steuerle and Spiro 1999.

policies are accommodating, labor force participation could increase substantially more than traditional predictions allow for the near-elderly in their sixties and early seventies. The notion that everyone wants to retire for one-third of his or her adult life, as current benefit programs suggest and promise, is a relatively new concept. In an information age, moreover, the meaning of retirement itself starts changing dramatically from what it was when one retired from physical labor that one could no longer perform. The future increase in the labor supply of the near-elderly could represent as big a shock to the labor forecasters of today as did the entry of women to the forecasters of a few decades ago.

One final note on labor supply. Increasing the work of the near-elderly does double duty. First, it decreases the percentage of the population receiving benefits. Second, it increases government revenues—not just Social Security taxes, but income and excise taxes as well. Thus, relative to other reforms, increasing the age at which individuals can retire generally allows for the smallest reduction in annual benefits or increase in tax rates.

Directly Controlling the Growth of Health Care Costs

A third approach to reforming the retirement and health programs attempts to control the costs of health care. Direct control methods try to limit one of three items: the quantity of health care consumed, the price of that health care, or the use of costly new technology. In the first two cases, controls are established either on the outputs (e.g., the coverage of some new procedure or the price of some services) or on inputs (e.g., the supply of doctors or the fees that they can charge).

To date, the federal government has not made many attempts to control quantities, although states have limited nursing home beds. Attempts to deny particular health services may fail for various reasons; for instance, technology firms switch their emphasis, or doctors adjust what they do and how much time they spend doing it. For the most part, quantity restrictions tend to emphasize mainly a few marginal or very expensive items that would be difficult to provide on a universal basis in any case. Attempts to control quantities by reducing inputs (for example, the supply of doctors) might entail some savings. Alternatively, it might lead to an increase in prices or the replacement of human services with more technology.

More efforts are usually made to control prices. Medicare, just like any other insurance, sets maximum fees and charges, and those rates are changed frequently. Like pushing on a balloon, however, the air pops out somewhere else. For example, doctors may upgrade diagnoses or divide what used to be one charge into two chargeable events.

So far, Medicare has not been required to operate under a fixed budget, although the sustainable growth rate formula for physicians' services attempts to limit spending for that category of services. Other countries have tried global budgeting, however, and it has been an element of various plans for comprehensive health reform in this country. CBO's approach to estimating the potential impact of limits on expenditures is to examine the proposal with respect to the stringency of the limits and the specified enforcement mechanisms. Based on its best judgment, CBO then assigns a rating for effectiveness, with a fully effective limit receiving a 100 percent rating and a completely ineffective proposal receiving a rating of zero. To be considered effective, the proposal must include specific details on the mechanisms for setting, monitoring, and enforcing the spending limits (CBO 1993, 11–12).

Some observers contend that as long as new health care services are going to be covered under insurance, new technology is always going to drive up costs. Thus, they argue that the only way to control health costs is to constrain technology itself. Controlling technology, however, would be difficult. One way would be to spend less on the National Institutes of Health. Alternatively, the prices at which new services are reimbursed might be cut, thereby reducing incentives to firms to develop new technologies. Requiring Medicare to operate under a fixed budget constraint with a fail-safe mechanism could curtail technological development.

Market Based Reforms and Defined Contribution Systems

One category of market based reforms involves imposing additional costs on recipients at the point of decision making over the purchase of health care. Higher deductibles and copayments have been among the mechanisms often proposed. More recently, proposals for Medical Savings Accounts would allow people to purchase health insurance with a very high deductible but provide an additional tax benefit for out-of-pocket medical payments. In general, estimators assume some reduction in demand for health services in response to higher charges, but advocates are often disappointed that the amount of response is estimated to be small. Typically, the amount of money to be charged is so modest relative to total health care spending that, even with a very strong response, the amount of saving would be limited. Now that health care spending exceeds $10,000 for the average household, even deductibles of $1,000 or $2,000 would cover only a modest fraction of total spending. They would have little impact on the very expensive bouts of illness, which comprise as much as 60 percent or 70 percent of total health care spending. People with Medical Savings Accounts would also generally be unable to benefit from the discounted fees that traditional insurers have negotiated with providers.

Most market based reforms being discussed today are some type of defined contribution or voucher system. In such a system, a fixed amount of money is paid to an intermediary or health maintenance organization in exchange for the provision of most or all health services to an individual. The notion is that the intermediary would be in charge of keeping total spending within the budget but would be allowed flexibility to make decisions about prices and quantities.

One of the biggest issues in designing a voucher system for Medicare is establishing the size of the voucher. Under the present structure of Medicare+Choice, the size of the payment to capitated plans is based (according to a complicated formula) on the average cost of traditional Medicare. Healthier people are more likely to join a capitated plan, where they may receive additional benefits, whereas the less healthy often remain within traditional fee-for-service Medicare, where they feel they will have easier access to the services they need. As long as traditional Medicare is available at no extra charge to the beneficiary, allowing beneficiaries to choose the plan that is best for them will tend to saddle the taxpayer with higher costs.

If traditional Medicare was phased out, the amount of the voucher could be set by law, regulation, or the market. If the amount was determined by a clearly specified formula, estimators would typically assume that spending per capita would be what is stated in law. Even if there is a strong belief that political pressures would lead to much higher fees in the future, those fee increases would be determined by future legislation and would not be included in the initial cost of the proposal. If the amount of the voucher was established by competitive bidding, estimation would be more difficult, and estimators would be unlikely to show substantial savings without strong evidence (Reischauer 1999).

CONCLUSION

As federal policy becomes increasingly dominated by entitlements that automatically grow faster than revenues, long-run budget projections will be crucial. These projections are not intended to provide an accurate forecast of the economy of tomorrow. A major reason is that over the long term, the law itself is not external to the economy but is one way in which society adjusts to new requirements and possibilities.

Budgetary projections do, however, provide a sense of the amount of slack in future federal budgets. They also demonstrate the pressure of past promises on net government saving or dissaving. And they indicate the extent to which future policymakers may have to alter old promises to fit new circumstances.

ACKNOWLEDGMENTS

The authors thank Laura Haltzel for helping prepare this chapter for publication. The views expressed are those of the authors, not their institutions.

REFERENCES

Board of Trustees, Federal Hospital Insurance (HI) Trust Fund. 2001. *2001 Annual Report of the Board of Trustees of the Federal Hospital Insurance Trust Fund.* Washington, D.C.: U.S. Government Printing Office.

Board of Trustees, Federal Old-Age and Survivors Insurance and Disability Insurance (OASDI) Trust Funds. 2000. *2000 Annual Report of the Board of Trustees of the Federal Old-Age and Survivors Insurance and Disability Insurance Trust Funds.* Washington, D.C.: U.S. Government Printing Office.

———. 2001. *2001 Annual Report of the Board of Trustees of the Federal Old-Age and Survivors Insurance and Disability Insurance Trust Funds.* Washington, D.C.: U.S. Government Printing Office.

Burtless, G. 1984. Effects of Social Security Benefits on Labor Supply. In H. J. Aaron and G. Burtless, eds., *Retirement and Economic Behavior.* Washington, D.C.: Brookings Institution.

Congressional Budget Office (CBO). 1985. *The Economic and Budget Outlook: Fiscal Years 1986–1990.* Washington, D.C.: U.S. Government Printing Office.

———. 1993. *Estimates of Health Care Proposals from the 102nd Congress.* Washington, D.C.

———. 1995. *Budget Estimates: Current Practices and Alternative Approaches.* Washington, D.C.

———. 1997. *The Economic and Budget Outlook: An Update.* Washington, D.C.: U.S. Government Printing Office.

———. 2000. *The Long-Term Budget Outlook.* Washington, D.C.: U.S. Government Printing Office.

———. 2001. *An Analysis of the President's Budgetary Proposals for Fiscal Year 2002.* Washington, D.C.

Friedman, J., R. Kogan, and R. Greenstein. 2001. *Final Tax Bill Ultimately Costs as Much as Bush Tax Plan.* Washington, D.C.: Center on Budget and Policy Priorities.

Gruber, J., and D. A. Wise, eds. 1999. *Social Security and Retirement around the World.* Chicago: University of Chicago Press.

Reischauer, R. 1999. Medicare Vouchers. In C. E. Steuerle, V. Ooms, G. Peterson, and R. D. Reischauer, eds., *Vouchers and the Provision of Public Services.* Washington, D.C.: Brookings Institution.

Smith, S., S. Heffler, M. Freeland, and the National Health Expenditures Projection Team. 1999. The Next Decade of Health Spending: A New Outlook. *Health Affairs* 18, no. 4: 86–95.

Social Security Administration. 2000. *Social Security Bulletin, Annual Statistical Supplement.*

Steuerle, C. E. 1990. Federal Policy and the Accumulation of Private Debt. In J. B. Shoven and J. Waldfogel, eds., *Debt, Taxes, and Corporate Restructuring.* Washington, D.C.: Brookings Institution.

Steuerle, C. E., and J. M. Bakija. 1994. *Retooling Social Security for the Twenty-First Century.* Washington, D.C.: Urban Institute.

Steuerle, C. E., E. M. Gramlich, H. Heclo, and D. S. Nightingale. 1998. *The Government We Deserve.* Washington, D.C.: Urban Institute.

Steuerle, C. E., and C. Spiro. 1999. *Nonemployment: A Necessary Economic Indicator.* Straight Talk on Social Security and Retirement Policy, no. 2. Washington, D.C.: Urban Institute.

U.S. Office of Management and Budget. 2001. *Budget of the United States Government, Fiscal Year 2002, Analytical Perspectives.* Washington, D.C.: U.S. Government Printing Office.

5

Increased Public Spending on the Elderly

Can We Afford It?

Wendell E. Primus, Ph.D.

One of my tasks twenty years ago, as a junior staff economist–budget analyst on the Ways and Means Committee, was to understand federal budget trends. One prediction that seemed safe based on this understanding was that by the year 2000, federal revenues, and especially spending, as a percentage of gross domestic product (GDP) would significantly exceed 20 percent. One needed only to examine current outlays plus projected health spending trends (Medicaid and Medicare outlays together increased by 1.8 percentage points of GDP since 1978) and the other promises that the federal government had made to the elderly. Given the political strength of the elderly, a presumed inability to arrest health spending trends, and the political power of the Appropriations Committee, a suggestion that both federal spending and revenues would be significantly above 20 percent of GDP was entirely reasonable.

As Table 5.1 clearly illustrates, I was wrong. Instead, decreases in discretionary spending and other entitlement programs have offset the increases in Medicare and Medicaid spending and the increase in net interest costs. Back in 1978, total discretionary spending was 9.9 percent of GDP, and defense spending was 4.7 percent of GDP. Since then, discretionary spending has decreased by 3.6 percentage points of GDP. Those reductions in expenditure levels were much greater than anyone

Table 5.1. Spending Outlays as a Percentage of GDP by Sector

	1978	2000	Average 2001–2010
Discretionary	9.9	6.3	5.8
Medicare and Medicaid	1.6	3.4	4.0
Social Security	4.2	4.1	4.2
Net interest on debt	1.6	2.3	0.7
All else	3.5	2.1	1.9
Total outlays	20.7	18.2	16.8

Source: CBO 2001.

predicted or could have imagined and are not likely to be repeated. By 2000, revenues were 20.6 percent of GDP and expenditures were 18.2 percent of GDP. Under the assumption that taxes will decrease and spending will increase to produce a balanced budget (not counting the Social Security reserves), the Congressional Budget Office (CBO) projects that over the next ten years, revenues will fall to about 19.2 percent and spending will decline from 18.4 percent of GDP in 2000 to 17.3 percent of GDP in 2010.[1] Long-term CBO projections estimate that expenditures will not significantly exceed the 20 percent barrier until some point between 2020 and 2030.[2] This presents a difficult political problem for policymakers today, who may be seen as ignoring their constituents' present-day needs to solve a problem that might not arise for another thirty years.

This chapter first addresses the important question of how the total burden on the economy of a nonworking elderly population should be measured and then considers how reforms to programs such as Social Security and Medicare, which are financed on a pay-as-you-go basis, impact total savings in the economy and the work effort of the population near retirement age.

The consumption burden that a nonworking elderly population places on the economy is not measured simply by the amount of total public expenditures on elderly persons. The Medicare and Social Security programs are not particularly generous and, in my view, are not a major problem. The services covered under Medicare, the copayment and deductibles, and the lack of catastrophic protection and a prescription drug benefit all suggest that Medicare is not nearly as generous as most private health plans. Similarly, for most high- and average-income families, Social Security alone does not produce an adequate income compared to their incomes just before retirement. One must consider how the public programs (both cash and health) and program rules interact with the private pension and other tax subsidized saving programs to obtain a complete picture of the burden the elderly population places on the economy. The interaction of these different programs on behavioral decisions about work versus leisure and when to collect benefits needs to be more fully understood. Why, for example, given the existence of Medicare and Social Security, do Americans buy earlier retirement benefits rather than deeper coverage (provision of long-term care services, payment for services not covered by Medicare, and more cash benefits) at older ages? How do these interactions vary for different segments of the elderly population, for example, in terms of blue-collar versus white-collar employment?

Perhaps the most important question has to do with the allocation of resources implied by these government programs and the growing elderly population. For example, given real or perceived revenue limitations, does the provision of long-term care services by states for the Medicaid program reduce the level of states' investment in education, particularly for children from low- and moderate-income families?

This chapter discusses the measurement of the economic burden of the elderly population and the impact of that burden on savings and work effort, the impacts on the economy if federal spending significantly exceeds 20 percent of GDP, recent developments in policies toward the elderly, and some budget rules.

MEASURING THE ECONOMIC BURDEN OF ELDERLY PERSONS ON THE ECONOMY

Simply calculating the amount of money spent on government programs or the contributions levied to finance those programs is not a good measure of the total burden of a nonworking elderly population on the economy. Lawrence Thompson (1998) answers this question and offers one of the best explanations in his book *Older and Wiser*. Henry Aaron and others have made similar arguments. Accurate measurement of the economic cost should be based on the consumption of goods and services by the nonworking elderly. What elderly persons consume is not available to the nonelderly population. The actual cost or burden of elderly persons is the percentage of the total national economic activity for any given year that is devoted to supplying the goods and services that the retired population consumes. The actual cost is the total amount of money spent by the nonworking elderly on consumption, since whatever part of the economy's capacity is used for this purpose cannot be used for anything else, such as consumer goods for nonretired people or investments for increasing productivity:

> The share of total economic activity devoted to the consumption of the retired—the actual economic cost—is influenced by a variety of economic, demographic, and public policy developments: the aggregate consumption ratio, which is the fraction of economic activity that is devoted to producing consumer goods and services for domestic use; the retiree dependency ratio, which is the fraction of the population that is retired; and the living standards ratio, which is the ratio of the average consumption of the retired population to the average consumption of all persons. (Thompson 1998, 6–8)

The only way to reduce the cost of supporting the retired population is by decreasing one or more of these three ratios. If the responsibility of providing support for elderly persons is shifted from public to private sources, without an accompanying shift in the number of retirees or the standard of living of the retired, the public to private shift will have no beneficial effect on the nonelderly population. If no changes in the retirement system are made, the economic cost will be driven up by a steady increase in the retiree dependency ratio.

There are at least two changes that would have an impact on the economic cost. Changing the statutory retirement age might reduce the dependency ratio if not offset by private pension or saving plans. Reducing the level of benefits provided to the retired population would also lower the living standards ratio. But these options do not have much political support.

Some analysts believe that economic growth policies will enable society to meet the demand of an aging society. Economic growth is a desirable policy for many reasons, but accelerated economic growth will only lower the relative costs of supporting elderly persons if economic growth causes increases in the living standards for the working-age population relative to the retired population or if it lowers the aggregate consumption ratio. If economic growth primarily encourages earlier retirement, the burden of the aging population may increase. Future alternatives for supporting elderly persons should be evaluated based on their ability to decrease the total economic cost of supporting the retired population (Thompson 1998).

We do not know to what extent the aggregate savings rate has been diminished as a result of the pay-as-you-go Social Security and Medicare programs. To some extent, that is not an important public policy question. Politically, the Social Security and Medicare programs are here to stay. The relevant question is what policies we should adopt now and in the future to increase our overall national savings rate (and lower the aggregate consumption ratio), increase investment, and thereby increase the size of the overall economy.

Conceptually, one can use the short-term Social Security program surplus to reduce our national debt,[3] to cut taxes or increase government expenditures, or to finance private retirement accounts. Paying down the national debt should result in increased savings and investments and produce a somewhat larger economy over time. This larger economy would then bring in more Social Security payroll tax revenue without raising the payroll tax rate and would enable us to better afford modifications in the Social Security benefit or revenue structure, or both, that are needed to restore the system to long-term balance.

Using the Social Security surplus to reduce the debt would also drive down the costs of interest payments. Funds that would otherwise have been spent on interest would be available to meet future fiscal policy challenges of the baby boom generation as it retires and requires Social Security and Medicare benefits.

As Table 5.2 illustrates, the budget surplus is not permanent. CBO has projected that if we spend the non–Social Security surplus now, deficits in the unified budget will return sooner and subsequently grow faster.[4] If the surplus is preserved in the form of debt reduction, the point at which deficits will return can be delayed. Social Security and other programs will not need to be reduced as much in the long-term.

Table 5.2. Projections of Federal Expenditures as a Percentage of GDP under CBO's "Save Off-Budget Surpluses" Assumption, 2010–2040

	2010	2020	2030	2040
Medicare and Medicaid	4.6	6.5	8.7	10.4
Social Security	4.3	5.2	6.0	6.4
Net interest on debt	0.9	−0.5	0.4	4.6
All else	9.4	8.0	4.1	−2.2
Total outlays	19.2	19.2	19.2	19.2
Total revenues	17.3	18.7	22.5	28.7

Source: CBO 2000.

Tax burdens on future generations will not be as great if the surplus is used to bring down the debt now.

There is a distinct possibility that the federal government may need to borrow large amounts of money in the future due to continued rises in health care costs or due to other factors that cannot be foreseen. Shrinking the national debt now will give us more room to borrow in the future, if necessary, when the baby boom generation retires. The economic burden of elderly persons on the economy is lowered permanently if the aggregate consumption ratio is lowered each year into the future.

Conversely, if a portion of the Social Security surplus is used to cut taxes or increase government expenditures, some of the surplus will be used for current consumption rather than investment that can boost economic growth and income. The national debt and the interest paid on it will be larger than they would be if the surplus were preserved. Higher interest payments will mean fewer resources for meeting other needs. Deficits will return earlier and the debt will begin to rise sooner if the surplus is forfeited, ultimately creating greater pressure to cut programs or increase taxes. A large national debt will place the government in a weaker economic position to borrow in the future if borrowing is necessary to meet pressing needs when the baby boomers retire.

Decisions that Congress and the White House make now about taxes and spending will affect how well prepared the country is to meet future needs of elderly and disabled citizens. Increasing national savings by using the surplus to pay down the debt should improve economic growth and place the government in a stronger position to honor its promises of Social Security and Medicare benefits to retirees and workers who have contributed in good faith.

Proponents of individual accounts often compare the potential rate of return on such accounts to the rate of return on Social Security contributions. They conclude that workers would enjoy a higher rate of return under a system of individual accounts. But, as explained in detail in chapter 12, creating individual accounts out of existing Social Security payroll tax reductions without any additional advance funding does not raise the rate of return. It is the additional funding, not the individual accounts themselves, that is crucial to producing the higher rate of return. Depending on the details of the proposal, some beneficiaries may be worse off because of the administrative costs of managing individual accounts, the increased risk, and annuitization cost. Furthermore, the burden on the economy could be increased if individual accounts raise the overall benefit level.

ECONOMIC IMPLICATIONS OF SUBSTANTIALLY INCREASED FEDERAL SPENDING

I have great faith in the ability of our economy to adjust to a higher spending level. First, any economy that has absorbed an increase in the labor force participation of women from 38 percent in 1960 to 60 percent in 1999, that constantly responds to changing technology and consumer demands, and that has adapted to a decline in federal defense spending from 9.4 percent of GDP in 1968 to 3.0 percent in 2000 should be able to absorb an increase of several percentage points in spending as a percent of GDP. Indeed, between 1965 and 1968, federal spending increased by three percentage points of GDP. Many times during recessions, federal spending has increased sharply. Consider also that national health expenditures went from 10.2 percent of GDP in 1985 to 13.6 percent just ten years later. If the economy can make these adjustments, why shouldn't it be able to absorb an increase in public spending of a few percentage points over a period of years without any undue effects?

Second, spending in the federal sector must exceed 20 percent if that is what the public wants. If we do not let spending increase, constituencies that are much weaker politically and more disadvantaged will bear the burden of artificial limits on spending. The increase in federal expenditures projected between 2010 and 2030 primarily results from increased health expenditures. The expenditure levels in Table 5.2 are probably understated. Discretionary spending probably will be greater than CBO baseline projections, and the resulting budget surplus and interest savings will probably be significantly less. The chances are also great that a recession will occur at some point, which also will increase net interest costs. If government spending was to be reduced further, it would probably not come from reduced health expenditures. The public appetite for increasing services under Medicare and providing access to a greater percentage of uninsured persons will probably mean a greater increase in health expenditures, not a lesser one. Thus, the only place to trim spending is from less politically popular programs. Furthermore, additional reductions in overall discretionary spending are not likely.

A third argument is directed to my conservative colleagues. Less public spending is not always the best. Consider the following examples. The concept of assuring every family a livable income could be regulated by demanding that all employers pay wages of at least ten dollars per hour, provide full reimbursement for child care expenses, and offer adequate health insurance. Alternatively, one could provide for a much lower wage level and enact earning subsidies (such as the Earned Income Tax Credit) and other publicly provided benefits to achieve the same objective of a livable income. Most economists probably would agree that the regulatory approach, which probably has the least tax and expenditure effect, is not the preferred approach to the public policy objective.

Another example is the public health implications of consuming too much tobacco, drug, and alcohol products. One can attempt to regulate the consumption of these products or, alternatively, one could create a tax structure that finances the social cost of this consumption behavior—by increasing the price of the product sufficiently to cover the social cost. The point of these examples is to simply illustrate that the approach with the least public budget impact is not necessarily the best public policy alternative.

Even if we succeeded in lowering government spending on elderly persons through reductions in Social Security and Medicare relative to current law in exchange for requirements that private spending on elderly persons be increased through private accounts, universal savings plans, or other methods, the overall burden of a growing elderly population would not change. In addition to issues previously discussed, these proposals raise economic questions that need to be addressed. What is the impact of private accounts on administrative costs? What are the distributional aspects of this exchange? Who are the winners and losers? Will financing pension and health costs privately decrease our ability to slow the growth in overall health expenditures?

RECENT DEVELOPMENTS IN POLICIES TOWARD ELDERLY PERSONS

In an era of budget surpluses, it will be extremely difficult to modify promised Social Security and Medicare benefits to elderly persons. The Clinton administration studiously avoided any mention of trimming benefits. But it did propose expansions of benefits to cover prescription drugs, to provide Medicare coverage to certain early retirees, and to provide better protection to low-income elderly widows. It also proposed a significant loss of revenue to promote universal savings plans, particularly for low-income workers. Indeed, the major Clinton administration proposals meant to extend the life of the trust funds were significant infusions of general revenues and investment of a small percentage of Social Security trust fund balances in equities. The Bush administration also has avoided any discussion about benefit reductions—indeed, the mandate to the Social Security Commission is that benefit reduction to elderly persons and those about to retire must be avoided.

The major congressional plans in the late 1990s also went to great lengths to avoid benefit reductions. In fact, most politicians hoped the problem could be solved without tax increases or benefit reductions of any kind. The most prominent conservative plan was the one advanced by Martin Feldstein. This proposal provided significant expansions of cash retirement payments for elderly persons. It would not have lowered the economic burden of elderly persons, and the plan had other substantial negatives as well (Greenstein, Primus, and Kijakazi 1998; Aaron and Reischauer 1998).

The most unfortunate aspects of the recent Social Security debate are the "privatization debate" and the political polarization that has resulted. This polarization may mean that the political system will be paralyzed and incapable of making a decision that would bring long-term benefits in close approximation to long-term revenues in the Social Security and Medicare programs. Reaching consensus on this decision was difficult enough, given the presence of huge budget surpluses, but now may be nigh impossible. The Social Security policy differences in the late 1970s and early 1980s could be compared to the difference between Bob Meyers and Bob Ball—a comparatively short distance. Now the difference is between privatization (creation of individual accounts) on the one side and closing the entire Social Security gap through revenues—such as increasing taxes on high-income wage earners or dedication of a portion of the existing federal funding surpluses to Social Security—and collectively investing Social Security trust reserves in equities, as states are currently doing with their public pension monies, on the other side. Reaching consensus on difficult programmatic proposals to reduce the overall burden on society of an aging population when most Americans do not want benefit reductions will be extremely challenging; it will require bipartisan cooperation and a significant amount of public education.

From the perspective of a twenty-year observation of the federal budgetary process, some aspects of recent budgetary decisions can be celebrated. First, the fact that the political system was able to turn a deficit equaling 6.0 percent of GDP in 1983 into an actual surplus in fiscal year 1999 suggests that the political system was able to make some difficult budgetary choices. These choices were primarily made in the fiscal year 1990 and 1993 budget deficit agreements, which, when combined with a long period of economic growth, will probably continue to produce budget surpluses over the next five years. That accomplishment deserves recognition.

In addition, many observers of federal budgetary policy believe that unified budget surpluses could not be set aside and would automatically lead to revenue reductions or increased spending. There is now considerable evidence that many politicians on a bipartisan basis will allow

Social Security surpluses to be used only for purposes of reducing the public debt and not for tax cuts or spending increases. Instead of spending 100 percent of the Social Security surplus on other government programs, as was done during the 1980s and 1990s, they are insisting that not one dime can be spent on other government programs. This is a bit ridiculous and is causing some unnecessary withdrawal pains (Greenstein and Horney 1999).[5] The Clinton administration deserves a substantial amount of credit for extolling the virtues of debt reduction and using the political power of the Social Security program to protect these budgetary surpluses and use them for public debt reduction.

SOME SUGGESTIONS REGARDING THE BUDGET PROCESS

One of my prouder moments as a congressional staffer was when I made a small contribution to the budget process legislated as part of the 1990 budget agreement. That agreement broke new ground by legislating a pay-as-you-go rule for mandatory spending or revenue reductions and discretionary caps for the appropriations process. Although any budget process rule can be overturned by a majority or supermajority vote of the current membership of Congress, it provides cover and discipline to those who want to restrain federal spending or revenue reductions. It was a way of codifying the simple notion that in an era of deficits, new spending or revenue reductions should be "paid for" by reducing existing spending or adding new revenues. Those rules have served Congress well. They isolated spending decisions that Congress could readily control and did not demand radical policy changes for events the Congress could not control (e.g., imbalances caused by recessions). The 1990 budget agreement also recognized that budget discipline needed to be organized by committee jurisdiction. The appropriations process was controlled by discretionary caps and enforced by reductions in discretionary programs. The process governing entitlements and taxes was the simple rule that any new spending or revenue reduction had to be paid for. If the rule was violated, an automatic across-the-board reduction in mandatory spending was enacted.

Changes to Social Security benefits and revenues were not supposed to be legislated in reconciliation bills. Decisions to change entitlement programs such as Medicare and Social Security are fundamentally different from other annual appropriations decisions. Revenue, retirement, and other entitlement program rules should be changed less frequently because individuals and businesses need to make choices about retirement and investments. Those business investment decisions should be made in an environment where tax rules that influence the decisions are not constantly changing. Providers of health services need to understand reimbursement rules and tax laws in order to make appropriate decisions. These program rules should change occasionally, but not every year. Budget rules need to reflect the different nature of different government programs.

The trust fund nature of many of our programs serving the elderly population has served us well. Reports by the Social Security actuaries that trust fund reserves would soon be exhausted led to reforms in the program both in 1977 and 1983. The fact that the Hospital Insurance program (until very recently) has never had more than a four- to ten-year time frame before exhaustion has led to constant congressional scrutiny. It is hard to find a program with more pages of enacted legislative language than Medicare over the past twenty years.

Many "pure" budget analysts do not like trust funds or dedicated revenue streams. However, they are a political fact of life, and no economic analysis is going to change the use of trust funds. Trust fund constituencies are usually politically strong. That is why spending was protected in the first place. In return for having a dedicated funding stream, these programs should not be allowed to dip into general funds when they get into financial trouble or need further financing unless there are true surpluses in the remainder of the budget. One of the worst violations of that rule occurred with the transportation act that should have financed more highway construction with increased revenues dedicated to transportation; instead, the Social Services Block Grant, a program with a very weak political base, was reduced by 40 percent on a permanent basis to finance the "highway bill."

It is appropriate to fund Social Security and Medicare in advance. But the real danger is that rather than increasing taxes or reducing benefits to improve trust fund solvency, a greater portion of existing revenues will be dedicated to elderly program trust fund programs in the name of solvency without appropriate recognition of the needs of others in our society.

The following proposed changes to the budget process rules might assist Congress and the administration in reaching appropriate budgetary decisions. "Appropriating" implies balancing the needs of the elderly population with other spending needs and tax priorities. However, budget process is only a tool. Any budget process procedure can and should be overridden if that is the will of the majority of Congress. Budget process rules are not an end in themselves. They should assist the resource or budget allocation process.

The most important budget tool is the pay-as-you-go rule. That rule without exception should be applied to every new revenue reduction and new spending program (even despite the earlier unfortunate result of the rule). This rule implies that when (and only when) new entitlement or tax legislation is enacted, there should be enough budgetary resources in each of the next ten years to finance new spending or tax cuts assuming that Social Security and Medicare trust funds (other trust fund reserves could also be set aside) are not used and discretionary spending grows with inflation and population growth (or with the economy). This rule should be permanently extended in the budget act, should be part of both House and Senate rules, and should be enforced by automatic spending reductions and revenue increases if it is violated. Programmatic changes that enhance the solvency of the Medicare and Social Security programs should not be used to finance other government programs. To a large extent, lockbox rules are only a restatement of pay-as-you-go rules. Within trust funds, Social Security and Medicare changes also should be subject to pay-as-you go rules that would forbid any short-, medium-, or long-range benefit increase or revenue reduction that would diminish overall trust fund solvency.

Another budget rule that could be adopted is combining Medicare Part B with Part A and creating a true trust fund instead of allowing an uncapped amount of general revenue financing. Capping in some future year the amount of general revenues that flow into the trust fund and indexing this flow to increases in the nominal level of GDP would force us to evaluate periodically how much we should spend on health care for elderly and disabled persons. Congress could then appropriately consider changes in reimbursement rules, coverage or eligibility, and revenues.

The implication of the pay-as-you-go rule (including the trust fund pay-as-you-go rule) would be that discretionary spending would no longer be squeezed out, and decisions about tax cuts or mandatory spending increases could be balanced against long-term needs. For example, the estate tax could be repealed or dedicated to the Social Security trust fund. Other programmatic issues could be brought to bear on whether this is a meritorious proposal, but the proceeds could be dedicated to Social Security only if the current non–Social Security surplus is large enough. If the decision was made to dedicate the proceeds to Social Security, these revenues could no longer be used to finance other spending decisions. If the estate tax was dedicated, and sometime later the estate tax was proposed for repeal, the proponents of the repeal would have to replenish by tax changes or spending rules governing the Social Security trust fund. The pay-as-you-go rule, if applied to the Social Security and Medicare trust funds, also would imply that within the trust fund, revenue and spending changes must not produce short-, medium-, or long- run increases in actuarial deficits.

If Congress cut discretionary spending below the levels of inflation and population growth, this would free up only a finite amount of resources for tax reductions, spending increases, or changes to trust fund reserves. Long-term discretionary caps would not be recognized for purposes of increased mandatory spending, tax reductions, or allocation of resources to trust funds.

CONCLUDING REMARKS

From my perspective, five major issues involve the intersection of politics, economics, public choice, and individual freedom. Reaching consensus on these will be extremely difficult.

Extending Work Lives. Under the current Social Security retirement system, an individual has a choice to start collecting benefits anywhere between age 62 and age 70. Benefits are adjusted so that overall benefits remain approximately equivalent. Many Americans want to retire early and have been voting so with their individual choices. As shown in chapter 13, the trend toward earlier and earlier retirement is no longer evident. These choices have been made in the context of current Social Security rules, private and public pension systems, and tax subsidized savings vehicles. To ease the overall burden on society of an aging population, the entire system will probably need to encourage or mandate later retirement. In a free market, prices would change enough to make the necessary adjustment. Compensation packages for older workers would increase, and retirement ages would adjust automatically.

However, the retirement decision is not a free market decision; it depends on program rules across a wide variety of institutions and programs—Medicare, Supplemental Security Income, Social Security, pensions, and other retirement plans. Unless changes are coordinated, rules governing the private programs can counteract the policy changes made in the public programs. The problem cannot be solved by incentives that make the entire retirement system more expensive. Increasing the retirement age across institutions will be difficult to achieve politically. Workers with disabilities or other impairments that truly impede work probably should be exempted from any retirement age increase.

Having Elderly Persons Pay for Increased Benefits. One way of improving elderly benefits (e.g., long-term care, prescription drugs) without imposing additional burdens on the overall society would be to insist that those additional services be financed primarily from the incomes of the elderly population. Unfortunately, that device for reducing the economic burden of elderly persons was tried in financing Medicare catastrophic benefits and was a political failure. As an adviser to Ways and Means Committee Chairman Daniel Rostenkowski, I still firmly believe Congress made the right decision by choosing to finance those additional benefits from elderly persons. The chief problem that led to the repeal was that the financing was too progressive, and it was the high-income elderly that insisted on repeal. The easy way out would have been for Congress simply to have changed the financing to a more broad-based revenue stream. In my judgment, total repeal was the right decision, given the alternative.

In retrospect, communication and implementation could have been improved. Perhaps prescription drug benefits should have been added and the financing changed so that it was not quite so progressive. But this example illustrates how politically difficult these decisions will be.

The Free Rider Problem. As mentioned earlier, Medicare and Social Security are not particularly generous programs. And as a society, we will not tolerate having old or disabled individuals not receive medical care and other needed necessities of life, regardless of whether they have paid for those services. However, many individuals will not purchase the necessary insurance unless they are required to do so. How many people would forgo fire insurance if mortgage companies did not require it? How many would forgo automobile insurance if the state did not require it? Individuals would rather spend their money retiring at an earlier age than work additional years and acquire deeper coverage such as long-term care insurance.

Coordination among Different Programs. We need better coordination between Medicare, Medigap, and provisions of employer retiree health plans and between Social Security and private pension plans. For example, Medigap plans increase spending by removing cost sharing requirements. This cost should be reflected in the price of Medigap or employer health plans.

Another example of needed coordination is that withdrawal of pension plans and other tax subsidized retirement vehicles should not be permitted until eligibility for Social Security benefits is obtained and health, long-term care, and other needs are addressed adequately.

Difficult political choices about extending retirement age or increasing financing from elderly persons can be made only with some "political" sweeteners. Financing long-term care services, adding prescription drug benefits, or lowering the Medicare eligibility age could provide those sweeteners and allow the overall burden of the elderly population to be reduced.

Prioritizing Resource Allocation. Finally, there is a real resource allocation problem. If there is a perceived limit to public resources, and elderly persons (using political power unmatched by any other group of voters) lay claims to those resources at the cost of spending or investment for children or the poor, we will have a serious misallocation of resources. There is no legitimate public reason why the goals of the elderly citizens should take priority over the needs of other Americans.

Our economy can afford elderly persons. It is less clear whether our political system can appropriately weigh the short-run benefits and costs of a tax cut or expenditure increase versus the long-term financing needs or burdens of the elderly population. If the current tax debate is primarily concerned with reducing taxes to squeeze future spending, then we as a society may underfund by a considerable margin the optimal level of public investment in children. Very few elected federal policymakers are seriously considering either reducing long- or short-run budget expenditures affecting elderly persons. Most are considering increases. Yet they feel compelled to reduce taxes significantly rather than fund the promises (or reduce the size of those promises) that have been made to elderly persons. Reaching a consensus on those trade-offs is the difficult decision-making process that must be undertaken.

NOTES

This chapter does not necessarily reflect the views of the Center on Budget and Policy Priorities.

1. The projections in Table 5.2 differ from the information presented in Table 5.1 in several important ways. The first two columns in Table 5.1 reflect the actual total of outlays in 1978 and 2000. The third column is projected using the current baseline for government expenditures adjusted for projected rates of inflation and other specified factors. In contrast, the projections in Table 5.2 are based on the assumption that the off-budget surplus will be saved. The assumptions for the projections in Table 5.2 are politically much more realistic. The two tables also differ in that Table 5.1 reflects the treatment of receipts and expenditures in the unified budget. In Table 5.2, receipts and expenditures are measured in the official national income and product accounts (NIPAs) produced by the Commerce Department's Bureau of Economic Analysis. There are some major differences in the treatment of federal receipts and expenditures in the NIPAs compared to their treatment in the unified budget. Because they offset each other, these differences do not affect overall totals significantly. See CBO 2001, appendix D, for a detailed description of these differences. The advantage of using NIPAs for this estimate is that they recast the government's transactions into categories that affect GDP, income, and other macroeconomic totals, thereby helping to trace the relationship between the federal sector and the economy.

2. These projections assume that the off-budget surplus will be saved. For this estimate of revenues, only about 70–75 percent of the Bush administration tax cut can be enacted with no change in the alternative minimum tax.

3. The use of the term *surplus* is problematic in this context. It suggests that one has too much of something, and that clearly is not the case here. All of the short-term Social Security surplus will be needed to pay future benefits.

4. In testimony before the Senate Budget Committee, Peter Orszag estimated that real GDP will be about $125 billion larger in 2011, the net debt of the federal government about $2.4 trillion smaller, and the capital stock about $1.8 trillion larger if the Social Security surpluses are saved rather than spent on tax cuts or spending increases. If the Social Security surplus, the Medicare (more specifically,

the Hospital Insurance trust fund) surplus, and one-third of the on-budget surplus were saved, real GDP would be $193 larger and the capital stock would be about $2.8 billion larger in 2011, compared to a scenario where the entire unified surplus is spent on tax cuts or spending increases.

5. Greenstein and Horney (1999) explain that a non–Social Security deficit would not affect the solvency of Social Security, since Social Security surpluses are never used directly in the payment of benefits. Instead, the surplus money is used by the Treasury to pay down the national debt. A $20 billion or $30 billion non–Social Security deficit in fiscal year 2000 is too small to have much effect on long-term economic growth and would not have any adverse effect on the Social Security program.

REFERENCES

Aaron, H. J., and R. D. Reischauer. 1998. *Countdown to Reform: The Great Social Security Debate.* New York: Century Foundation Press.

Congressional Budget Office (CBO). 2000. *The Long-Term Budget Outlook.* Washington, D.C.: U.S. Government Printing Office, October.

———. 2001. *The Budget and Economic Outlook: Fiscal Years 2002–2011.* Washington, D.C.: U.S. Government Printing Office, January.

Greenstein, R., and J. Horney. 1999. *A Small Non–Social Security Deficit in Fiscal Year 2000 Would Not Adversely Affect Social Security.* Center on Budget and Policy Priorities, September.

Greenstein, R., W. Primus, and K. Kijakazi. 1998. *The Feldstein Social Security Plan.* Center on Budget and Policy Priorities, December.

Thompson, L. 1998. *Older and Wiser: The Economics of Public Pensions.* Washington, D.C.: Urban Institute Press.

6

The Economic Consequences of Funding Growing Elderly Entitlements

Rudolph G. Penner, Ph.D.

What will happen to the welfare of the nation if public pensions and health expenditures on elderly persons are allowed to grow rapidly relative to GDP as baby boomers retire and life expectancy continues to rise? In Congressional Budget Office (CBO) long-run projections, Social Security, Medicare, and Medicaid spending grow from 8 percent of the GDP in 1999 to 12 percent in 2020 and to 17 percent by 2040.[1]

Economists know a lot about some of the issues related to a relative increase in government spending. But in a democracy, the most important welfare question is, What do the people want? It is not clear that economists know much about that. Obviously, there is nothing wrong with allowing Social Security and Medicare outlays to rise relative to GDP considerably above current levels if people like the result and are willing to bear the cost. Few begrudged the huge increase in the government's command over economic resources in World War II, even though the war was probably fought very inefficiently according to criteria favored by economists.

In this chapter I discuss briefly the extreme difficulty of discerning people's tastes in matters related to Social Security and Medicare reform. I then consider issues that economists know a bit more about—the sustainability of current policy and the economic efficiency implications of rising tax burdens and transfer payments.

PUBLIC CHOICE

Social Security and Medicare are two of the most popular public programs in the United States. The key question is whether they will remain popular as the relative cost of health care continues to rise and lifetime Social Security benefits are associated with higher and higher lifetime payroll tax bills. Something will have to be done eventually, or Social Security and Medicare benefits will continue to rise relative to GDP. That cannot go on forever. But it can go on for a good long time, and it can go on at a faster or slower pace.

When contemplating reforms, we generally assume that they will stay in place for a very long time. This is appropriate, because abrupt changes in the program wreak havoc on those trying to develop a long-term retirement plan. But that means that reforms will have important impacts on future generations. It is difficult enough to discern the tastes of the present population, let alone the tastes of those not yet born.

During the recent Social Security debate, public opinion polling was often used to see if there was a consensus building around any particular reform option. The polls revealed that the public, and indeed the pollsters, are not well informed about the characteristics of the program as it exists today or the effects of particular policy options.[2] For example, only 19 percent of respondents knew that current law began to increase the normal retirement age for people turning 62 in 2000.

More disturbing, evidence shows that prominent pollsters do not understand the issues either. One pollster asked the public whether they preferred "raising the retirement age or cutting Social Security benefits."

Public ignorance may imply that public opinion will be volatile as people react to new bits of information. Public ignorance also enhances the power of interest groups to influence and distort the decision-making process. Groups representing elderly persons are extremely powerful, especially the AARP. Indeed, the constituency of such groups is so broad that I hesitate to call them "special" interest groups. Among those with an intense interest in protecting the benefits promised to elderly persons are the elderly themselves, the near-elderly, and the children of the elderly. Many in the corporate sector also worry that if public support is reduced, they may have to fill the gap for former employees.

Although not well informed on the issues, people do seem to sense that the system needs to be changed. A sizable majority (58%) agree that "big changes will be needed to correct [Social Security's] problems," but that majority breaks down into a number of feuding minorities when asked which reform options they favor. In general, a majority of respondents oppose tax-increasing options. The one exception is raising the payroll tax base to $100,000, which gets majority support but would finance a relatively small portion of the increase in benefits promised by current law. Benefit-reducing options that would reduce the rate of growth of benefits relative to GDP are also opposed by clear majorities, although 52 percent favor investing some portion of payroll taxes in individual accounts.

Not only is a majority of the public aware of the need for reform, but they also seem tolerant of reformers. Although Social Security used to be known as the third rail of politics, legislators who have put forward relatively painful reforms have not suffered electorally. Senators John Breaux and Judd Gregg survived the election of 1998, as did Representatives Jim Kolbe, Charles Stenholm, and Nick Smith, along with several others who had the courage to tackle the problem. That does not mean that the public favors the plans put forward by these legislators—only that voters are tolerant of those willing to debate the issues. Clearly, the public does not agree on how much Social Security and Medicare should be allowed to grow over time, and without that consensus one cannot say whether such growth is desirable. Those who study the problem can only fall back on their own judgments, hoping that the debate among them will lead the public to a conclusion.

The issue of what people know and do not know about the relevant programs permeates the rest of this analysis. People's understanding of program characteristics will determine their economic reaction to the growth of the programs and help determine the size of the burden imposed on the economy.

THE SUSTAINABILITY OF POLICY

Whatever reform option people choose, they must be willing to pay for it. Under current policy, future tax revenues are not sufficient to cover future promised benefits. Although the nation now enjoys a substantial budget surplus, that surplus will eventually wither away under current policy and become a deficit. The deficit will grow relative to GDP, and eventually the national debt will grow relative to GDP. The growth in the deficit will accelerate both because interest on the debt will grow faster and because revenue growth will slow. Revenue growth will slow because the growth rate of the economy slows as the government absorbs more and more saving that would otherwise finance productivity-enhancing investments. In the long run, the government debt will explode and the economy will collapse, either because the capital stock declines when saving becomes negative or because the government tries to capture resources through hyperinflation.

Put another way, governments face budget constraints even though they have a monopoly over the creation of money and can compel people to pay taxes. In the long run, revenues must at least equal non-interest expenditures if the average interest rate on the public debt equals the growth rate of the economy. Otherwise, the debt ultimately explodes. If the average interest rate exceeds the growth rate, revenues must be higher relative to noninterest spending.

A debt explosion is virtually certain under current policy, because that policy implies that expenditures will continually grow faster than revenues. It is, however, highly uncertain when the catastrophe will occur and how much of a policy change is necessary to avert it. As recently as March 1997, CBO's long-term budget projections implied that the economic collapse would come as soon as the 2030s. The same projections implied that the disaster could be avoided and the long-term debt / GDP ratio seventy years later could be held to 1997 levels with some combination of immediate tax increases and expenditure cuts equal to 4.1 percent of the GDP. That would require a very large policy change. If all of that adjustment was made on the tax side, every tax in the system would have to be raised 20 percent. If all of it was made by focusing spending cuts on Social Security and Medicare, benefits would have to be immediately reduced by more than half.

By January 1999, less than two years after the 1997 projection was completed, the short-term surplus outlook was much improved. Because analysts make long-run projections by extrapolating recent trends at compound rates of growth, short-run changes radically change long-term projections. The date of the economic collapse was pushed off to the 2060s, and the necessary change in tax and expenditure policies was reduced to 0.6 percent of the GDP, about one-seventh of the necessary change implied earlier. CBO's long-run assumptions were last updated in October 2000. The projections assumed that medical costs would grow more rapidly in the future than according to earlier projections, but the effects of this change were offset by the assumption of a higher rate of economic growth. The necessary change in tax and expenditure policies remained about the same at 0.8 percent of the GDP.[3]

Such erratic long-run projections cannot be taken very seriously, especially when the current view implies that serious problems are more than fifty years away. However, there are reasons to worry:

- No politician today is talking about tax increases and spending cuts. The only question is how large tax cuts will be and by how much the spending constraints adopted in 1997 will be violated. Policy is moving in the wrong direction.
- The longer we wait, the larger the necessary correction. If nothing is done until 2020, the necessary correction about doubles relative to GDP. Because policy is moving in the wrong direction in the short run, the necessary correction by 2020 is likely to be far in excess of twice the 0.6 percent of GDP needed currently.
- Although 0.6 percent of the GDP seems like a small amount, it is almost 9 percent of current expenditures on Social Security and Medicare. But if cuts focused on these programs, they could not be implemented immediately. To allow people a chance to adjust their retirement plans, cuts must be phased in slowly. But then, they have to be much larger relatively. One option that would solve the entire problem would be to phase in an increase in the normal retirement age (NRA) to 70 beginning with people who are now 32 and to increase the eligibility age for Medicare concomitantly. The NRA would be increased one month every two years after 2011. The poll results discussed above imply that this option would be extremely unpopular politically.

If the nation moved to a sustainable policy immediately by raising taxes, we would face a practical problem. Although the demographic problem in the United States is less severe than in most other developed countries, the aging of the population will impose a bigger shock, because the budget problems that it causes come more rapidly. Demographics are now highly favorable to the budget because Depression babies are now retiring and there are not many of them. But they are followed by a larger cohort born during World War II and then by the baby boom that followed. Consequently, we go from a good budget situation to a bad budget situation over a relatively short time period.

As a result, moving to a sustainable policy immediately implies paying off the entire public debt over the next ten years or so while the budget is in good shape and then buying substantial amounts of private, state and local, or foreign assets. The notion of the federal government buying a substantial amount of private assets makes many people, including Alan Greenspan, very nervous. They fear that the government would use its investment decisions to reward friends and punish enemies. Moreover, the private assets would have to be sold after a relatively short time when the budget situation begins to worsen quickly.

EXCESS BURDEN

There is a long-standing proposition in public finance that a general expansion of government spending financed by anything other than a lump sum tax imposes an excess burden in the sense that the taxes used to finance the expansion distort individual behavior in ways that reduce efficiency and welfare. This burden must be added to the direct cost of moving resources from the private to the public sector. Some estimates suggest that the excess burden is very large relative to the direct burden. For example, Ballard, Shoven, and Whalley (1985) calculate the marginal efficiency loss from an additional dollar of taxes at $0.365.

I know of no quantitative estimates of the efficiency costs of expanding Social Security and Medicare using payroll tax increases or any other means of finance. Consequently, we cannot say with certainty whether the proportionate excess burden exceeds or falls short of that of a general expansion of government. However, the following discussion indicates that the benefit or expenditure structure of these programs has the potential to significantly distort choices regarding work and saving. In other words, distortions come from both the tax and the spending sides of the programs, and as a result their expansion could very well create more inefficiency per dollar than a more general expansion of government.

Estimates of how Social Security affects private saving behavior differ wildly. Some consensus exists regarding the effect on the timing of retirement. The effect on work effort during a career is more mysterious.

Two fundamental issues are important in analyzing the effects of Social Security and Medicare on saving and work behavior. The first question asks what is replaced by public support for the elderly. Are the public programs substitutes for private saving that would otherwise finance pensions and medical costs in retirement, or are they substitutes for transfers from children and other pay-as-you-go mechanisms for supporting elderly persons? If the former, the programs' effect on private saving could be huge and could have caused a significant reduction in our standard of living. If the latter, the effect on saving would be negligible as a socialized pay-as-you-go mechanism substituted for private pay-as-you-go mechanisms. The difference between the two approaches was the topic of a debate between Barro and Feldstein (1978) about twenty years ago, in which Feldstein argued that the effect on saving was massive while Barro argued that it was negligible. Both sides provided empirical evidence supporting their points of view.

It is not easy to resolve the dispute. If one looks at mechanisms for supporting elderly persons that preceded Social Security, it is true that only the most affluent saved to finance their retirement. The rest were supported with pay-as-you-go mechanisms. Transfers from children were very important, but so were Civil War pensions, charities, fraternal organizations, local governments, and union pensions. Corporate pensions grew in significance after the turn of the century, but they were destroyed by the Great Depression.

At first sight, it may seem as though current public programs for elderly persons are mainly substitutes for traditional pay-as-you-go mechanisms and therefore have little impact on private saving. However, Social Security and Medicare are very different from traditional pay-as-you-go mechanisms. Traditional mechanisms did not treat elderly persons very generously. The elderly constituted one of the poorest groups in society, and they may have been treated even more harshly by traditional mechanisms as life expectancy at age 65 continually increased. In recent decades, the poverty rate among elderly persons has fallen drastically with the expansion and increased generosity of Social Security. Elderly persons now experience a lower poverty rate than children.

The key question is whether private saving for retirement would have increased with rising affluence and life expectancy if Social Security and Medicare had not been invented. Although one cannot say for sure, it is hard to believe that private retirement saving would not have become somewhat more common and that therefore the programs do have a significant impact on saving. Put another way, if people are rational and well informed and have adjusted their saving, borrowing, and work plans to provide an optimum level of retirement income in the presence of the programs, one would expect them to respond to a reduction in expected benefits by increasing private saving. Given the affluence of elderly persons relative to their economic status historically, one would not expect modest reductions in benefits to be offset by equivalent increases in transfers from children, although smaller transfers from elderly persons to children could be possible.

But all this assumes that people are well informed and rational, and as we saw earlier, it is apparent that they do not understand the details of the public pension and health insurance systems. That makes it very difficult to discern the effects of changing the system on private saving. There is a sufficient diversity of empirical estimates to sustain any prejudice; the economics profession has much left to do in resolving the issue.

It seems clearer that the existence of Social Security and Medicare have reduced labor force participation rates among older workers. Medicare is especially important in reducing the retirement age, especially among those who have no employer health insurance. The average age at which people claim their first Social Security benefit has decreased through time, but it fell especially rapidly after the early retirement age was created for women in the late 1950s and for men in the early 1960s (Steuerle and Spiro 1999).

The impact of Social Security on people's desire to work was undoubtedly lessened in 2000 when Congress eliminated the retirement test on recipients aged 65 to 69. The test reduced benefits substantially for those who continued working beyond age 64, and it is still in effect for those aged 62 to 64. Not many elderly choose to work beyond age 64, but recent studies suggest that the retirement test had significant effects on the relatively small group that remained in the labor force (Friedberg 1997). Indeed, the effect seemed too large given that those who lose benefits because of the retirement test will receive larger benefits later that are increased by an amount that is gradually rising toward an actuarially fair amount. However, empirical research has failed to find that this delayed retirement credit had any effect. That is probably because few people realize that it exists, whereas the earnings limit was much better known.

The effect of Social Security on work effort during a career depends on a second fundamental issue regarding the way people understand Social Security. That is, do people view the payroll tax as being independent of eventual benefit levels, or do they take account of the fact that they are earning additional benefits as they work? Obviously, the payroll tax will have a less negative impact on work effort and job opportunities if people associate it with increased benefits.

It is not easy for people to figure out how much eventual benefits are increased with the payment of each dollar of payroll taxes. Aside from the possibility that benefit rules will be changed in the future, the ratio of the present value of benefits to the present value of payroll taxes depends on such things as the level and timing of lifetime earnings, marital status, the lifetime earnings of a spouse, one's tax status during retirement, and the growth of average wages in the economy.

However, the fact that the benefits associated with the payment of an extra dollar of taxes are difficult to determine does not mean that no benefit is attributed to the tax payment. I know of no empirical evidence that sheds any light on the extent to which people link tax payments and eventual benefits.

OTHER CONSIDERATIONS

Improving Efficiency

One could infer from the discussion thus far that a reduction in the growth of Social Security and Medicare expenditures implied a reduction in benefits. Many believe, however, that Medicare benefits could be delivered more efficiently if the system was opened up to competition. Obviously, if the same benefits could be delivered with fewer resources, or if increased benefits could be delivered with the same resources, social welfare would improve.

Individual Accounts

A number of proposals for reforming Social Security would create a system of individual accounts. Deposits in these accounts would be either mandated or 100 percent subsidized by income tax credits or reductions in the payroll tax. After retirement, income from the accounts would fully or partially replace traditional Social Security benefits. Many of the economic impacts of such accounts are discussed by Geanakoplos, Mitchell, and Zeldes (chapter 12 in this volume).

Because of that discussion, I do not consider the economic effects of individual accounts here. However, since my chapter is about the impact of increased public spending one should note that some experts in budget accounting think the contributions of income to individual accounts should be counted as government receipts if they are mandated or 100 percent subsidized. The immediate deposits in individual accounts would then be counted as government outlays (Committee for a Responsible Federal Budget 1997). Those who argue for including individual accounts in the government's budget do so because they consider a mandate to save to be identical to a tax. If a mandated contribution is considered to be a tax, then a voluntary contribution that is 100 percent subsidized must also be considered to be a tax by budget documents, because the effect of this reform on future retirement income will be virtually identical to that resulting from a mandate.

The choice of approaches to accounting for individual accounts may seem an arcane matter, but it will have a major impact on the policy debate. If deposits in accounts are considered to be government receipts, government and the tax burden that it imposes will appear larger. This will make individual accounts appear less desirable to many politicians and make the reform harder to enact.

My own view is that it would be foolish to allow the debate over Social Security reform to be complicated by this accounting dispute.

There are many mandates that require private outlays for things like safety devices and antipollution equipment where the outlays are not considered to be tax receipts in the budget, even though they have many of the attributes of taxes. A mandated deposit in a retirement account should, in my view, be treated like these other mandates. The debate should make it clear, however, that a mandated deposit imposes a burden on those who can only satisfy the mandate by reducing consumption. Those who can reduce other saving or increase borrowing are affected less severely.

Relative Costs and Absolute Living Standards

This chapter focuses on the share of GDP going to Social Security, Medicare, and Medicaid. It is, of course, possible for that share to grow while the absolute amount of GDP left for other uses also continues to grow.

The CBO projections of October 2000 imply that the GDP left for other uses grows by 3.0 percent per year between 1999 and 2010. That is faster than the rate of GDP growth because of the favorable demographics associated with the retirement of Depression babies. After 2010, worsening demographics cause the annual growth in the GDP left for other uses to slow below the growth of total GDP. The rate is 2.1 percent per year between 2010 and 2020, 1.8 percent between 2020 and 2030, and 1.7 percent between 2030 and 2040.

On a per capita basis, the residual GDP grows at a rate of 2.1 percent annually between 1999 and 2010. The per capita rate of growth falls to 1.3 percent annually between 2010 and 2020 and to 1.0 percent between 2020 and 2040.

These numbers imply a major reduction, compared to past history, in the per capita growth of GDP remaining after the federal government takes its share. For example, over the twenty years from 1978 to 1998, the nonfederal GDP per capita grew at a rate of 1.7 percent per annum. The political implications of an abrupt slowdown in the growth in the amount of resources left for nonfederal purposes are hard to predict. Whether it strengthens the resolve to reform programs for elderly persons remains to be seen.

CONCLUSIONS

This chapter is not rife with definite conclusions. No public consensus has formed regarding appropriate reforms for Social Security or Medicare, and without knowing what people want, it is difficult to judge the desirability of continually increasing the share of the nation's resources devoted to supporting elderly persons. My conclusion is that supporting elderly persons in longer and longer retirements as expected life increases should not be a high priority of the nation. This makes increasing the normal retirement age an appealing option; but if anything is clear, it is that there is little public support for this approach. Those of us who favor this option can only fall back on the hope that people do not understand its implications. Some seem to believe that they will get no benefits at all if they retire earlier than the new higher normal retirement age. In fact, the proposal would simply reduce benefits by an actuarially fair amount at any specific age of retirement, say 65.

If the share of GDP going to elderly persons is increased, it is of paramount importance that the cost be financed by raising the overall tax bill. Like the rest of us, government is subject to budget restraints, and currently the long-run budget restraint is not being satisfied. The implication is that public debt will explode in the long run with dire consequences for the economy. The timing of this disaster is not easy to estimate, but currently it appears that it will not occur for a very long time. Unfortunately, policy is now moving in the wrong direction and is hastening the day that the economy will face severe difficulties.

The expansion of support for elderly persons may have important effects on work effort and saving and therefore reduce the efficiency of the overall economy. Clearly, generous benefits hasten retirement. The effects on work effort during a career and on saving are less clear. The size of these effects is hotly disputed in the literature—especially the effect on saving—and it may be a long time before the economics profession reaches a consensus on such issues.

In any case, a continuation of current policy implies an abrupt slowdown in the growth of nonfederal resources after 2010. Whether this provokes dissatisfaction with programs for elderly persons and a call for reform remains to be seen.

NOTES

1. Medicaid is included because it supports long-term care for indigent elderly persons.

2. The results described here are from a poll published September 30, 1998, and sponsored by Americans Discuss Social Security. Polling results for Social Security reform seem to be particularly sensitive to the exact wording of the questions, so one can find polls that imply more or less support for some of the options.

3. This gap is compared to a baseline in which all projected surpluses are saved. In their most recent projection, CBO also computes the higher gaps implied by assuming that only Social Security surpluses are saved or that the budget is balanced during the period in which current policy implies a surplus.

REFERENCES

Ballard, C. L., J. B. Shoven, and J. Whalley. 1985. General Equilibrium Computations of the Marginal Welfare Costs of Taxes in the United States. *American Economic Review* 75:128–38.

Barro, Robert J., and M. S. Feldstein. 1978. *The Impact of Social Security on Private Saving: Evidence from the U.S. Time Series.* Washington, D.C.: American Enterprise Institute for Public Policy Research.

Committee for a Responsible Federal Budget. 1997. *Social Security Reform: Economic and Budget Concepts, Enforcement, and Scorekeeping Perspectives.* Washington, D.C.: Committee for a Responsible Federal Budget, December.

Congressional Budget Office (CBO). 1999. *The Long-Term Budget Outlook.* Washington, D.C.: U.S. Government Printing Office, October.

Friedberg, L. 1997. The Labor Supply Effects of the Social Security Earnings Test. Discussion paper 97-01, University of California, San Diego.

Steuerle, C. E., and C. Spiro. 1999. *The Many Reinforcements for Retiring Early.* Straight Talk no. 7, The Retirement Project. Washington, D.C.: Urban Institute.

7

The Entitlement Crisis That Never Existed

Joseph White, Ph.D.

The first step in any policy analysis is to define the problem. That is also the first step in political debate about supposed solutions.

In recent years, political debate in the United States about future costs of federal programs for the aged has been dominated by a tone of hysteria. Establishment commentators in the mainstream press set this tone. Joe Klein wrote in *Newsweek* (1996) that, while the press "harps on the entitlement monster," President Clinton was ducking the issue. David Gergen, a senior aide in the Ford, Reagan, and Clinton administrations, declared in *U.S. News and World Report* (1996) that reform of entitlements was a matter of "national character and honesty" that demanded "immediate, significant changes not only in Washington but in our own personal lifestyles as well." As President Clinton was inaugurated for his second term, *Time*'s cover article declared, "No Guts, No Glory," and referred to Social Security and Medicare as "the middle-class entitlement monsters that will consume the budget if left unchecked" (Pooley 1997). On an only somewhat happier note, reporter Jackie Calmes in the *Wall Street Journal* (1997) praised politicians for recognizing how "unprecedented fiscal and demographic pressures could push the deficit to unthinkable depths." She added that, "as in any chronic addiction, publicly acknowledging the problem is an important step, but there is no consensus about how to cure it." Much less optimistically, David Broder (1996) warned of "fiscal calamity" and "all-out generational war" and argued that if the two parties did not solve the problem, one could be realigned out of existence by the year 2000.

Such rhetoric on the part of centrist reporters and commentators makes anything short of radical change appear not just inadequate but cowardly and immoral. It begs explanation. A large part of that explanation must include how long-term forecasts of the federal budget and economy have commonly been made and interpreted. Claims about the eventual effects of entitlements for the elderly on the budget, and of the budget on the economy, were used to argue that action must be taken immediately to slash commitments to entitlements for the elderly and thereby save the economy.

Those claims are largely wrong. Parts of my argument to that effect are at least implicit in Henry Aaron's debunking of the relevance of long-term budget forecasts to policy choice. The estimation uncertainties on which I remark are noted by Steuerle and Van de Water, Aaron, and others. And my analysis of economic effects is not really contradicted by Primus or Penner. But by taking a different view of the meaning of "responsibility to future generations," I come to a conclusion that, even if it may be shared by some analysts, is rarely stated so bluntly. Much of the challenge posed by estimated future costs for Social Security, Medicare, and Medicaid can and should be left to future politicians and citizens to address. Incremental policy choices that will make these programs easier to finance in the future but do not pretend to "solve" the "crisis" are not only all that is needed now but also all that is justified.

A responsible approach to the future cost of entitlements justifies careful budget policies in the short run, more careful than many current politicians seem to prefer. Some savings or reforms in those programs seem modest and fair; others might be more controversial but could be justified and, in order to be fair and effective, should be adopted far in advance. Some measures that I view as ways to give future decision makers better information, such as experiments with competitive bidding by Medicare managed care plans, clearly are highly controversial. All of these policy measures should be pursued and would make the programs easier to finance in the future. But there is no economic basis for radical structural change or drastic cuts in Social Security and Medicare. They are not "entitlement monsters" but programs that make this a more decent country and that should be preserved in order to respond to the real challenges of an aging society.

THE BUDGET AND ECONOMIC PERFORMANCE

The campaign to create a political sense of crisis is exemplified by Peter G. Peterson. The former secretary of commerce and leader of the Concord Coalition has written extensively about the "momentous question" that "looms over America's economic future." In his account, how Americans "prepare and pay for the growing dependency of our rapidly aging population" will "determine whether your children will participate in the American dream of rising affluence." Americans' "addiction to universal entitlements—welfare for all, in effect," and the "projected explosion in entitlement costs" could cause "the nation's wealth-producing engines" to "fail" because America is "undersaving." Dollars cut from entitlements would instead fuel investment and growth, restoring the American dream (1996, 3–10).

National Savings

Peterson's concern with national savings resonated with the nonexpert opinion leaders whom I quoted to begin this chapter because many of the nation's most eminent policy economists, associated with both political parties, saw "the need to increase the nation's anemic savings rate as the paramount issue" in economic policy (Passell 1996). From around 1983 on, they used arguments that economic growth required higher savings to criticize budget deficits, provide an alternative to other proposals to revitalize the economy (such as tax cuts, deregulation, public investment, or protection) and even, beginning in the mid-1980s, to argue against cuts in Social Security.[1]

This is not the place to discuss the political logic of some of the connections made by these mainstream economists. Nor need we discuss alternative economic theories. It seems reasonable to conclude that the economic effects, other things being equal, go in the direction that the argument for savings claimed.[2] The problem for the savings campaign is that mainstream economists' own estimates of the size of the effects have not been large.

Estimated effects are much smaller than Peterson's rhetoric suggests because positive changes in the federal government's net savings position do not translate so dramatically into extra investment. The effects are slow to begin with, accumulating over perhaps thirty years. Some of the money is offset by individuals' reducing their own personal savings when their taxes are raised or government benefits are cut. Some of the extra savings displace foreign investment in the United States, rather than increasing total investment. Further, the benefits eventually top out, because a larger capital stock creates more depreciation, and eventually the new rate of savings is needed to pay for the higher level of depreciation (CBO 1993, 1997a; Aaron, Bosworth, and Burtless 1989). As a result, mainstream estimates, though they vary a bit, center around the 1993 estimate by the Congressional Budget Office (CBO) that "for each percentage point of permanent increase in the ratio of national saving to GDP, consumption will eventually be permanently raised by about 1 percent above what it would have been without the savings increase" (CBO 1993, 74–75). But CBO's own estimates have said that at least 20 percent of any increase in federal government savings would be offset (CBO 1997a). So CBO is saying, in essence, that changing the federal government's savings position by 3 percent of GDP would eventually increase the GDP available for consumption by 2.4 percent.

To put that in perspective, consider that if productivity grew even by 1 percent per year, total output per worker would grow by 40 percent over thirty-five years (Eisner 1996). If the savings rate did not change, consumption would increase by the same amount. By CBO's standard, a 3 percent of GDP swing in the federal budget balance—which would be quite large in budget terms—would make consumption 43.4 percent bigger instead. The future of the American dream does not lie in the difference between 40 and 43.4 percent. Other effects are much larger, including the unexpected economic growth of the second Clinton term, CBO's revision of its long-term productivity growth assumption to 1.7 percent annually, and even the effects of technical changes that the Bureau of Labor Statistics made to its calculation of the Consumer Price Index in the late 1990s. If you do not like Social Security and Medicare, then the possibility that cutting them would produce a small amount of extra growth is an extra reason to cut them. But if you believe the programs are important, then the economic benefits of cuts could well not seem worth the pain.

National Dissavings

Budget policy could have severe economic effects in the long term, but only if policymakers ignored obvious signs of trouble. If the government's deficit was to trend upward and nothing were done in response, then each year's deficit would increase the debt relative to the national economy; the cost of servicing the debt would rise accordingly; this would drive deficits higher, and deficits would balloon further. Deficits would soak up larger and larger shares of the combined pool of Americans' savings and foreigners' investments in the United States, until eventually the funds available for investment would be less than each year's depreciation. The nation's capital stock would decline, and whether the government would be unable to sell its bonds or the economy would totally crash first is hard to say.

This doomsday scenario depends above all on the logic of compound interest. Responsible budget policy would involve acting soon enough to prevent interest costs from getting out of control. Long-term budget estimates became a major factor in policy debate when the U.S. General Accounting Office (GAO), and then other agencies, began extrapolating current law to the point of total irresponsibility and then modeling the results.

Table 7.1 displays long-term budget forecasts made between 1992 and 1999 by GAO, CBO, and the presidential Office of Management and Budget (OMB). Each model assumed that the economy would implode at a level of deficit somewhere over 20 percent of GDP. Our real concern should be the level at which it would become quite difficult to stop the accumulation of interest toward doomsday.[3]

The table shows that the projections are extremely unstable. The forecasting agencies' models and assumptions differ, but even a single agency's projection can change dramatically in a short time. The forecast deficit as of 2020 was cut in half between GAO's 1995 and CBO's March 1997 projection, even though there had been little antideficit legislation. More economic good news, and some small effects from the Balanced Budget Act of 1997, meant that by February 1998 the pro-

Table 7.1. Estimates of Long-Term Budget Shortfalls in the United States, 1992–1999

	Estimated Surplus or Deficit as a Percentage of GDP					
	2000	2010	2020	2030	2040	2050
GAO June 1992 (a)	−5	−8	−20			
GAO April 1995 (b)	−3	−7	−15	>−23		
CBO March 1997 (c)	−2	−3	−7	−17		
GAO October 1997 (d)	0	0	−2	−7	−13	−20
OMB January 1998 (e)	0	2	2	2	1	1
GAO February 1998 (f)	0	1	−1	−5	−10	−16
CBO May 1998 (g)	0	1	−1	−5	−10	−23
CBO January 1999 (h)	1	3	1	−1	−3	−6
GAO May 1999 (j)	1	3	2	−1	−2	−4

Sources: GAO 1992 and 1997 are from U.S. General Accounting Office 1997, fig. 2. GAO April 1995 is author's estimate from U.S. General Accounting Office 1995, fig. 2. GAO February 1998 and May 1999 are from spreadsheets kindly supplied by the Office of the Chief Economist, U.S. General Accounting Office. CBO March 1997 is from CBO 1997b, with economic feedbacks and discretionary spending growing with the economy after 2007, table 5. CBO May 1998 is from CBO 1998, summary table 2. CBO January 1999 is from CBO 1999, table 2-1 and summary table 3. OMB January 1998 is from U.S. Office of Management and Budget, *Analytical Perspectives: Budget of the United States Government, Fiscal Year 1999* (Washington, D.C.: U.S. Government Printing Office, January 1998), table 2-2. I report only this OMB forecast because OMB assumed that the accounts known as "discretionary" spending would grow only with inflation to the end of time. This assumption is highly improbable. But the figures are worth including to show how much such assumptions matter. For more extensive discussion, see White 2001.

jected deficit in 2020 had practically disappeared. In CBO's and GAO's 1999 estimates, the deficit was projected to be manageable for the next half century. The improvements between October 1997 and 1999 occurred even though there were no budgetarily positive policy changes.[4]

These projections are so volatile because relatively small changes in either initial conditions or assumed trends can compound, over many years, into large differences in final totals. The effects of differences in underlying health care spending, or revenue growth, or other factors, then are exacerbated by their feedbacks on federal costs for debt service. The good news is, small policy changes can *look* as if they are doing a huge amount of good. But that good can disappear—or be doubled—by small changes in reality or underlying assumptions. In short, policymakers cannot know what the true long-term budget situation is. And ignorance is not a good basis for policy choice.

These analyses do demonstrate the difference between what one of their authors called "sustainable" and "unsustainable" policies. Doomsday involves not the benefits of savings but the risks of dissavings.[5] Since the real problem is to avoid letting deficits get so large that they would feed on themselves, and the forecasts are uncertain, a responsible approach would be to have a budget policy at any given time, given available information, that does not threaten serious movement along the doomsday spiral within the next two decades. Serious movement could be defined as deficits of 10 percent of GDP or more. By this standard, GAO's 1992 projections justified worry. CBO's and GAO's 1999 projections did not.

In fact, both the more negative and the more positive forecasts were unrealistic. Long-term forecasts must assume that policy will be on some form of automatic pilot, but that assumption is so unrealistic that even the forecasters fail to follow it consistently.

FISCAL CAPACITY AND LONG-TERM BUDGET ESTIMATES

How hard will it be for future politicians to fund something close to current promises for Social Security, Medicare, and Medicaid and still avoid a doomsday deficit spiral? Any government's ability to pay for particular programs depends on those programs' own costs and the government's fiscal capacity. Fiscal capacity depends on the size of the economy, the proportion of national product that citizens are willing to devote to government spending, and the size of preexisting spending obligations. Increased expenses for some programs relative to GDP will be affordable if voters are willing to pay the extra costs, if other obligations can decline enough to offset those costs, or if some combination of those two effects occurs.[6]

Steuerle and Van de Water's chapter in this book (chapter 4) shows that long-term projections make assumptions about each of those factors. Those assumptions are presented as continuations of current law, but they are actually presumptions about future policy choice.

We have seen that, *until* the deficit gets totally out of control, budget policy is not likely to have large effects on the size of the economy.

Therefore, economic effects can be only a small factor in *whether* the deficit becomes unmanageable. Turning to the size of government that citizens will pay for, the logical question is whether a greater need for spending on entitlements for the elderly, defined as higher costs due to an aging population and medical advances, will raise the acceptable level of taxes.

Revenue Prospects

The estimates in Table 7.1 assume that revenues will never rise. But one would expect some relation between revenues and what the government is buying. The federal government has raised taxes in wartime, kept them high by previous standards to finance the Cold War against the Soviet Union and, not incidentally, raised them significantly in order to reduce the deficits that burgeoned after the tax cut of 1981. Revenues in 1997 were 2.1 percent of GDP higher than in 1986, in part because of the substantial tax hikes in the 1990 and 1993 deficit reduction packages. Local and state governments raised revenues to educate the baby boomers.

It is at least arguable that the public is more willing to pay to finance Social Security and Medicare than to reduce budget deficits. For instance, polling data has consistently shown strong majorities more willing to tolerate deficits than Social Security cuts (Page 1999). As a statement about political conditions at the turn of the century, it was fair to say that "the anti-tax mood is so strong that Congress is not likely to close the projected long-term Social Security deficit primarily by raising taxes" (Aaron and Reischauer 1998, 153). But the situation when the bills come due may be very different.[7]

Costs of Pension and Health Programs

Ability to pay for programs also depends on how much they cost. Rather than cover the same ground as chapters 3 and 4, I want to suggest some judgments.

First, demographic assumptions, while surely imprecise, are more reliable than the others. There is good reason, therefore, to expect program costs to increase significantly as a share of GDP.

Second, differences in economic assumptions are more significant for how we conceive of burdens as a social matter than for the federal budget. To borrow an analogy from Henry Aaron and Lawrence Thompson (1987), the economy is the donut, and the cost of social insurance for elderly persons is the hole. If the donut is much bigger, then a larger hole is not a major social problem. The difference between a 1 percent per year and a 1.7 percent per year growth in productivity will have only small effects on eventual costs of Social Security as a share of GDP, but it will have large effects on what workers have left over after paying Social Security taxes.[8]

Third, as Henry Aaron also argues in this volume, there is no reliable way to forecast the nondemographic component of future costs for Medicare and Medicaid. Some analysts seem to believe that costs balloon because of technological advances, that only drastic choices are likely to constrain costs significantly, and that large increases can be expected based on the more inflationary periods during the past few decades (Fuchs 1999). Others, represented in this volume by Theodore R. Marmor, believe that costs can be significantly affected by policy choices and that much of the "pain" of cost control can be allocated to the income stream of the medical business, including the incomes of the vast superstructure that is built on top of medical providers. Both recent experience in America and variation in experience across countries suggest that policy choices matter greatly. There is no reason to believe that "technology" per se varied between countries or periods except inasmuch as policies affected the availability of new procedures or services. So policy seems primary. But that does not tell anyone what cost control policies will be followed in the future or what the results might be.

For three reasons, forecasts cannot simply assume that recent medical cost control policies will be continued. First, many cost control provisions, as a matter of law, are not permanent. Second, the targets of cost control policy are a very large number of extremely intelligent people. It is wishful thinking to imagine that they could not find a way, over time, either to break through or to foment powerful public dissatisfaction with any set of cost control measures. Third, we do not know what level of benefits the health care providers will be offering, so it is uncertain what level of cost control will seem desirable in the future. So there is no good basis for projecting future costs from current law or policy.

In practice, the estimating agencies have followed two procedures. For the first ten to twenty years of forecasts, they have made assumptions based on extrapolations of current law. When savings measures are projected to expire, for example, CBO has expected costs to increase more rapidly afterward. Why politicians would allow that is not explained. For the longer term, they have adopted an arbitrary figure for the annual growth of per capita medical costs relative to per capita GDP. How politicians would attain that (generally lower) cost trend also is not explained.[9]

I have argued elsewhere that the political system is quite capable of holding the growth of Medicare costs per enrollee to about 1 percent per year above the growth rate of per capita GDP and that more stringent cost control is certainly possible (White 1999). We can use such arguments to critique individual projections. The 1 percent standard provides a basis for assessing the future difficulty of controlling costs more or less stringently. But it does not tell us what costs will be.[10]

Other Spending

Future costs for social insurance for elderly persons will be either more or less affordable, depending on costs for other programs. In the doomsday scenario, increasing interest costs eventually bankrupt the federal government. In the positive periods of the forecasts in Table 7.1, declining costs (as a share of GDP) for the accounts termed "discretionary spending" combine with the elimination of federal interest payments to largely pay for increased social insurance costs through at least the next two decades.

Unlike projections for entitlements or revenues, discretionary spending estimates cannot be phrased as what will happen if Congress does not change existing law. Discretionary programs, funded by annual appropriations, would disappear when those appropriations expired. So those estimates are explicitly guesses about action by Congress in the near as well as the distant future. The discretionary spending estimates in the 1998 and 1999 projections in Table 7.1 seemed to critics at the time, and have proven to be, unrealistically low (Reischauer 1997b; Horney 1999; CBO 2000a).

Forecasts of interest costs follow directly from the rest of any given projection.[11] The catch here is the assumption that politicians and citizens will not respond to interest trends by changing policies on revenues or program spending. It is unrealistic to assume that costs will be allowed to rise at the rate assumed in doomsday scenarios. Conversely, the positive portions of recent long-term projections include periods during which the federal government retires its debt, reducing interest spending to zero, and then accumulates a nest egg of some sort of assets, on which it earns interest. As Penner argues in chapter 6 of this volume, the political prospects for that development are rather dicey.

It is more likely that accumulation of some fund could be made part of Social Security policy, as "diversification" of the trust funds.[12] Even that policy has fervent opponents; it is likely to be more politically plausible if the total accumulation is limited to an amount similar to other investments, such as the largest private funds or state and local government funds. I argue elsewhere that an accumulation of about 10 percent of GDP would be a reasonable compromise (White 2001). In terms of overall budget policy, any significantly larger accumulation is unlikely.

Some forecasts therefore have likely overstated the extent to which future costs for entitlements for the elderly can be met by reducing discretionary spending and turning interest into revenue instead of an expense. Nevertheless, budgetary trends when this book's chapters were being written were highly favorable. Continuation of the budget policies of President Clinton's second term would help finance future expenses for Social Security, Medicare, and Medicaid by greatly reducing spending for net interest and likely somewhat reducing discretionary spending.

Long-term budget estimates inherently must make questionable assumptions about future politics; and by seeming to say what "will" happen, they can distract attention from a more complex, but more appropriate, discussion in terms of future fiscal capacity. Yet estimates can be useful not only as warning flags when a vicious cycle of increasing debt and deficits becomes foreseeable but also as the basis for a more nuanced discussion of fiscal prospects. The most recent forecast available at the time of writing, CBO's long-term projections in October 2000, can be used to provide that kind of understanding.

ONE VIEW OF BUDGET PROSPECTS

The figures in Table 7.2 should provide some perspective on the extent of the economic and political challenges posed by the projected aging of the U.S. population. CBO's policy baseline assumed massive federal surpluses both within "off-budget" (mainly Social Security) and "on-budget" (most other spending and revenue) accounts. CBO therefore prepared three different scenarios, according to whether policy would be unchanged from its baseline ("Save Total Surpluses"), all surpluses would be eliminated ("Save No Surpluses"), or policy changes would eliminate only the on-budget surpluses ("Save Off-Budget Surpluses"). "Save Off-Budget Surpluses," which I refer to hereafter as SOBS, is the most plausible of the scenarios and so is the best approximation of the current American budget situation.

In the SOBS forecast, the American federal budget is in excellent shape through 2020, and its condition looks tolerable in 2030, with a deficit of 3.3 percent of GDP. Deficits and debt spiral out of control in the 2030s, however, as the debt feeds on itself and negative economic feedbacks develop.[13]

If we look more closely at the components of the SOBS forecast, in the second half of Table 7.2, we see that spending for Social Security, Medicare, and Medicaid is projected to grow by 4.2 percent of GDP between 1999 and 2020 and by another 5 percent of GDP between 2020 and 2040. The first increase does not produce budget difficulties because it is assumed to be offset by reductions in interest and other categories of spending. But those favorable dynamics cease after 2020, as there are no further savings and the federal government shifts from a net creditor to a net debtor position.[14] In essence, then, the forecast assumes that no effort is made to pay for the 3 percent of GDP increase in spending on Social Security, Medicare, and Medicaid during the 2020s.

The forecast in Table 7.2 is substantially more negative than the most recent CBO forecasts in Table 7.1, for three reasons. First, CBO is assuming much greater growth in health care costs after the year 2020 than it did before. Previously, CBO adopted the Health Care Financing Administration's projection that after 2020 there would be no excess medical cost growth beyond demographics and (roughly) per capita GDP. Now CBO is projecting an excess of 1.1 percent per year

Table 7.2. U.S. Congressional Budget Office Alternative Long-Term Forecasts of Federal Surpluses or Deficits as Shares of GDP on National Income and Product Accounts Basis as of October 2000

	Calendar Year				
	1999	2010	2020	2030	2040
Scenario 1: "Save Off-Budget Surpluses"	1.2	1.9	0.5	−3.3	−9.5
Scenario 2: "Save Total Surpluses"	1.2	4.3	3.9	1.8	−0.4
Scenario 3: "Save No Surpluses"	1.2	0	−2.4	−8.4	−23.9
Memorandum: Scenario 1 details, as percentage of GDP					
NIPA Receipts	20.2	19.2	19.2	19.2	19.2
Social Security	4.1	4.3	5.2	6.0	6.4
Medicare	2.2	2.9	4.1	5.6	6.6
Medicaid	1.2	1.7	2.4	3.1	3.8
Subtotal	7.5	8.8	11.7	14.7	16.7
Other programs	8.6	7.6	7.5	7.5	7.5
Net interest	2.8	0.9	−0.5	0.4	4.6

Source: CBO 2000b and backup table supplied by CBO in December 2000. CBO staff bear no responsibility for how I have manipulated and interpreted their data.

above those factors. Second, CBO is assuming that revenues will fall by a full percent of GDP, due to policy choice, over the next decade. Third, the most recent forecast eliminated the previous assumption that discretionary spending would be held through fiscal year 2002 to the levels that were legislated as budget "caps" in the Balanced Budget Act of 1997. Nevertheless, CBO still assumed that these accounts would increase only by the rate of inflation from fiscal year 2001 through fiscal year 2010, so discretionary spending would decline by 1 percent of GDP over the next decade.

How realistic were these assumptions? The forecast that revenues would fall quickly might seem to have been confirmed by the tax cut legislation enacted in 2001. But one should not assume that revenues would be set at CBO's estimated level to the end of time; indeed, many of the provisions in the tax cut expire after ten years, leaving doubt as to what the law will be in 2011, as the first baby boomers reach age 65.[15]

CBO's forecast for Medicare is arguably pessimistic in two signifi-cant ways. First, CBO assumes that costs per enrollee will grow by 2 percent above per capita income for at least ten years before trending down to the lower eventual level. Although one can find periods of even faster growth within Medicare, that is much faster than recent experience and represents a significant speedup before the eventual slow-down. Second, CBO treats Medicare Part B premiums as revenues. Those premiums are currently set, legislatively, at 25 percent of the Part B program's costs. Therefore, the premiums should grow as program costs grow, which means the national government's net expenses for the pro-gram do not rise as quickly as its gross expenses. Yet, by capping fore-cast revenues as a share of GDP, CBO assumes that other taxes will be cut as Part B premiums rise! That is simply unreasonable. The net ef-fect on the federal budget of these two assumptions could be as much as 1 percent of GDP in 2040—excluding interest and economic feed-backs.[16]

Even before September 11, 2001, it was quite unlikely that spending on all "nonmandatory" activities, such as national defense, education, research, federal law enforcement, and natural resources, would in-crease by no more than the rate of inflation from 2002 to 2010, as CBO assumed. Real wage growth, for example, likely should be at least somewhat reflected in spending levels. So should the effect of popu-lation increase when programs deliver services to individuals. Yet not all such factors should be reflected in all spending; a larger population, for example, would require neither more weather forecasts, more space exploration, nor more submarines. Therefore, a more reasonable trend would have this spending, in total, increasing by more than the rate of inflation, though perhaps marginally declining as a share of GDP. This criticism implies that CBO's forecast for the next decade is, on the discretionary spending side, too low. But it also suggests that the gap might narrow after 2010, because CBO's further assumption, that this spending will be a constant share of GDP after 2010, should not be taken for granted.

Aside from these details, the SOBS forecast may be argued to be a reasonable guess about the period from 2000 through 2020 because it assumes that the federal government will eliminate its debt and accu-mulate a net reserve of about 7 percent of GDP. Given diversification of the Social Security trust funds, a net result approaching that may be possible. We may expect that, compared to "Save Total Surpluses," some policy changes will produce something resembling the SOBS trend over the next two decades. Yet the details matter because they will shape the underlying political dynamics as budget conditions worsen.

Because avoiding a vicious cycle of interest cost increases is far more important than the effects of budget position on national savings and through that on the economy, so long as interest costs are not out of control, it is possible to analyze the underlying budget situation in the SOBS forecast in relatively static terms.[17]

Imagine that the SOBS forecast was altered by raising revenues as necessary to prevent accumulation of more than a few percentage points of GDP in national debt after 2020. That would require a tax increase of about 5 percent of GDP, from 19.2 percent of GDP to 24.2 percent, over the following twenty years. Relative to the year 2000, U.S. federal taxes would have to be 4 percent of GDP higher. Is such an increase in the government share of the economy unreasonable or severe? More precisely, are social insurance programs for elderly persons the kind of government activity that justifies higher spending as a share of the economy? The answer is clearly a matter of political values, not economic necessity.

Should health care costs be constrained further? Policymakers certainly should do better than CBO's assumptions over the next two decades. Yet it is not at all clear that we should decide now what growth rate will be right for citizens in 2025 or 2035. Nor is it clear that we would know the right way to control costs even if we wished to. Should other programs be cut further? Again, beyond the level of discretionary spending restraint that seems appropriate at present—likely less than in the forecast—it is hard to see why we should make that decision. Some constraint beyond whatever the figure may be in 2010 or 2020 may well be appropriate, but it is absurd to pretend we know the right figure for conditions that far in the future. The fairest answer is that some savings in other programs will be possible, but we cannot determine now the proper balance among new revenues, savings in other programs, and reductions in spending for Social Security, Medicare, and Medicaid.

PROTECTING "OUR GRANDCHILDREN" WHILE RESPECTING THEM

Future voters can probably cope with the bills for entitlements for the elderly when they come due. They will know both their own values and the facts of the situation better than we can. Yet current citizens and politicians should consider those future challenges in our own actions, in two ways.

First, we should recognize that our actions now can make future challenges greater or smaller. Most evidently, although it is unreasonable to expect the federal government to build up a huge fund of private assets with no earmarked purpose, there are good reasons to reduce debt and thus interest significantly and perhaps to create a fund of private assets to help finance Social Security in particular. Those actions depend on budget policies in the immediate future and whether there is legislation over the next few years to create such Social Security trust fund diversification.

Similarly, budget policies in the near future may make action in the more distant future more or less difficult. Careful restraint of Medicare spending now would lower the baseline that needs to be controlled later. All things being equal, more modest tax cuts are safer. Discretionary spending should exceed the levels in the CBO baseline of the SOBS forecast, but commitments to very expensive and long-term projects also should be viewed with skepticism.

Second, there is a case for relatively incremental reforms of both Medicare and, more particularly, Social Security. Most evidently, Medicare costs in the medium term should be controlled better than in the SOBS scenario.

In addition, proposals for structural Medicare reform have focused on creating some sort of voucher system. The evidence that such a reform would actually save money is strikingly weak.[18] But both sides of the debate ought to recognize that any functioning voucher system would be facilitated by some innovations that have their own merit. For example, Parts A and B should be combined; experiments in competitive bidding to determine premiums in the current Medicare+Choice system should be implemented; subsidies for medical education could be removed from the Medicare payment structure and replaced by a new system; and the Part B premium might be replaced with an income-related premium.

On the Social Security side, there is a set of modest reforms in benefits and taxation, most of which were endorsed by the 1994–96 Advisory Council on Social Security, that could be adopted in the near term. Some of these reforms would lose value in other years, but a package could well net, in value, at least another 0.2 or 0.3 percent of GDP in 2020.[19] If Social Security trust funds are to be diversified, that too should be done as soon as possible, both in order to maximize the period of accumulation and in order to work out the likely significant administrative and governance issues.

There are also strong arguments for addressing *some of* the effects of increased life expectancy *beyond or in addition to the retirement of the baby boomers.* Any such measures should begin to take effect after the age of normal retirement, for the purpose of benefit calculations, has been increased to 67, which means after 2022. Such measures should not be limited to increases in the retirement age. They could include higher taxes, because, to the extent that people still might want to retire earlier than policy experts prefer, they should be willing to pay somewhat higher payroll taxes (just as they would have to save more if they were on their own). In addition, there should be some way to address the probable class differences in ability to work to a later age. I would change entitlement to Social Security from a basically age-based system to a mix of age and years in the workforce. Blue-collar workers enter the workforce earlier than professionals, so would be able to retire at a younger age. The design of such a system requires serious study and debate, and any such alteration in the basic terms of entitlement should be adopted well before it would affect individuals' retirements. Both are reasons to begin consideration and aim for action sooner, rather than later.

The measures suggested above would not come close to eliminating the projected return of budget deficits in the mid-2020s. Yet they would produce a less difficult baseline for policy choice at that time and so would represent responsible efforts to make the challenge faced by future voters easier.

The whole exercise of "planning for the future" presumes that we have a right to make policy choices for others who will have to live with them. Policies always depend in part on past choices. But when a choice is between, say, workers paying significantly higher taxes or elderly persons having much better protection in 2050, it is not clear that we, in the early years of the century, should make that decision. Maybe workers in 2035 will have a different opinion than we would—depending, for example, on how much standards of living grow between now and then or on the extent to which medical costs are believed to have paid for real increases in the patients' welfare. Policy discussion at present should recognize the tension between our supposed obligation to *protect* our "grandchildren" and our equal obligation to *respect* them.

A common argument asserts that future retirees need to know in advance about any benefit cuts, so they can begin planning to compensate for those reductions (Board of Trustees 1998, 5; Aaron and Bosworth 1997, 271). This argument is well-meaning but, on closer examination, may seem rather backward.

Most evidently, the argument assumes that the future changes will be benefit cuts. If the programs instead were financed by revenue increases, future retirees would not need to adjust in advance.

Nor, according to the advocates of such positions, would workers have to adjust their plans for the future if Medicare were replaced by a voucher system or Social Security were partially privatized. Voucher advocates claim that their approaches could even improve benefits (Aaron and Reischauer 1995; Wilensky and Newhouse 1999). Social Security privatizers also assert that benefits will be increased (Feldstein 1998; Weaver 1999). Therefore, the supposed need to give ample warning is irrelevant to the case for those approaches.

Nor could many people do much to adjust even if they were given warning. Consider the effects of traditional reductions in Social Security and Medicare spending. What could a person do to replace reduced Social Security benefits? An important alternative is private pensions, but the average worker cannot say, "Now that my Social Security has been cut, I'll demand a higher pension from my employer." More precisely, the worker may say that, but it is unlikely to get him or her anywhere. Employers are showing little interest in increasing their pension obligations (Schieber 1997). Individuals would have more opportunity to increase their private savings, but there are reasons why individuals with low incomes, in particular, tend not to save much. They could be compelled to save, but that would not be a matter of planning to compensate for cuts; it would just be another form of tax increase. On the Medicare side, the effects on patients of tighter constraints on medical payments to providers are ambiguous. But if those measures did affect available services— for instance, if there was less investment in medical technology because hospitals had lower incomes, and therefore there was less high-tech equipment available in 2030—it is hard to see what most individuals could do about that.

Even if individuals could adjust, the evidence that the average person actually behaves in the way that forewarning is supposed to help them behave is, to put it mildly, meager. Economists and public opinion experts who study retirement savings and expectations continually report that people do not save "enough," do not know how much they need to save, do not know what their Social Security benefits will be or what Medicare will cover, and so on (American Academy of Actuaries 1998; Bernheim 1991; Bernstein and Stevens 1999; Burtless 1996; Rovner 1995; Schieber 1997). If these reports are true, how would some benefit cuts change them? In fact, political realists argue for policy changes far in advance precisely because they are unlikely to be noticed. They can point to an excellent example: the fact that the normal retirement age was raised, beginning nearly two decades later, back in 1983, and voters paid hardly any attention to such a long-term effect.

For all these reasons, the argument that it is only fair to future workers to cut their future benefits now is less than compelling. Most workers might consider it much more fair not to cut their benefits at all.

Ultimately, the notion that future costs of entitlements for the elderly will be unaffordable is a value choice, not an economic fact. Three value issues are primary.

First, do we care more about the effects of aging or health care costs on government budgets or their effects on the nation and its citizens? If Social Security and Medicare did not exist, then, other things being equal, the fact that people live longer would produce lots of miserably impoverished old people. Burdens would fall even more unequally on individuals and their families, rather than being shared collectively. But they would still be burdens. So the primary question is not whether "entitlements" will be a burden but whether citizens should believe social insurance would provide the most acceptable form of finance in terms of adequacy, equity, reliability, and broader economic effects. Readers may believe that government is inherently inefficient, or that social insurance represents a vision of equity that they do not share, or that the difference between 20 and 25 percent of GDP flowing through the federal government has major economic effects. But those readers should object to Social Security and Medicare now, when they represent the same vision of equity, are part of the same supposedly inefficient government, and eliminating them would reduce government spending by as much as the projected eventual increases. Costs grow with a larger beneficiary population, but so should benefits.

Second, do we care about the effects of policies on individuals at one point in time or over a lifetime? Most evidently, taxpayers who might have to pay more in the future due to an aging society also would be likely to receive more as retirees for the same reason.[20] In essence, individuals would sacrifice more consumption during their working years, but, since they would have longer lives in retirement, they would also consume guaranteed pensions and more extensive Medicare benefits for a longer time. Government spending would grow as a share of GDP because government programs would be the means by which individuals would divert a share of their personal consumption to their retirement years. Opponents of such an increase in government's share of GDP need to establish either that social insurance does not have the advantages its proponents claim or that future citizens neither will nor should want to allocate a larger share of their longer lives to retirement, with decent health care. The first issue brings us back to the point that the merits of social insurance are not evidently affected by budget figures. The second seems almost entirely a value choice—hardly an evident "crisis."

Third, what values do we want to be dominant in the future? Critics of current programs worry that if the programs are not reformed soon, the large number of voters who will be dependent on those programs in the future will prevent future reform. Therefore, current policies risk forcing future citizens to accept commitments that they might not have chosen on their own. But the same criticism would be true if the "reformers" got their way. Once Medicare is turned into a voucher system, that will be very hard to reverse. Social Security privatization should be impossible to reverse, because that would require converting personal "savings accounts" into taxes. Demands that other people be "responsible" about the future are really arguments that they should accept our preferences, now.[21]

The bottom line is, whether the challenges of paying for current commitments to the elderly in an aging society represent a crisis, or even a severe difficulty, is far more a matter of values than objective reality. Neither the political realities of budgeting nor the economics of budget policy suggest that they are unmanageable. Long-term budget estimates, interpreted correctly, show the value of cautious budget policies and incremental programmatic reform in the immediate future. The commentators who were led, in the 1990s, to believe that these estimates showed the need for drastic change became caught up in a policy hysteria that treated a partisan position, dislike of social insurance, as if it were clearly the national interest.

ACKNOWLEDGMENTS

I would like to thank the Robert Wood Johnson Foundation for commissioning this chapter; I especially thank the Century Foundation for its support of the study that provided the basis for the chapter. Neither the officers, the staff, nor the trustees of either organization bear any blame for my conclusions.

NOTES

1. Readers interested in the details or history of these arguments could consult chapter 5 of White 2001 or, for a somewhat more critical discussion, White 2000b. The seminal article that redefined the budget deficit problem in terms of national savings is Gramlich 1984. Another good statement is Schultze 1989. For a prime example of the national savings argument being compared to other economic policies, see Schultze 1997. The history and prominence of the argument that increased national savings could finance Social Security can be seen in Aaron 1990. For extension of this argument to entitlement finance more generally, see Aaron and Bosworth 1997.

2. "Other things being equal" means when the economy is not in terrible short-term shape, so that cyclical adjustments can be left to the Federal Reserve, through monetary policy. When conditions become bad enough, attempts to stimulate growth through increasing the money supply or lowering interest rates may be like "pushing on a string," and more traditional Keynesian measures, even though they would decrease savings in the short run, may be necessary.

3. A deficit of more than 20 percent of GDP can, has, and likely should be sustained in the right circumstances, such as World War II. But major wars make

eventual budget adjustments relatively easy: the war ends and a large part (but not all) of the expenses stop.

4. See also Henry Aaron's discussion of the volatility of estimates in this volume (chapter 3).

5. CBO's long-term analyses continually show that there is little difference between "sustainable" policies, meaning those with different levels of government savings but no interest spiral. One good example is the analysis of the difference between balancing the budget and running a permanent deficit of 1.7 percent of GDP, presented in CBO 1997b. Another is the difference as of 2030 between the three scenarios presented in Table 7.2. Only after the deficits begin to spiral out of control, after 2030, do we see substantial differences in forecast GDP. See CBO 2000b, tables 4, 6, and 7.

6. I refer to citizens' willingness here as shorthand, understanding that the political process does not necessarily reflect those preferences. If the advocates for radically reforming Social Security and Medicare want to claim that those cuts will be made contrary to citizen preferences, they are free to do so.

7. As I argue in more detail elsewhere, I am not saying simply that payroll taxes can be raised. See White 2000a. That article provides a much more extensive discussion of some of the issues in this chapter.

8. I have criticized this "hole and the donut" argument when it has been used as an argument for greater national savings through near-term budget deficit reduction or surplus increases, because the evidence cited earlier in this chapter suggests that the donut would not be enough larger to make much difference. But the differences among economic assumptions can be much larger than the savings effect.

9. For an extensive discussion of particular Medicare estimates, see White 1999.

10. Any uncertainties about Medicare cost are more than matched for Medicaid. As an intergovernmental program, both Medicaid's enrollment and its payment rates depend greatly on state policies, and there is surely no good way to project those far into the future.

11. They also depend on assumed interest rates. There is good reason to believe that the assumed return in the scenarios where the government accrues a positive balance is too low, but since those balances are themselves probably overstated, the understated interest can be a minor concern.

12. For a good discussion of the policy merits, see Aaron and Reischauer 1998.

13. In addition to the data provided in the published CBO report, my analysis uses a backup spreadsheet kindly supplied by CBO staff in December 2000. These figures show GDP growth slowing very gradually through the 2030s and then declining substantially as, in the model, deficits balloon during the 2040s.

14. Interest earnings as a share of GDP begin to decline, in the model, in 2022; by 2029 the federal government is beginning to pay interest again, and that expense then burgeons over the following decade.

15. Like the other authors in this volume, I prepared my analysis using as a baseline the long-run projections made by CBO in October 2000. Both economic

conditions, before and after the terrorist attacks of September 11, 2001, and legislation, including the tax cut and later spending to cope with the effects of those attacks and limit the threat of further attacks, dramatically changed the short-term budgetary conditions that were included in the CBO 2000 long-term projections. The long-term forecasts, however, assume that there should be occasional economic slumps; so, unless the results of the economic shocks of 2001 are unusually extensive and long-lasting, they should not change the underlying budgetary dynamics very much. The amount of extra spending after the immediate repairs should also be a small fraction of previously projected totals. And the bizarre provisions of the 2001 tax legislation, under which the cuts would disappear in 2011, only confirm my point that it is not a good idea to assume that revenues will be cut indefinitely. As of October 2001, my own guess is that budgetary prospects with careful policies would be more negative than the text describes but not so much as to change the conclusions.

16. CBO 2000b estimated that Medicare spending would rise from 2.2 percent of GDP in 1999 to 6.5 percent in 2040. I adjusted CBO's figures downward on a spreadsheet calculation by reducing the increase by 1 percentage point for ten years and then phasing up to the CBO figure over the following ten. That would reduce Medicare spending in 2040 to about 5.7 percent of GDP, about 0.8 percent less than in CBO's forecast. Part B is smaller than Part A but has generally been expected to grow more quickly. If spending increased from a total of 2.2 percent of GDP to 5.7 percent, the net increase would be 3.5 percent. Assume that 1.6 percentage points are in Part B. Then the premium increase should be 0.4 percent of GDP. So the two effects sum to 1.2 percent of GDP. Since my calculation is exceedingly rough, I recognize that the adjustment could be smaller; nevertheless, this gives a sense of the importance of CBO's assumptions that spending will increase more quickly in the short run and that premium increases will, for no intelligible reason, be offset by tax cuts.

17. The economic feedbacks from interest costs spiraling upward are, of course, relevant to any attempt to analyze the effects of policy changes after 2040. But the following paragraphs emphasize conditions before then.

18. For example, readers might note the absence of such evidence in Aaron and Reischauer 1995 or Wilensky and Newhouse 1999.

19. These proposals were (1) making a technical change in taxation of Social Security benefits, (2) raising the number of years of contributions included in the calculation of benefits from thirty-five to thirty-eight, (3) including all new state and local employees in the Social Security system, and (4) raising the threshold below which wages are subject to Social Security payroll tax so as to increase the proportion of total payroll subject to the tax by two or three percentage points. I have made very rough spreadsheet calculations of the possible effects of this set of measures on a pay-as-you-go basis; I would much prefer that somebody else, such as CBO or the Social Security actuaries, do a better job.

20. The argument here does not apply to the effects of differences in "genera-

tion" size. There is a case for making the baby boomers prefund a portion of their own costs, whereas that would not be required of smaller groups. Note, however, that the policy of retiring most or all of the national debt, thereby eliminating interest expenses, already serves that purpose: baby boomers would be improving the fiscal position of later birth cohorts by running budget surpluses in the decade leading up to the first boomers turning 65, in 2011. I discuss other aspects of this issue in White 2001.

21. I do not consider myself remotely exempt from this charge.

REFERENCES

Aaron, H. J., ed. 1990. *Social Security and the Budget.* Proceedings of the First Conference of the National Academy of Social Insurance, December 15–16, 1988. Lanham, Md.: University Press of America.

Aaron, H. J., and B. P. Bosworth. 1997. Preparing for the Baby Boomers' Retirement. In R. D. Reischauer, ed., *Setting National Priorities: Budget Choices for the Next Century.* Washington, D.C.: Brookings Institution.

Aaron, H. J., B. P. Bosworth, and G. Burtless. 1989. *Can America Afford to Grow Old?* Washington, D.C.: Brookings Institution.

Aaron, H. J., and R. D. Reischauer. 1995. The Medicare Reform Debate: What Is the Next Step? *Health Affairs* 14, no. 4: 8–30.

———. 1998. *Countdown to Reform: The Great Social Security Debate.* New York: Century Foundation Press.

Aaron, H. J., and L. H. Thompson. 1987. Social Security and the Economists. In E. D. Berkowitz, ed., *Social Security after Fifty: Successes and Failures.* Westport, Conn.: Greenwood Press.

American Academy of Actuaries. 1998. *Financing the Retirement of Future Generations: The Problem and Options for Change.* Washington, D.C.: American Academy of Actuaries.

Bernheim, D. 1991. *The Vanishing Nest Egg: Reflections on Saving in America.* New York: Twentieth Century Fund.

Bernstein, J., and R. Stevens. 1999. Public Opinion, Knowledge, and Medicare Reform. *Health Affairs* 18, no. 1: 180–93.

Board of Trustees, Social Security and Medicare Trust Funds. 1998. *1998 Annual Report of the Board of Trustees of the Federal Old Age and Survivors Insurance and Disability Insurance Trust Funds.* Washington, D.C.: U.S. Government Printing Office.

Broder, D. 1996. The Party's Over: By 2000, the GOP or the Democrats Could Fade in Favor of a Third Party. *Washington Post,* August 11, C1.

Burtless, G. 1996. Will American Workers Be Ready for Retirement? Testimony for the Subcommittee on Aging, Committee on Labor and Human Resources, U.S. Senate, June 13. Draft copy in possession of the author.

Calmes, J. 1997. Fiscal Fitness: Washington Wants Discipline in Budgets to Carry beyond 2002. *Wall Street Journal,* February 27, A1.

Congressional Budget Office (CBO). 1993. *The Economic and Budget Outlook: Fiscal Years 1994–1998.* Washington, D.C.: U.S. Government Printing Office.

———. 1997a. *The Economic and Budget Outlook: Fiscal Years 1998–2007.* Washington, D.C.: U.S. Government Printing Office.

———. 1997b. *Long-Term Budgetary Pressures and Policy Options.* Washington, D.C.: U.S. Government Printing Office.

———. 1998. *Long-Term Budgetary Pressures and Policy Options.* Washington, D.C.: U.S. Government Printing Office.

———. 1999. *The Economic and Budget Outlook: Fiscal Years 2000–2009.* Washington, D.C.: U.S. Government Printing Office.

———. 2000a. *The Budget and Economic Outlook: An Update.* Washington, D.C.: U.S. Government Printing Office.

———. 2000b. *The Long-Term Budget Outlook.* Washington, D.C.: U.S. Government Printing Office.

Eisner, R. 1996. What Social Security Crisis? *Wall Street Journal,* August 30, A8.

Feldstein, M. 1998. Savings Grace. *New Republic,* April 6.

Fuchs, V. R. 1999. Health Care for the Elderly: How Much? Who Will Pay for It? *Health Affairs* 18, no. 1: 11–21.

Gergen, D. 1996. When the Baby-Boomers Retire. *U.S. News and World Report,* October 28, 100.

Gramlich, E. M. 1984. How Bad Are the Large Deficits? In G. B. Mills and J. L. Palmer, eds., *Federal Budget Policy in the 1980s.* Washington, D.C.: Urban Institute.

Horney, J. 1999. *Spending a Non-Existent Surplus.* Center on Budget and Policy Priorities Issue Brief, October 20. Washington, D.C.: Center on Budget and Policy Priorities.

Klein, J. 1996. Pretty Close to Awful: Dole's Fading Campaign Makes It Less Likely the Next President Will Break the Entitlement State. *Newsweek,* September 16, 51.

Page, B. I. 1999. Is Social Security Reform Ready for the American Public? Paper presented at the annual conference of the National Academy of Social Insurance, Washington, D.C., January 27–28.

Passell, P. 1996. Trying to Slice the National Pie and Mend Social Security, Too. *New York Times,* December 27, D1.

Peterson, P. G. 1996. *Will America Grow Up before It Grows Old?* New York: Random House.

Pooley, E. 1997. No Guts, No Glory. *Time,* January 20, 23–26.

Reischauer, R. D. 1997a. The Unfulfillable Promise: Cutting Nondefense Discretionary Spending. In R. D. Reischauer, ed. *Setting National Priorities: Budget Choices for the Next Century.* Washington, D.C.: Brookings Institution.

———, ed. 1997b. *Setting National Priorities: Budget Choices for the Next Century.* Washington, D.C.: Brookings Institution.

Rovner, J. 1995. Congress' "Catastrophic" Attempt to Fix Medicare. In T. E. Mann and N. J. Ornstein, eds., *Intensive Care: How Congress Shapes Health Care Policy.* Washington, D.C.: American Enterprise Institute and Brookings Institution.

Schieber, S. J. 1997. Retirement Security Income at Risk. In S. J. Schieber and J. J. Shoven, eds., *Public Policy toward Pensions.* Cambridge, Mass.: MIT Press.

Schultze, C. L. 1989. Of Wolves, Termites, and Pussycats: Or, Why We Should Worry about the Budget Deficit. *Brookings Review* (summer).

———. 1997. Is Faster Growth the Cure for Budget Deficits? In R. D. Reischauer, ed. *Setting National Priorities: Budget Choices for the Next Century.* Washington, D.C.: Brookings Institution.

U.S. General Accounting Office. 1995. *The Deficit and the Economy: An Update of Long-Term Simulations.* GAO/AIMD/OCE-95–119, April. Washington, D.C.: General Accounting Office.

———. 1997. *Budget Issues: Analysis of Long-Term Fiscal Outlook.* GAO/AIMD/OCE-98–19, October. Washington, D.C.: General Accounting Office.

Weaver, C. 1999. Personal Security Accounts: A Means of Strengthening and Securing Social Security. In U.S. Senate, Committee on Finance, *Retirement Security Policy: Proposals to Preserve and Protect Social Security: Hearing before the Committee on Finance.* 105th Cong., 2nd sess., September 9, 1998.

White, J. 1999. Understanding Long-Term Medicare Cost Estimates. A Century Foundation White Paper. Century Foundation, New York.

———. 2000a. Budgeting for Social Security; or, When Are Savings Really Savings? *Public Budgeting and Finance* 20, no. 3: 1–23.

———. 2000b. Savings and "Saving" Social Security and Medicare: A Tale of Elite Opinion. Paper presented at the annual conference of the American Political Science Association, Washington, D.C., September.

———. 2001. *False Alarm: Why the Greatest Threat to Social Security and Medicare Is the Campaign to "Save" Them.* Baltimore: Johns Hopkins University Press.

Wilensky, G., and J. Newhouse. 1999. Medicare Reform: What's Right, What's Wrong, What's Next? *Health Affairs* 18, no. 1: 92–106.

III

POLICY

ALTERNATIVES

8

The Case for Universal Social Insurance

Theodore R. Marmor, Ph.D., and Jerry L. Mashaw, Ph.D.

Universal social insurance programs are preconditions for a workable system of industrial or postindustrial capitalism and political democracy. Basic protection against common risks—illness, disability, death, and involuntary unemployment—make a dynamic, entrepreneurial economy an acceptable social and economic institution. To mimic Jefferson, we find these statements self-evident—political and social axioms that should be plain to all.

Imagine for a moment an America without social insurance. This is an America where middle-aged, middle-income Americans bear the burden of supporting, or helping to support, their aged parents. Where they risk financial disaster from corporate downsizing, the vagaries of the business cycle, their own incapacity from illness, and their parents' potentially catastrophic medical costs. Help, in the form of private or public charity, may be available, but only through the demonstration of destitution. Many will escape most of these risks, of course, and many more will believe they will—until disaster strikes. Those who receive aid will be a minority. The majority will not always, perhaps not often, believe that the poor are blameless for their plight. The skeptical might well give aid, but they will do so grudgingly.

This would be an America that manages to combine high anxiety about personal security with the self-righteous belief that whatever one has, has been individually earned. Its likely politics would oscillate between attempts to entrench the status quo by regulation—tariffs, plant closing laws, job guarantees, employer mandates, and the like—and bitter contests over who among the poor are sufficiently "deserving" of aid.

Without the security of social insurance, it is hard to imagine how American workers would be brought to accept the desirability of an ever changeable market with flexible and modest legal constraints. And to the extent that workers managed to get protections for their own group, locality, industry, or profession, they would inevitably see those protections as their just reward. Those without protection who ended up seeking public financial assistance in their time of need would be the undeserving "others." They would become the Americans who, by participating (and failing) in a truly free market, were a "drag on the economy." Without social insurance, the most reasonable scenario is the collapse of any strong sense of national social solidarity, fueled by the contentious interest group politics of economic regulation. It would not be a society that most Americans would say they want for their families.

Since the 1970s, however, Americans have heard a very different— and unnerving—story about social insurance. They have been taught to doubt both the financial affordability and the operational manageability of universal programs that literally hold our economy and society together. Critics have portrayed solutions as problems. In many quarters, dread of the future and excitement about "entitlements" have replaced good sense.[1]

Against this backdrop of confusion and misplaced anxiety, we propose to do three things. First, we restate the basic case for social insurance. Second, we discuss the realities of the twin pillars of social insurance in the nation: Social Security pensions and Medicare. We describe the ways in which these programs were unfairly maligned in the 1990s and what the broader options are for their defensible adjustment. We then turn briefly to the unfinished agenda of American social insurance: the coverage of medical care expenses in a universal health insurance program during a period when political attention continues to focus on regulating the new and often disturbing world of American medical care.

THE CASE REVIEWED: AFFIRMATIVE AND
CRITICAL ARGUMENTS

American social insurance rests on the premise that we should protect workers and their families from dramatic losses of economic status through programs that are socially respectable, economically sensible, and politically stable. For virtually all Americans, a socially respectable protection against economic loss means one that is earned through participation in funding the insurance pool. Whatever the details of particular programs—whether disability insurance, Medicare, unemployment insurance, life insurance, or Social Security pensions—social insurance rejects safety nets made of means-tested welfare programs as stigmatizing and unreliable. The social insurance recipient is neither pauper nor supplicant.

The contributor's Social Security card—not a poverty level, means-tested safety net—is the central metaphor of social insurance. Rather than catching those who have fallen through the net, the social insurance card symbolizes the collective effort to prevent a radical decline in a family's living standards. Modeled after the fringe benefits that economic elites take for granted, U.S. Social Security is meant to protect citizens against the statistically certain, but individually unpredictable, risks of loss of income in a modern capitalist economy. Social insurance represents a social ideal of economic security, one guaranteeing a sense of deservingness and individual dignity through participation while working in a cooperative social enterprise.

This social ideal has political consequences. It produces an us-us rather than a we-them political dynamic. The question is not what "we" (the affluent) should do for "them" (the impoverished). Rather, it is how we should manage the risks of economic misfortune that will befall some of us at any one time and threaten all of us over the course of our lifetimes. This perspective both helps to stabilize the politics of particular programs and helps to dampen the fires of class conflict that might otherwise destabilize the political order more generally. The latter concern—class conflict—was prominent at the beginning of American social insurance in the 1930s. The former—the destabilization of long-standing commitments—can hardly be lost on anyone who has witnessed the ravaging of antipoverty programs and the corrosive politics of "welfare" from the mid-1970s to the end of the twentieth century.

The economic rationale for universalistic social insurance has several parts. Assuring retirement security and insuring against the loss of family income through premature death or disability confronts the acknowledged myopia and excessive optimism that, along with low income, limit family saving for events like retirement. It also recognizes the economic difficulties of insuring against the loss of earning capacity when work life has just begun, earnings are relatively low, and other family obligations are relatively large. Collective insurance against these risks also protects the prudent against the "free riding" of the imprudent, who would ultimately claim social support from "pools" (general taxation) to which they had not contributed.

Moreover, some financial risks are extremely difficult to insure against through private markets, even if all Americans were responsible, reasonably well off, and farsighted. The moral hazard inherent in disability insurance, along with the tendency of courts to rewrite contracts, makes market provision for disability risks very inefficient for virtually all who really need it. Similarly, rational risk selection by private insurers will exclude from reasonably priced health insurance pools just those persons or families who are most at risk. And no insurance executive worth her or his stock options would even propose attempting to provide private unemployment insurance. In these situations universal insurance programs are not just socially and politically desirable; they are, economically, the only game in town.

These social, political, and economic advantages notwithstanding, critics can be heard to complain of the "unfairness" of social insurance arrangements. The character of these complaints reveals the ideological chasm that separates the social insurance vision of economic security from its individualist, libertarian antagonists—critics who, out of a sense of charity, are anxious to help the "truly needy" by reducing the benefits to middle-class Americans.

Talk of fairness is, of course, a staple in political conversation. The debate over Social Security is no exception. Many critics of Social Security claim that their real objection to the program is its financial unfairness. Workers who make more and put in more, they say, do not get the same rate of return as the lower-paid workers who put in less.

This claim of unfairness presumes that if government addresses the economic security of families at all, it should build a system around the idea of the individual "saver investor." Under such arrangements, governments mandate that individuals put aside some percentage of their income for retirement purposes and to insure against death, disability, and unemployment. Payments made when or if any of these events materialized would reflect the accumulation in each individual's account. Even if such a system was economically feasible—which is true only for retirement pensions—it fundamentally misunderstands the social contract that social insurance entails.

U.S. Social Security pensions treat retired persons as "worker-contributors," all of whom have participated in the same insurance pool. Ignorant at the outset of who will have high or low earnings over a working life, all those who pay FICA taxes receive a reasonable base pension in retirement. The aim is simple: a guarantee of an amount that, when combined with some private saving and private pensions, will provide an adequate retirement income for everyone. But to make good on that aim requires some redistribution from those who turn out to have had higher wages to those who have had lower wages.

American workers can rightly expect that the larger their Social Security contribution, the greater their retirement benefits. Larger "contributions" (our euphemism for the taxes that private insurance would call premiums) mean that higher-wage workers receive larger pensions than lower-wage workers. But the degree of financial hierarchy in Social Security is reduced by another of its purposes—the commitment to a minimally adequate income for lower-wage workers. The ratio of benefits to former wages is higher the lower a worker's average wages. (In the jargon of the program, Social Security aims at "minimal adequacy" and does so with a "kinked benefit curve.") In this way, the United States has constructed a worker-contributor, not a saver-investor version of fairness. The "every boat on its own bottom" ethos of the market economy is tempered by the "everybody in the same boat" ethos of social insurance.

The clash between individualistic and collective visions of fairness properly frames the debate about universalism. We believe that the social, political, and economic arguments for universalism are persuasive. And opinion polling concerning support for social insurance suggests that most Americans have little taste for running the risks that "privatizers" of various stripes believe they should prefer.

The attack on social insurance has therefore taken a different form. It has not directly and openly confronted issues of fairness, uninsurable risks, and failures in the private insurance market. Instead, opponents repeatedly assert the unaffordability or ungovernability of the social insurance programs we currently have. Without contesting the desirability of social insurance itself, critics have urged us to believe that the collective provision for economic security simply cannot be organized successfully. Criticisms of "entitlements," "big government," and "deficit spending" have been blended in a litany that buries the truth about social insurance programs in the atmospherics of more generalized anxieties.[2]

The attacks of the 1990s were hardly all new. Over the period since 1973 we have heard persistent claims of a crisis in U.S. government—with social policy deeply implicated in these troubles. Stagflation after the oil crisis of 1973–74 provoked distress about the government's capacity to manage its operations, let alone improve social conditions. Shrinking public revenues, it was argued, made it impossible to satisfy the expectations generated by the Great Society programs of the Kennedy-Johnson years. Others claimed the excessive expenditures from the programs themselves helped produce the economic difficulty in which we found ourselves. These years of doubt and dismay were followed by the antigovernment politics of the Reagan era. Strategically induced fiscal anemia and hyperappreciation of "government's limits" inaugurated a school of "tough choice" commentary. These critical streams converged on an image of American social policy as a failed enterprise we could neither manage nor afford.

We live with the legacy of this rhetoric of failure. Nowhere is this clearer than in the misguided pessimism with which Social Security and Medicare were discussed from the beginning of the 1990s. The task for progressive commentators is not only to attack criticism where it is unjustified but also to recognize that adjusting and improving our social insurance programs is central to sustaining a humane America in the twenty-first century. Unless we do so—and renew the inclusive and adaptive dream of Social Security's birth in the 1930s and its continuous adjustments since that time—conservatives will triumph in their decades-long efforts to derail social insurance programs that serve the nation's middle class as well as its poor.

SENSE AND NONSENSE CONCERNING SOCIAL SECURITY

Debates over Social Security pensions are generally presented as a response to fiscal crisis. But these are merely occasions for replaying in differing chords the profound opposition that social insurance has always generated among economic conservatives. The 1990s provided ample illustration of this.

In the early 1980s, when public officials announced that the Social Security accounts would be "bankrupt" without adjustment, Americans accepted without commotion the changes made by the 1983 Greenspan Commission. These changes bolstered rather than revamped Social Security; they involved a combination of modest reductions of benefits and small increases in social insurance taxes. The public's confidence in Social Security's financial future gradually returned to normal; opinion polls reported that support remained (and remains) very high.

Then, as a result of the early 1980s reforms, surpluses grew in Social Security's accounts. Oddly enough, this too awakened critics. Some fiscal gurus—including the *New York Times* economic columnist Peter Passell—complained then that growing surpluses constituted a "crisis in slow motion." (Collectors of oxymorons take note: a "crisis in slow motion" is hardly urgent.) The interpretive point is obvious: when both deficits and surpluses bring cries of alarm, the evidence points toward ideological opposition, not episodes of programmatic crisis.

The Great Social Security Scare

The rhetoric of imminent disaster reemerged in the 1990s. It was primed by the prophets of doom and gloom in the Concord Coalition, supported by the high anxiety of the 1995 Entitlements Commission, and reinforced by financial interests anxious to gain new business from mandated individual savings accounts for retirement. The case for big changes in U.S. public retirement arrangements shouldered its way back onto the broader national agenda. Extrapolating short-term trends into

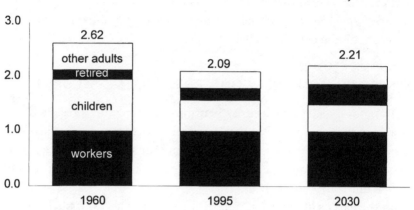

Fig. 8.1. Population support ratios: How many people does each worker support, counting everybody (workers themselves, children, retirees, and other adults), in the past, now, and in the future? *Source:* calculations provided by the Office of the Actuary, Social Security Administration, using 1995 Trustees Report demographic assumptions, the National Academy of Social Insurance.

the indefinite future, critics once again portrayed Social Security pensions as uncertain promises, unlikely to be fulfilled and requiring a strong dose of market medicine to put things right. They used the demographic certainty of an older population to make the unwarranted claims that the country cannot afford that degree of population aging and that Social Security will not be able to pay its bills without draconian tax increases or benefit reductions. Although it is true that the ratio of workers to retirees will, in the absence of major immigration changes, fall from about 3 to 1 down to 2 to 1, it is not the case that the number of Americans dependent on the workforce will sharply increase over the first decades of the twenty-first century. The composition will change, but, as Figure 8.1 shows, the increase in older Americans will be balanced in part by decreases in the number of children Americans will be raising.

The Claim of Crisis: A Revealing Clash in the 1990s

As the former commissioner of Social Security, Robert M. Ball, observed in 1995, moderate adjustments in the pension benefit formula would stabilize the system. The system was accruing substantial surpluses, and total income was then expected to exceed outlays until about the year 2020. Thereafter, Social Security reserves would be retired to pay current benefits. By 2070 benefits were projected to exceed taxes by about 5.5 percent of taxable wages. So unless some adjustments were made in benefit levels, taxation levels, or trust fund earnings, Social Security's retirement program would not be able to pay all its bills by 2020. From this perspective, critics like Peter Peterson were at that point technically correct: without adjustment the current system was "unsustainable."

Nonetheless, the critics' assertion that something very like the current system cannot be financed was nonsense. Indeed, by gradually shifting to a partially funded system that invests in equity securities, there were ways to close the projected gap in future funding without tax increases and with extremely modest changes in current benefit levels. To illustrate these contentions, we discuss the reform proposals that emerged from the 1996 Social Security Advisory Council.

Maintaining Social Security: The Ball Plan

Under the Social Security Advisory Council's option proposed by Ball and five other members, the total seventy-five-year deficit could have been eliminated, and then some, by six modest adjustments:

1. Extend Social Security coverage to currently excluded state and local employees.
2. Increase the length of the computation period for workers' average earnings from thirty-five to thirty-eight years.
3. Tax Social Security benefits that exceed already-taxed contributions, as with private defined benefit retirement plans.
4. Correct the current overstatement of the consumer price index used to calculate cost of living increases in accordance with the Bureau of Labor Statistics March 1996 proposal.
5. Credit income taxes on Social Security pensions to the pension rather than to the Medicare trust fund.
6. Shift approximately 40 percent of the Social Security trust funds, now invested in Treasury securities, into equity securities.

Not only would Ball's proposal have sustained the present system, but also financing it would not have been very hard. So proposals for more radical revisions must reflect other aims, as illustrated by the doctrinaire privatizers on the 1996 Social Security Advisory Council.

Competing Remedies for Social Security: The Attempt of the Privatizers

A faction of five within the thirteen-person Advisory Council proposed a major overhaul that would really privatize our Social Security program. Every worker would be required to create a personal security account (PSA) financed by returning five percentage points of the payroll taxes that finance Social Security pensions. Workers could invest the money however they pleased. On retirement, they would receive the accumulated value of their PSAs, plus a small base pension financed the old-fashioned way.

This base pension—$410 a month—would be paltry, far lower than the poverty threshold. On retirement, workers would receive this basic pension, and whatever had accumulated in their PSAs would be available for lump-sum payment, investment, or annuitization. Still, the PSA proposal requires the diversion of so much money from the Social Security trust funds that privatization would require a hike of 1.52 percent in the FICA tax, plus other benefit reductions and public borrowing, to make good on that guarantee and to fund the transition to individual retirement accounts. (These other changes are substantial: increasing the retirement age to 67 by 2011 and borrowing an additional $1.2 trillion over the next thirty-five years.)

According to the Office of the Actuary at the Social Security Administration, each of the Advisory Council proposals satisfied the statutory requirement that the scheme be in long-term (seventy-five-year) actuarial balance. But if that is true, why go beyond the Ball solution? The real debate was (and still is) between those who view social insurance as worth saving and those who want to reduce government's role in retirement security in favor of market outcomes. Although the rhetoric of the Social Security debate in the U.S. presidential campaign of 2000 hardly got beyond charges of arithmetic incompetence, the two paths developed in the Advisory Council report more informatively defined the contested terrain. Al Gore emphasized maintenance of public control over finance and expenditure in the interest of universal provision; George W. Bush pushed partial privatization as a means of giving individuals more control over how to achieve their own economic security in old age. Because the Bush and Gore proposals were ideological cousins to the Advisory Council positions but without the discipline of working within identical budget constraints, the Ball Plan and the PSA proposal provide superior vehicles for illustrating the true stakes in this continuing debate. To simplify matters, we will concentrate on these proposals.

The Advisory Council Proposals Compared: Risk and Reward

Both of these plans link Social Security's fortunes more closely to the performance of private capital markets. The Ball plan would retain a collective system, whereas the PSA proposal would create individualized, funded accounts. Over the last sixty years (the life of the Social Security pension system), capital markets have out-performed real wage growth by several percentage points. In principle, this change would improve the intergenerational equity of the system by allowing future retirees (who will collect less of a windfall than their parents) to receive higher returns.

Nevertheless, there are risks. Tying Social Security retirement pensions to the performance of the capital markets would have looked quite bizarre in 1935, when the Social Security system was constructed. And even if we do not experience another Great Depression, the events of October 1987, and most recently the boom and bust of 2000, should remind us that the stock market can make quite precipitous "corrections." Although on average, over long periods of time, one may do better by investing in the market, some individuals and some cohorts of individuals will do substantially worse.

This concern about smoothing out the vagaries of market returns underscores the first striking difference between the Ball plan and the PSA model. In effect, the Ball approach puts the market risk on the government—on all of us collectively. The PSA model puts that risk on individuals. The choice between these proposals is thus similar to the choice between a defined benefit and a defined contribution retirement program. Private savings, whether in IRAs or otherwise, are the equivalent of a defined contribution pension plan. Workers save a certain "individual defined" amount and have assets at retirement equal to the performance of their portfolio.

Social Security, by contrast, has always been similar to a defined benefit scheme. The federal government makes long-term promises to pay certain pension benefits and bears the risks that the performance of the economy will make those promises either harder or easier to fulfill. Historically, many private firms have also provided defined benefit retirement plans. But only about 30 percent of Americans now retire with a company pension, and companies are rapidly shifting from defined benefit to defined contribution pension arrangements. In short, Social Security is the only vehicle available to most Americans in which they do not bear market risks to their basic retirement income.[3]

The Ball proposal allows pensioners to capture the higher returns of financial markets, while keeping the risk collectively shared rather than individually borne. The projections for the PSA plan show it, on average, outperforming the Ball proposal. This has nothing to do with privatizing the investment choices and everything to do with adding 1.52 percent to the tax rate and hence the total amount invested. If we added the same tax hike to the Ball plan, the returns would be even greater than the average PSA because of lower administrative costs.

Economics or Ideology

The real issue here is not economics but political ideology. Most privatizers want to privatize because they do not trust the government, or because they believe the American people do not trust the government, or because they assume that Social Security depresses savings rates.

The lack-of-trust argument takes two forms. In one incarnation it asserts that Americans prefer market risk to political risk. Hence, to preserve the political acceptability of a mandatory retirement program, Americans will demand that they, rather than a government agency, should control investment decisions. The second form of the argument is that the government cannot be trusted to invest in the private capital markets without meddling with them as well. Neither argument is persuasive.

To give the first argument its due, privatization can be seen as an attempt—indirect, to be sure—to shore up confidence in the pension system. Americans who have "ownership" of an individual or personal security account might view their investment as more secure than a claim on Social Security. If so, this surely has more to do with the drumbeat of criticism from the media than any reasonable judgment of the program. The Social Security program avoids inflation risks, bankruptcy risks, and market risks. It has been running since 1935 without ever missing a payment. It continues to have the overwhelming support of the American populace, and Americans say that they are quite willing to pay some additional taxes to ensure the financial soundness of the system into the distant future. Nevertheless, it is conceivable that Americans will come to prefer risky over nonrisky investments. Nor can we fully discount the Lake Wobegone effect—excessive optimism among young workers that their lifetime earnings will be above average. If their earnings do turn out to be above average, they will be increasingly susceptible to the argument that Social Security provides an inferior return on their contributions.

The real risk, however, is that partial privatization will lead to inexorable pressure for full privatization. Investment of some Social Security funds in stocks rather than Treasury bonds will likely improve the investment performance of Social Security over the long run. But if this investment is done in a privatized form, it will appear that the improvement has come through privatization of accounts rather than from a simple shift in investment holdings. And because most workers tend to ignore the life insurance, dependents' benefits, and inflation protection that are a part of the Social Security pension package, this argument may be persuasive.

Even more importantly, workers may ignore the crucial protection that social insurance provides to everyone against low average lifetime earnings, against poor performance of their individual investments, against higher taxes, and against the need for intrafamily transfers to support those who do have these experiences. The less stake American workers believe themselves to have in the collective provision of retirement benefits through Social Security, the more likely political support for the system is to erode. Partial privatization in this scenario would be destabilizing rather than anchoring. It could lead to the destruction of the very economic security that "reform" is supposed to preserve.

The argument about government "meddling" in capital markets is even less compelling. Maintaining the soundness of and confidence in financial markets by massive governmental "meddling" is one of the great success stories of U.S. public policy since the 1930s. Investing Social Security funds in equity securities will not roil capital markets, so long as investments are limited to broad "index" funds, these funds are managed solely in the interest of beneficiaries, and government is a passive shareholder. These constraints are not difficult to construct, as the experience of the Federal Employees Thrift Plan, the Tennessee Valley Authority's and the Federal Reserve Board's defined benefit retirement programs, and many state retirement funds illustrate.

In short, workers would not, on average, be better off investing privately for retirement than having those investments made through Social Security. Because private investing exposes beneficiaries directly to temporal fluctuations in the financial markets, privatizing accounts will make many worse off. There is no reason, other than ideological antipathy to government money management, for Americans to prefer the PSA to the Ball approach. There are obvious reasons for private money managers to prefer PSAs.

Distributional Fairness

Critics of Social Security make much of the supposed burden that retirees place on the working young. By the 1990s, the image of the affluent old enjoying a secure retirement on the backs of hard-pressed wage earners had become an established cliché. But data on the income of the aged in the mid-1990s revealed that 56 percent of persons over 65 would be below the poverty line without their Social Security payments. Three-quarters of all recipients have total income, including their Social Security benefits, of less than $25,000 per year. Fifty percent have income of less than $15,000 per year. Families with an income of $50,000 or more represent only 9 percent of Social Security beneficiaries. In short, most elderly Americans are not rich.

Reform of Social Security really poses two distributional issues—

fairness between generations and fairness within age cohorts. The intergenerational equity issue is mostly a distraction. The first generation of pensioners indeed enjoyed a windfall, but that is history. Both proposals aim to put Social Security pensions into long-term actuarial balance. Given that the burdens on current and future generations under the two schemes will be equivalent, the real issue is fairness within generations. Here an ideological chasm separates the two proposals.

The Ball approach maintains the worker-contributor model of equity that currently undergirds Social Security. Distributional fairness in this social insurance model is straightforward but not always well understood. First, workers are insured against a lifetime of relatively low-wage work by a guarantee of a minimally adequate pension in old age. Second, recognizing that the level of wages includes some combination of personal circumstance and effort, the size of the pension increases with a worker's level of contribution. But it redistributes by giving lower-wage workers a better "return" on their lifetime earnings.

In other words, everyone signs up at the beginning of their working lives for a system that makes two promises: a minimally adequate retirement income for all workers and a guarantee of higher returns (in absolute dollar amounts) to those who make higher contributions over their working lives.

The serious privatization approach proposes significant distributional changes. Under the PSA conception, the pensioner is viewed as an investor. Supposedly, higher-wage workers who save more (and those who make more fortunate investments) are fully entitled to their better retirement situation. As a matter of individual deserving, the "investor" notion of fairness seemingly rewards individual prudence and self-denial—the decision to give up current consumption as a hedge against an uncertain future. Yet a mandatory requirement to save a fixed percentage of wages rewards neither prudence nor self-sacrifice. The saver, after all, did not choose to save. And sacrifice is inversely related to affluence.

The fairness of this shift is even more doubtful when placed within the context of America's overall retirement policy. Tax policy already offers greater subsidies to the retirement savings of higher earners than lower earners. The home mortgage interest deduction and the nontaxability of IRA, Keough, 401(k), and defined contribution plans provide much more assistance for wealth accumulation to high earners than to low earners. The current structure of Social Security pensions somewhat reduces this imbalance. A shift to PSAs would eliminate an important equalizing feature of the overall retirement system. Given that "personal circumstances" as a determinant of lifetime earnings includes being born black or white, male or female, able-bodied or impaired, and into a rich or a poor family, the unfairness of this approach seems manifest.

The imposition of substantial stock market risks on lower earners is also objectionable. The lower one's earnings over a lifetime, the more Social Security pensions matter to one's bedrock protection against destitution in old age and the less likely one would be to prefer having that protection subject to market risks of the sort contemplated by the PSA proposal. After all, if one's investments went south under the PSA plan, one would be left with a guaranteed benefit of only $410 per month in 1994 dollars—less than current Supplemental Security Income payments and much less than the poverty threshold.

The PSA scheme also trades a portion of Social Security's protections—survivor benefits—for ownership of the PSA, which passes to one's heirs at death. Security for younger workers and lower-wage workers' families is again being traded for increased benefits to higher-wage workers, and particularly to the survivors of those who do not outlive the value of their PSAs. This is not a trivial trade. Social Security currently provides life insurance valued at $1.3 trillion, more than all private life insurance policies currently in force in the United States. In short, the PSA proposal piles stock market and other risks on families who are poorly positioned to bear them.

Although it seems clear that the Ball plan is vastly superior to the PSA approach, there is no reason, in principle, to adopt the Ball proposal. Technical changes agreed to by all members of the Advisory Council, plus some acceleration in the phase-in of later retirement ages, would solve virtually all of the pension fund's fiscal problems. We could increase FICA taxes by the monumental 0.8 percent (0.4% on workers, 0.4% on employers) now and solve the whole projected fiscal problem. Or we could wait awhile to see whether anything more really needs to be done. In short, there is nothing that could responsibly be called a fiscal crisis in Social Security pensions. The problems that exist are easily manageable. And the remedies are so affordable that if no one had mentioned them, they could probably have been implemented without many people noticing the changes. But make no mistake about it: crucial values of social solidarity, political stability, and economic fairness are at stake in the proposals to privatize Social Security pensions.

Beneath the surface of the technical debate about Social Security's tax rates, benefit schedules, and long-term financial future, there is a deep ideological divide between defenders and opponents of social insurance. Defenders, like us, see necessary adjustments as a natural and inevitable evolution of a prized public institution. Opponents see these occasions as opportunities for radical revision—times for convincing Americans, especially the young, that social insurance is an unfair, unsustainable sham. But privatizing Social Security is a contradiction in terms. It would change the dynamics of the program in order to fit the imperatives of private markets. Markets can supply a marvelous array of investment vehicles, but they cannot supply social insurance.

THE FIGHT OVER MEDICARE

Medicare, largely ignored in the battle over health care reform in the early 1990s, returned to American politics' center stage following the Republican congressional victories of 1994. Given bipartisan calls for reductions in the nation's budget deficits and Republican hostility to Medicare's social insurance roots, it was almost certain that the Medicare program would once again generate intense and very public conflict. Moreover, unlike Social Security pensions, the projections for Medicare expenditures suggested real worries about unsustainable budget outlays.

A somewhat longer view reveals, however, that these projections present a puzzle rather than a crisis. For most of Medicare's history, its expenditures grew about as rapidly as outlays in the private medical economy. Indeed, from 1983 to 1993, those outlays increased less rapidly than private health expenditures. (On a per enrollee basis, private health insurance grew on average 12.2 percent annually between 1969 and 1994, compared to 10.9 percent for Medicare.) In the mid-1990s, Medicare's expenditures grew at a more rapid rate than the private medical economy, as Figure 8.2 suggests. And it is this atypical feature—a more rapid rate of inflation in Medicare rather than the other way around—that, in combination with projected early deficits in the Medicare trust fund, set the stage for fearful debates in the 1995–97 period about what should be done.

Once again, privatization was touted by some as the solution to Medicare's problems. Privatizing here came in at least two quite different forms. One was a broad proposal for Medical Savings Accounts (MSAs). Instead of participating in group insurance at the place of employment or paying the health insurance portion of FICA taxes, Americans would be required to contribute (tax free) to MSAs to cover their medical needs. Presumably, the buildup in these accounts would provide sufficient reserves for medical care both during employment and during retirement.

There are major transitional problems with this scheme, but those need not distract us from the main line of argument. For the young, the healthy, and the affluent, the MSA approach is a great deal—particularly so if, as is virtually certain, this tax-free saving could be tapped for other purposes once a sufficient cushion was achieved. What happens to the remainder of the population is only slightly less clear, but it is broadly predictable. With the "good risks" now not contributing to the insurance pool, the bad risks must be "insured" by general taxation. In short, instead of medical care as an aspect of social insurance, the system would move rapidly toward segmentation: private insurance for the relatively well off and welfare medicine for everyone else.

The alternative privatization approach retains social insurance coverage for elderly persons but attempts to save money by having private health insurance plans compete for Medicare's patients. This alternative poses no direct threat to social insurance. Rather, the worrisome question is whether these plans can both save money and deliver decent medical care to elderly persons—or anyone else. These are crucial questions for the whole of American medicine, not just Medicare. They only distantly connect with whether medical care for elderly persons should continue to be provided under American social insurance principles.

Indeed, the controversies over Medicare's financing divert us from the more fundamental issue of whether the insurance risks of ill health should be dealt with in a universal program or left to a patchwork system of private payment, private insurance, and diverse public pro-

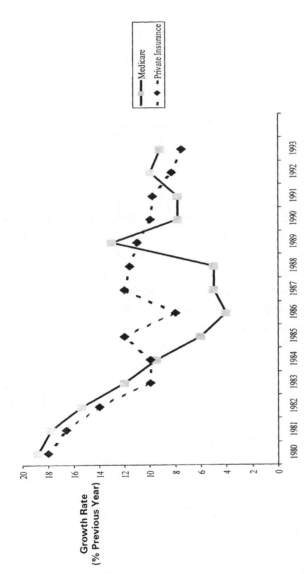

Fig. 8.2. Growth in Medicare and private health insurance spending per enrollee, 1980–1994. *Source:* Office of the Actuary, Health Care Financing Administration, 1996.

grams. For although we think of Medicare as the socialization of health risks—which it is—we often forget that it is an incomplete social insurance program. It emerged from the failure of universal health insurance proposals, not from their success.

Understanding Medicare's Origins and Character

Medicare is, of course, not universal health insurance. It is a program for Social Security retirees (and recipients of disability insurance) whose political origins lie in the nation's rejection of national health insurance. First discussed before World War I, national health insurance fell out of favor in the 1920s. When the Great Depression made economic insecurity a pressing concern, the Social Security blueprint of 1935 broached both health and disability insurance as controversial items of social insurance that should be included in a reasonably complete scheme of social protection. From 1936 to the late 1940s, liberals called for incorporating universal health insurance within the emerging social insurance package. But the conservative coalition in Congress defeated these attempts at expansion despite their public popularity.

The original leaders of Social Security, well aware of this frustrating opposition, reassessed their reform strategy during President Truman's second term of office. By 1952 they had formulated a plan for incremental expansion of government health insurance. Looking back to the 1942 proposal that medical insurance be extended to Social Security contributors, the proponents of what became known as Medicare shifted the category of beneficiaries to elderly retirees while retaining the link to social insurance financing and eligibility.

Medicare thus became a proposal to provide retirees with limited hospitalization insurance—a partial plan for the segment of the population whose financial fears of illness were as well grounded as their difficulty in purchasing health insurance at modest cost. With this, the long battle to turn a proposal acceptable to the nation into one passable in Congress began, stretching from its strategic birth in the early 1950s to a fully developed legislative plan by 1958.

These origins determined the initial design of the Medicare program and created expectations in its proponents concerning how it was to develop over time. The incrementalist strategy assumed that hospitalization coverage was the first step in benefits and that more would follow under the common pattern of Social Security financing. Likewise, proponents presumed that eligibility would be gradually expanded. Eventually, they believed, it would take in most if not all of the population, extending first, perhaps, to children and pregnant women. And they thought of Medicare as national health insurance for a population group, "universally" covering retirees and, later, the disabled. Like much of the U.S. welfare state (but not education), inclusiveness meant workers and their families, not literally every citizen or person in the land. But there was no mistaking the aspiration of broad coverage that the Medicare strategy reflected. All Medicare enthusiasts took for granted that the rhetoric of enactment should emphasize the expansion of access, not the regulation and overhaul of American medicine. The clear aim was to reduce the risks of financial disaster for elderly persons and their families. And the clear understanding was that Congress would demand a largely hands-off posture toward the doctors and hospitals providing the care that Medicare would finance. Decades later, that vision seems odd. It is now taken for granted that how one pays for medical care affects both the care given and the amounts paid. But in the buildup to enactment in 1965, no such presumptions existed.

The incrementalist strategy of the 1950s and early 1960s assumed not only that most of the nation was concerned with the health insurance problems of the aged but also that social insurance programs enjoyed vastly greater public acceptance than did means-tested assistance programs. Social insurance in the United States was acceptable to the extent that it sharply differentiated its programs from the demeaning world of public assistance. "On welfare," in American parlance, is regarded as a term of failure, and leaders within the Social Security Administration made sure that Medicare fell firmly within the tradition of benefits "earned," not given as charity. The aged could be presumed to be both needy and deserving because, through no fault of their own, they had lower earning capacity and higher medical expenses than any other age group. The Medicare proposal avoided a means test by restricting eligibility to persons over age 65 (and their spouses) who had contributed to the Social Security system during their working life. The initial plan limited benefits to sixty days of hospital care and excluded physician services in hopes of softening the medical profession's hostility to the program.

The form actually adopted—Social Security financing and eligibility for hospital care and premiums, plus general revenues for physician expenses—had a political explanation, not a consistent social insurance rationale. The very structure of the benefits themselves, providing acute hospital care (Part A of the legislation) and physician treatment as an unexpected afterthought (Part B), was not tightly linked to the special circumstances of elderly persons. Left out were provisions that addressed the problems of the chronically sick elderly—those whose medical conditions would not dramatically improve and who needed to maintain independent function more than triumph over discrete illness and injury. Viewed as a first step, the Medicare strategy made sense. But by the twenty-first century, with essentially no serious restructuring of the benefits, Medicare deserves a sober review, not a panicky one.

From the standpoint of universalism, Medicare is conceptually divided. It separates the retired worker from those still on the job, thus breaching one version of social solidarity. (The response to that, of course, is that all of us hope to become retired; Medicare taxes [Part A] on workers then become down payments on their own hospital insurance as retirees.) Because Medicare covers two groups of the population, it can take on the coloration of interest group politics, though not the us-them vitriolics of welfare policy. And by insuring those with the greatest risk, Medicare encourages cost shifting by providers from areas of tight to areas of lax fiscal control. In short, though it is critical to the well-being of the aged, Medicare cries out for expansion to make good on the social, political, and economic promise of universal provision. For now, however, we will concentrate on the debate over Medicare's finances.

Understanding the Current Debate over Medicare Reform

Coping sensibly with Medicare's problems first requires freedom from two misleading claims in the debates of the 1990s. One is the mistaken view that if Medicare faces financial strain, the program requires immediate and dramatic transformation. The experience of the 1980s and late 1990s demonstrated that Medicare administrators, when given appropriate tools and political support, can limit the pace of increase in the program's costs. Cost escalation is not a necessary feature of the Medicare program. It is an artifact of particular techniques of monitoring and reimbursement.

The second misleading notion has to do with the very language used to define the financial problems Medicare undoubtedly faces. Critics (and some defenders) continue to use the fearful language of insolvency to describe Medicare's future, a dreaded one in which the program's "trust fund" will literally run out of money. This language represents the triumph of metaphor over thought. Government, unlike a private household, adjusts its patterns of spending and fund-raising by fiat. The trust fund is an accounting term of art, one applied in this case to Part A of Medicare, the hospital insurance program. The term reflects the convention we have developed for describing earmarked revenues for spending both now and in the future. Congress can change the taxes that finance Medicare, if it has the will. Likewise, it can change the benefits and reimbursement provisions of the program. Or it can do some of each. Channeling the fiscal consequences through something called a trust fund changes nothing in the real political economy. Thinking so is the cause of much muddle, unwarranted fearfulness, and misdirected energy.

To view the crisis-ridden debate about Medicare's finances as misleading is not to suggest that the program is free of problems. Far from it. But it is important to understand that Medicare can be adjusted in ways that fully preserve the national commitment to health insurance for America's elderly and disabled.

What should be done? One place to start is the reduction of the growing gap between the benefits Medicare offers and the obvious needs of its beneficiaries. What Medicare pays for should be widened to include the burdens of chronic illness. That means incorporating prescription drugs and long-term care into the program, which is precisely what the Clinton administration hoped to do in connection with its ill-fated health insurance overhaul.

Widening the benefits package does not mean, contrary to what many claim, that total expenditures must rise proportionately. Expenditures represent the volume of services times their prices. Many other nations not only have universal coverage and wider benefits than Medicare but also spend less per capita than we do for their elderly. Canada, for example, is able to do this because it pays its medical providers less, spends less on administration, and uses expensive technology less often.

There is no reason that Medicare's outlays need to rise at twice the rate of general inflation—or more. To achieve lower rates of increase in Medicare's expenditures does not require change in the program's status as an entitlement. What does have to be changed is the amount of income medical providers of all sorts receive from the Medicare program. The restraint of costs necessarily means reductions in payments to those in the medical industry. The real question is whether the reduction comes from fewer needed services, fewer unneeded services, or lower payments for services, needed or not.

Medicare's financing also could use some overhauling. Raising payroll taxes will have to be part of the answer. For some this is simply ruled out of current discussion, a good example of fearfulness defeating evidence. The breadth of public support for Medicare suggests that it is possible to mobilize popular opinion in favor of tax increases when the problem is clearly defined and the justification convincingly offered.

We need debate over how Medicare should be improved. What we do not need is debate that scares the country about its future by disseminating false claims of Medicare's unaffordability. It would indeed be a crisis if the legitimate health costs of our aged and disabled were unaffordable. And it is true that a pattern of health expenditures increasing at twice the rate of national income growth is unsustainable over the long run. But there is no reason to believe that we must tolerate this future.

The politics of budget deficits, not the program's aims or operations, brought Medicare to renewed prominence on the nation's agenda. In the process, another highly misleading claim about reforming Medicare's "premiums" has arisen, one with profound implications for American social insurance. It is the view that Medicare's financial troubles require means testing the program in the form of income-related premiums for the Part B physician insurance coverage. Indeed, there is a constituency within the Washington political community that regards such a policy change as simply common sense. Defying hundreds of years of common usage, these actors have developed a new jargon, in which "means testing" does not mean what ordinary language suggests. Tests of means are normally understood as a way to settle issues of eligibility, who is in and who is out of some program. Such tests suggest the distinction between we (the generous) and they (the needy); means testing conveys exactly the connotation generations of Americans have associated with being "on welfare."

There is a quite different vocabulary in the world of public finance that is largely free of such associations. The language of public finance refers to progressive, proportional, or regressive ways to pay for government programs. Or one discusses the redistributive effects of either the financing or the benefits of a program.

Not so with the 1997 Congress, where Republican leaders suggested "means testing" Medicare in the sense of having premium levels rise with the income of retired beneficiaries. This appeal to "soak the rich" populism is dangerous. It represents a threat to social insurance principles and constitutes another road to unraveling the broad political support that social insurance programs have by virtue of their eligibility and financing. Here is why. The purpose of insurance is to spread the costs of a risk, not to concentrate them. Spreading costs over a lifetime of work is precisely what the current financing of Medicare's Part A hospitalization coverage does. Imagine now subjecting upper-income retirees to a premium for their medical insurance set at, to use a current idea, 50 percent of the average Medicare expenses for physician and related coverage (Part B). The sickness expenses of the elderly, as with any group, are wildly uneven. The top 10 percent of users have expenditures more then twenty times those of the cheapest 90 percent. Any benefits manager for any substantial firm with relatively healthy retirees will be able to find group policies for them that will compete with a "means-tested" Medicare Part B program financed by "income-related" premiums. This is an obvious road to undermining the broader risk pool that Medicare's social insurance roots express.

The appeal to "means testing" Medicare is but one of the misconceived approaches to dealing with the financial pressures on the program. If there were wide support for more progressively financing Medicare, it would be worth reconfiguring the sources of payment for Medicare's bills. One obvious possibility would be to increase the use of general revenues, including general income taxes that both the elderly and the nonelderly pay, or expressing the Part B premium as a small proportion of one's Social Security pension. But there is very little to be said for adjusting premiums as the means-testing enthusiasts suggest. First of all, it is dangerous as a matter of social solidarity. Moreover, such changes not only fail to raise significant funds but also are administratively cumbersome and costly to administer. Only in the world of the blinkered technocrat—without attention to linguistic sensitivities or implementation barriers—would such an idea appear appealing.

Medicare's early implementation stressed accommodation to the medical world of the 1960s. Its objective was to keep the economic burden of illness from overwhelming the aged or their children. It was assumed then that incorporating elderly persons into the wonders of American medicine was the welcome task at hand. The setting now is radically different. The difficulties of Medicare are those of an American medicine that has many troubles. We pay too much for some procedures, and we do too many things that either do some harm or do little good in relation to their costs. In the world of American private health insurance, cost control has now arrived with a vengeance. Medicare is unsettled and is likely to remain so in the context of budget politics unless we accept that limiting what we spend on Medicare need not mean eviscerating, or even radically transforming, the program. The price of cost control will undeniably have to be borne, but that burden should be borne, as social insurance would prescribe, proportionately.

AN EXEMPLARY CASE FOR EXPANDING
AMERICAN SOCIAL INSURANCE

Between exaggerated fears of unmanageable budget deficits and mindless incantations of the unsustainability of "big government," the sensible discussion of the American public household has been largely paralyzed. Presidents—Democrat or Republican—announce the end of big government. Fiscal elites wring their hands about the affordability of public budgets. A kind of collective amnesia blots out the reasons why the nation should have embarked on social insurance programs in the first place and obscures the remaining gaps that only social insurance can fill efficiently, equitably, and affordably.

The most prominent gap remains in medical care, where more than

40 million Americans lack health insurance despite the risks of unbudgetable expenses from unexpected illness or injury. The fact that most Americans will not tolerate refusal of treatment to the uninsured does not remove the insecurity the uninsured are bound to feel. Nor does the readiness to pay by some—through haphazard cross-subsidization— remove the increased pressure on hospitals, doctors, and health insurance plans as the growth of competitive pricing in health insurance has increased in recent years.

On economic grounds, the unwillingness to let people die or suffer from lack of health insurance is the premise that justifies universal coverage and the extension of health insurance "contributions" from those with income. On political grounds, the case for widening coverage and expanding the insurance pools from which the currently uninsured can draw payments is familiar and powerful. Most Americans are healthy most of the time; most health outlays are for the sickest 10 percent of the population. The impact of competitive pricing in health insurance— in the absence of legislative reform—will be to make the sick pay more or get less. And the race to the bottom will proceed relentlessly unless the principle of sharing the costs of illness widely is once again brought into prominence.

To understand this is to understand why the unfinished agenda of American social insurance in the first decade of the twenty-first century includes program expansion as well as program protection for Medicare and Social Security. This chapter has focused primarily on protecting the existing regime of social insurance against the twin attacks of unaffordability and unmanageability. The remaining emphasis has to be on fulfilling the promise to cushion modern citizens from both the expected risks of postindustrial capitalism (unemployment, forced retirement, and premature death from accident or bad luck) and the expected costs of modern medicine (large, unbudgetable, and concentrated on the few). Before the fact, all of us expect to live healthy, extended working lives. After the fact—where that fact is distress—all of us ought to have the financial cushion that collective provision can provide, even if we cannot ward off the predictable (old age and some illness and injury) and the unexpected (accidents, illness, and a longer life than we expected). That is the case for both stability and prudent expansion of social insurance.

The continued vitality of America's version of social insurance is uncertain. The contemporary debate goes beyond prudent tinkering to fundamental restructuring. A wider range of critics—conservative figures joining the libertarians and the neoliberals—are complaining about the "excesses" and worrisome future of entitlements. With monetary support from the financial services industry, the fears of the future are buttressed by those with the most obvious pecuniary stakes in a sharply curtailed public retirement program as well as in restructuring the Medicare and disability programs. To counter these ideological and economic interests will require the mobilization of ordinary Americans. And that will not happen without rediscovering why social insurance arguments made sense in 1935 and 1965 and clarifying the crucial difference between abandoning universal programs and adapting them to changing demographic and economic circumstances.

The case for universal health insurance is, to our minds, unanswerable. But the fact is that the contemporary struggles in U.S. health policy concentrate not on universal health insurance but on the regulation of what commentators call managed care. This is where American medical debates—other than those over financing Medicare and Medicaid—are (and will be) concentrated. The fate of managed care plans, as important as it is for Americans, is not distinctively linked to the social insurance features of Medicare. The effects of managed care—on patient choice, professional autonomy, and costs—will be debated heatedly as state after state confronts the conflicts over regulating the plans in which some 70 percent of Americans now receive their care. And they will arise as well in connection with claims that Medicare should adapt to managed care rather than the other way around. Our discussion, however, has emphasized the social insurance case for Medicare, not the full range of considerations that bear on the program's future.

AMERICAN EXCEPTIONALISM—AGAIN

Throughout this chapter we have viewed "universalism" through the lens of U.S. public provision. For Americans, *universal* means all workers or contributors, not all citizens or residents. We should not leave this discussion, therefore, without underscoring the profoundly traditional, indeed conservative and work-oriented, vision that American universalism embraces. It says not that you are entitled because you are a part of the nation but that you are entitled because of your contribution to the nation. Funding is linked to earnings, and entitlement is defined by years of work. Hence, for Americans, universalistic entitlement has always been a concept tied to, supported by, and supporting a market economy. That the protection of social insurance—and the demand for its expansion—should be thought to be the distinctive position of "liberals" is, to say the least, ironic.

More critically, this American version of universalism powerfully constrains our collective imagination concerning the potential reach and utility of universal provision. It cripples our attempts to provide adequate protections for children. And it has begun to infect the dialogue between present and past workers under the misleading label of "intergenerational equity." The problems of American social insurance are thus grotesquely miscast by current controversies. Our problem is not that we have attempted too much but that we have completed so little.

ACKNOWLEDGMENTS

Financial support for continuing research on social insurance has come from the Robert Wood Johnson Foundation. Both the Committee to Save Medicare and Social Security and AARP have supported the writing, editing, and dissemination of this work. An earlier version of this chapter was published in *The New Majority,* edited by S. Greenberg and T. Skocpol (Yale University Press, 1997).

NOTES

1. We elaborate on this argument in T. R. Marmor, J. L. Mashaw, and P. L. Harvey, *America's Misunderstood Welfare State: Persistent Myths, Continuing Realities* (New York: Basic Books, 1992). The mix of myth, mischief, and mistake incorporated in these claims of unaffordability and unmanageability is especially striking in the case of Social Security, the nation's premier example of a prudent program, run efficiently and widely accepted as legitimate. Peter Peterson, the Wall Street financier who for well over a decade has been rewriting the same article of gloom and doom, illustrates the problem. While conceding that rising medical costs are a far more important source of future strain, Peterson nonetheless has prominently used the Concord Coalition to claim Social Security's unaffordable costs. He has sponsored the formation of organizations supposedly speaking on behalf of the current young—the Third Millennium is the most recent

example. And he persistently confuses discussion by moving without notice between complaints about Medicare, concerns about Social Security pensions, and criticism of the unfairness of "entitlements," which is simultaneously a budgetary, a legal, and a cultural category.

2. These assaults arise from a variety of sources: right-wing libertarian organizations like the Cato Institute of Washington, less extreme antigovernment critics at the American Enterprise Institute, and advocates of the standard complaints about "excessive" government regulation like the Chamber of Commerce. In the late 1980s and early 1990s there was supplementation from budget deficit hawks like the Concord Coalition and elements within the financial services industry. In the particular case of Social Security, the publication of Marshall Carter and William Shipman's *Promises to Keep: Saving Social Security's Dream* (Washington, D.C.: Regnery, 1996), is a good example of the new combination of players. Carter was then the chief executive officer of the State Street Bank, and Shipman was a member of the Cato Institute's advisory panel on Social Security.

3. Herbert Stein, the former chair of the Council of Economic Advisers in the Nixon period, supported this argument in the most unlikely of places, the opinion page of the *Wall Street Journal*, February 5, 1997. "If the purpose of Social Security is to provide a certain benefit upon retirement," he wrote, "then an investment policy that yields a probable, even though possibly higher, benefit is not appropriate [referring to investments in stocks]."

9

The Moral Imperative of
Limiting Elderly Health Entitlements

Richard D. Lamm

You would be surprised at the number of years it took me to see clearly what some of the problems were which had to be solved. . . . Looking back, I think it was more difficult to see what the problems were than to solve them.

— CHARLES DARWIN

THE CHALLENGE OF AN AGING SOCIETY

One of the great challenges in America's future is to retire the baby boomers without bankrupting the country or unduly burdening future generations. This crisis is creeping up on America and could soon overwhelm American public policy. Yesterday's baby boom is tomorrow's grandparent boom. This demographic revolution presents us with some interrelated challenges. How do we fund present programs for the elderly, let alone expand those programs for twice as many elderly persons? How do we adapt and fund our retirement and health care systems for a country of many more elderly and fewer children? What are the social and political consequences of running a society whose average age will be approximately twice that of American society during our first two hundred years as a nation? How do we fund all the needed health care, long-term care, and income security? How do we provide the social infrastructure for an aging society? How can we accomplish this and still be fair to present and future generations who will fund these programs? How can this be accomplished politically? If we act soon, we can answer these questions rationally, prepare for our future, and avoid steep economic decline. But if we wait, the decisions we will be forced to make will be draconian. Age could well be as divisive in the next forty years as race and sex have been for the last forty years.

The average age of much of the world is going up as families have fewer children and life expectancy expands. Although good for us individually, this trend is undermining some of society's most popular programs. Medicare, Medicaid, Social Security, and our health care systems cannot survive the aging of our society without substantial change to many of our most politically popular programs. The dilemma is complex in its details but simple in its description: the industrial world has dramatically increased its life expectancy and reduced the number of children born to an average family. There are essentially two social policy ways to provide health care and retirement benefits for the elderly—society can prefund these programs in a way similar to how most of the private sector funds its retirement programs, or it can develop a social insurance scheme in which I am obligated to take care of my parents in turn for my children's obligation to take care of me. The United States chose social insurance, and it has worked well to date, but can it continue? Baron von Bismarck set up the first social insurance system in Germany in 1888 and set the retirement age at 65—a number that most of the rest of the industrial world adopted. The catch is that life expectancy in Germany in the 1880s was 42. It is no trick to retire people at 65 when they have lots of children and the national life expectancy is 42.

The developed world added approximately three months per year to life expectancy throughout the twentieth century. The United States, for instance, added approximately thirty years to average life expectancy during that period, and we continue to add life expectancy with no short-term end in sight. This is, bottom line, a great public policy victory. My 93-year old father toured Europe recently with his older brother. I am 65 years old, and I can reasonably expect to have more life and more health ahead of me than any previous generation in history. And my children can expect even more.

This success story has its price. Our retirement systems are now actuarially unsustainable, and our health care system has been growing during my professional lifetime at about two and one half times the rate of inflation and now consumes over 14 percent of GDP. Thoughtful people are realizing that, given our myriad of medical miracles, our aging bodies can bankrupt our children and grandchildren. The status quo in these two policy areas is not an option; the only question is the extent and type of reform.

Elderly persons account for approximately 13 percent of the U.S. population, yet they get over 60 percent of all federal social spending. We, as a nation, spend about three times more taxpayer funds on elderly persons than we do on our children; the federal government spending is even more disproportional. I would suggest that it is not a nation-building strategy to spend significantly more on the last generation than we do on the next generation. We face a massive, and I believe unsustainable, burden under current programs in caring for our elderly. We can still have compassionate and caring retirement in America, but only if we anticipate the full magnitude of change and act in time. Infinite needs have collided with finite resources in an aging society, and we must rethink many of our basic public policy assumptions.

The Demographic Trap

Extended longevity is clearly good news for us individually. Eighty percent of babies born today will live past their sixty-fifth birthday, whereas fifty years ago less than 40 percent lived to see that day (U.S. Bureau of the Census 1994, chart A1-3). Today's senior citizens have unprecedented opportunities for a dignified and active retirement. "This is the first time humans have altered the age structure of the population," says University of Chicago demographer Jay Olshansky (1994; see also Usdansk 1992). Sam Preston (1976) estimates that more than two-thirds of the improvement in longevity, from prehistoric times to the present, took place in the twentieth century.

The results of this demographic change are predictable in some ways and unknowable in others. The public policy dilemma is that we forged a majority of our politically sacred programs assuming a growing number of children and slowly increasing longevity. We thought that we had solved forever the age-old problem of support for the elderly. In 1967 Nobel Prize winner Paul Samuelson wrote in *Newsweek:* "The beauty about social insurance is that it is actuarially unsound. Everyone who reaches retirement age is given benefit privileges that far exceed anything he has paid in." How can this be? He explained: "The national product is growing at compound interest rates and can be expected to do so as far ahead as the eye cannot see . . . a growing nation is the greatest Ponzi game ever contrived" (quoted in Peterson 1993, 75–76).

Alas, the era of unlimited possibilities is over and the day of reckoning is upon us. We are a technologically inventive society living longer, demanding more, and yet having fewer children. One of America's greatest challenges is to resolve the difficulties of an aging society and then sell that resolution to our complacent society. We should take great care not to underrate the magnitude of this change to our age structure. It is a change in demography so fundamental that it alters the nature of both the problem and the historical solutions. One set of authors predicts:

> By the middle of the next century, when this revolution has run its course, the impacts will have been at least as powerful as that of any of the great economic and social movements of the past—movements such as the conquest and subsequent closing of the frontier, the successive waves of European immigration, the development of our great cities, or from more recent times, the post-WWII baby boom, the civil rights and women's movements, the massive influx of women into the paid labor force, the revolution in sexual mores, and the decay of many of our large urban centers. All these developments have had a profound effect on our nation, but the aging of the population will certainly have an equal, if not greater impact. (Phifer and Bronte 1986, 3)

Societies do not inevitably age; they can grow younger or older. Time ages our bodies, but an aging society is due to multiple factors, mainly life expectancy and the number of children born per woman. We are an aging society, and we must get ready for the implications to our society. We delay addressing these problems at our own peril.

Health Care in an Aging Society

The dominant issue in American medicine for the immediate future will be how we adjust to the demographic realities of our aging society. It will be politically and professionally painful. It will cause much agony in a medical profession trained to assume that there are virtually unlimited resources available and that cost is never a consideration. It will be a seminal issue, causing as much unsettling change as did the reform of medical education early in the twentieth century. It raises issues of limits in a society that has prided itself on having no limits. Yet adjust we must.

We cannot retire the baby boomers under the same thinking that has dominated American culture for the last sixty-five years. This is and will be a transforming event, and in transforming events, yesterday's solutions become today's problems. It will require more than an extrapolation of our old thinking—as the poet James Russell Lowell reminds us, "New occasions teach new duties, time makes ancient good uncouth."

We simply have invented and discovered more things to do to our aging bodies than our aging society can afford to pay for. We are on the threshold of the bionic body: medicine can have some positive impact on practically every organ in our body. Modern medicine has outrun the ability of any nation, even a rich nation, to pay for everything beneficial to everyone within its borders. We have created a Faustian bargain, according to which our aging bodies can and will divert resources that our children and grandchildren need for their own families and that public policy needs for other important social goods.

Americans now spend an average of four thousand dollars per capita on health care (Smith et al. 1999). Four thousand dollars is twice as much as an average American spends for *all* functions of state government and is more than the total yearly income of more than half the world's population. For most of us, our largest purchase in life is no longer our house but our health care. Many thoughtful people may worry that we are unbalancing our economy and that it is not wise national policy to spend one out of every seven dollars on health care, but polls show that Americans think health care is one of the most important priorities and that most Americans want to spend more, not less, on health care. That is politically important, because in a democracy we generally get what we want, but is it wise public policy? Do we really know what we are doing to our society and its institutions? What does it mean to our nation's future? What price my aging body?

The Next New Deal

The New Deal was so mesmerizing to my generation of public policy makers, so just, so right for the time, so politically stabilizing, that it has dominated our thinking for sixty-five years. It deserves to have dominated our thinking for many of those years, because the more we look at the Depression in hindsight, the more we recognize how prescient the New Deal was, how large the stakes, how appropriate the response. Germany got Hitler, Italy got Mussolini, Japan got Tojo, and the United States got FDR. No small feat, this.

But many of these institutions are demographically obsolete. We are living too long and having too few children to continue the New Deal programs without substantial amendment. They are no longer in the interest of the younger generations who increasingly fund them. These programs are from thirty-five to sixty-five years old. We must see realistically and address without nostalgia the new circumstances we are faced with. We must rethink, reevaluate, and reconceptualize.

Modernizing the New Deal will be much more difficult than initiating it was, due to the popularity of the programs in the United States. Both political parties support Social Security and Medicare and have a large stake in making the right decision concerning them. They are the most popular governmental programs in America. The sheer weight of a popular success and the drag of the status quo compounds the magnitude of what we are faced with. It is understandable why many people do not want to substantially amend this system. To admit that our system of funding health care is unsustainable requires us to give up the dream of a totally universal and egalitarian health care system. To many people this is the death of a dream. Like "take backs" in the union movement, it is unacceptable to many people that we should give back benefits painfully achieved, no matter what the evidence.

This means we will need leadership—bipartisan leadership. The public is already distrustful of the political process and wrapped up in their own lives. With the nation now politically divided almost equally, it will be hard to prepare the public for the type and magnitude of change necessary. Walter Lippmann once wondered how we could sustain a democracy when "the public will arrive in the middle of the third act and will leave before the last curtain, having stayed just long enough perhaps to decide who is the hero and who the villain of the piece. . . . He does not know how to direct public affairs. He does not know what is happening, why it is happening, what ought to happen" (1925, 65). Who will tell the people? How does a democracy downsize expectations? How do we make the unpalatable at least digestible?

SEEING THE BIG PICTURE

The Moral Art of Seeing

Proust once observed: "The real voyage of discovery is not seeking new lands but seeing with new eyes." We must look at these new demographic realities with new eyes. We must look fully and honestly at what it means to run "a nation of fifty Floridas." British philosopher and novelist Iris Murdoch writes, "Seeing is a moral art." She says our "moral quality functions in what we see and remember and know" (1970, 41), and a colleague of mine has asserted that "seeing" is, in fact, *the first and perhaps the most important* moral art. We have to see, recognize, know, become aware of, before we move to solve. The world has many problems that patiently await our ability to see that they need to be solved. We have to morally open our eyes.

Seeing the Problem of Intergenerational Equity

I am among those who claim that we must start to recognize a new equity in America, intergenerational equity. We must enlarge our concept of justice as we did for other forgotten or ignored people and interests and start to see and evaluate distributional issues in light of justice across the generations. What is the impact of today's policies on the future of our children and grandchildren and society? One great step forward taken by the New Deal was to see clearly the plight of the elderly and the poor, and perhaps today's challenge is to see what the solutions to past problems are doing to the future.

My generation has been credit card liberals. We got elected and re-elected partly by encumbering our children. However much wealth our generation has created, in public policy we have not fully paid our own way. I am not arguing any Iroquois duty to seven generations or other syrupy social or environmental goal—just the practical question of how we are treating our children and grandchildren.

In one of my life's iterations I was a certified public accountant, and to my eyes we have understated our governmental debt and overstated our assets. The real debt we leave our children is closer to $20 trillion than the $5.5 trillion federal debt we admit to. In addition, we have created an ocean of contingent liabilities that may come due if the economic dominos start to fall. We have also overstated the assets we have left to cover these obligations; for instance, many claim there is no meaningful value in the Social Security trust fund. If an individual inherits a million dollars of government bonds, that individual is truly enriched. If a generation inherits $4 trillion of government bonds, its members have inherited nothing of real value to the next generation. They have simply received an asset and an offsetting liability. You can "spend" an asset only once, and when we take today's payroll taxes and pay today's elderly Social Security and use the remainder on other governmental expenditures, we are consuming those assets, no matter what type of accounting tricks we play. Our debts are real and a burden to our children, but not all of our assets are real. Resources that are to be consumed in the future will have to be earned in the future. There is nothing "saved."

We need to recognize that however successful and however popular our entitlement programs are, they have become unjust to our children who are paying into them. This applies with special urgency to our health care programs.

Universal Coverage: Seeing the Forgotten Uninsured

We must also see that not only does the United States ration medicine but also that it is likely that we deny more people more health care than any other industrial country. A public policy definition of rationing is any allocation of medical resources that leaves some important medical need unmet. People forget that a health care system rations when it fails to deliver medically needed health care to the citizens within its jurisdiction. We don't mind people falling overboard, as long as we don't personally have to throw them overboard or listen to them splash.

We lack the moral imagination to see the "forgotten men, women and children" who don't have health coverage, who, even when they receive charity care for emergencies, do not get adequate care. All studies show that the uninsured are less able to get adequate care, and their health statistics in virtually every category are below (or far below) those who have insurance coverage.

One of the reasons we have failed to "see" unmet need is that my generation of policymakers has not adequately asserted the public interest. The uninsured are not on our public policy radar screen. We have relied too much on health professionals to define the problems and solutions in health care. Public policy has essentially subcontracted health policy to physicians. But the focus and genius of medicine is individual health, not societal health. No one has been promoting the interests of the total public. As one expert put it: "Professionals tend to believe that they are the only ones able to make informed choices. In fact, many of them are not trained to see the overall health situation of the whole population, but only the problems of the individual patients. The devotion of the physician to his/her patient may make it difficult for him not to seek an excessive share of available resources for them and to overlook the resulting loss to other patients" (Attinger 1987).

We try to tell ourselves that as long as we are not denying specific procedures to specific individuals, we are not rationing medicine. We have a constipated vision of both a just society and the real impact of our public policy. We know that we are the only industrial country in the world without universal health care, but we do little about it. Our moral maps are calibrated solely to the individual; none of us own the problem of the uninsured. Every man for himself and "God save us all," said the elephant, as he danced among the guinea pigs.

Certainly we can make Americans understand that rationing is not only an individual denial but a societal denial. Oregon sailed into *terra incognita* when it decided to limit benefit coverage rather than not cover medically indigent people. Health providers and most Americans did not recognize this new moral landscape because we had all been assuming that the proper and sustainable role of government was to fund the existing doctor-patient relationship. Whatever the dynamics that relationship demanded had to be paid—regardless of its impact on other social priorities.

Governor John Kitzhaber, a physician-legislator at the time, asserted the public interest. He recognized that legislators had a different and broader moral universe than a physician. A physician has a duty to a patient, but legislators are responsible for the whole state and its citizens. A physician in America can reasonably deny that he rations medicine when he treats a patient, but the state does not have the moral luxury to make such a claim. Governments are responsible for broad public policy. If they provide subsidized health care to some medically indigent citizens but not to others, they are rationing.

When a state attempts to maximize health, it is not making moral judgments. It has a different and broader moral radius than a physician. It is allocating resources where they will do the most good. Oregon decided to ration benefits rather than ration uninsured people. It was allocating limited resources using all the relevant considerations available, trying to achieve a just and equitable Medicaid system that maximized health benefits to Oregonians. It was an empirical process that should not be evaluated by the medical ethics of the doctor-patient relationship.

A sustainable, publicly funded health care system must look beyond the individual to the justice of the system. It must step above medical ethics and ask what is ethical public policy. It cannot be content to merely fund all doctor-patient relationships but must try to maximize the health of society using a variety of tools. It is a world of trade-offs, priority setting, and rationing. My argument is that an ethical health care system must, inevitably, do all three.

Do I forget that medical ethics contains the requirement of "distributive justice?" I do not. Distributive justice is among our ethical principles and urges universal coverage, but not, I submit, in a meaningful way. It is an orphan ethic to health policy. It is what the appendix is to the body, a nonfunctioning vestigial organ. An orphan ethic that nobody owns and nobody fights for. It is not functional in any real sense and is easily forgotten. Daily, all over the nation, we give a blank check to professional autonomy and only pennies to distributive justice, without protest or even recognition. We care more about giving a doctor everything than giving the uninsured anything.

But to public policy, "distributive justice" may be the most important ethic. You cannot build a modern health care system a person at a time. Some institution must ask, How do we keep a society healthy? We need a method of assessing health needs that looks not at individuals but at the broader health-producing possibilities. Public policy should not define *ethical* an individual at a time. It must quantify need cumulatively and relate that need to the real and limited world of resources. The public policy equivalent to nonbeneficence would be universal coverage.

Setting Limits: Seeing Infinite Needs and Finite Resources

We turn a blind eye to the necessity of setting limits in health care. Setting limits may have a strange sound to American ears, but we must have the maturity to recognize why it is necessary.

Government cannot and should not allow health care to crowd out all other important social spending. The predominant characteristics of state and federal health programs, almost the unifying factor, is that they have ended up costing five to fifteen times as much as anticipated. We are a compassionate society and can afford a lot, but we cannot afford everything. No publicly financed health system can ignore the law of diminishing returns. All systems must set up procedures to decide what health care is financially practical. It is necessary to find, among the myriad of things we can do, what practically in a budget we ought to do. The price of modern medicine is to honestly admit that all health care systems ration.

It is beyond the purpose of this chapter to argue the case that we have limited funds. David Eddy (1994a) asks the bottom line question: "The acid test for whether financial resources are limited is to simply ask those who are responsible for budgets of health plans whether they have enough money to do everything everyone wants to do. If not, then the budget is limited."

Once we admit that we must inevitably set limits, the whole nature of the problem changes, and so must our analysis of the problem we face. Limited funds must be budgeted and prioritized. Medical culture makes it hard for health providers to recognize that resources are limited, and it makes it hard to recognize that other people in the system are also entitled to their just share of these common resources or that those providers have any stake in or duty to other necessary social goods in their society.

Likewise, patients see so clearly their own self-interest but not how their needs fit into broader public policy. It is difficult to make a nation of individuals see their place in the broader community. Yet approximately 50 percent of health care is funded by taxpayer money. No one person or family feels responsible for the air or water pollution of the community, and all drivers plead "not guilty" to causing a traffic jam. People fail to see the cumulative impact of their individual demands. Likewise, few citizens who use one part of the budget see their funding as related in any way to other parts of the budget or other social needs. Our health care system thus lacks perspective and vision.

Seeing the Need to Broaden the Scope of Benefits

Just as we have to restrict, we also have to broaden. Health care cannot be seen solely through the eyes of allopathic medicine; we must see the needs for the total health and well-being of society. The total health care of a society, particularly of elderly persons, is much broader than we now cover under Medicare. I would argue that we have to spend some of the resources we gained by setting limits to provide some services that relate to the *quality* of life for seniors, not just biological life. More important to many seniors than many of the things we now provide through traditional medicine are

Meals on Wheels
Health education
Medical information and referral
Aging resource centers
Telephone reassurance
Personal emergency response systems
Homemaker services
Transportation
Wellness programs

Reforming U.S. health care is a two-front war. We must simultaneously restrict and broaden.

Seeing Contributive Justice

We also need to see in a new light the rules of sharing a joint pool of resources. Approximately 80 percent of health care is paid by commonly collected funds, taxpayer or insurance. All those who contribute to a common pool have a joint stake in that common pool. Not an equal share, but a *joint stake* in seeing that these resources are rationally and effectively spent.

Health care delivery systems employ two strategies to ration: they limit access or they limit availability. In the United States, we are sensitive to limitations on our personal health care but not that of our neighbors. Whoever determines what is "medically necessary and appropriate care" is the rationer. The federal and state governments have a macroallocation choice to ration the *who* or ration *what* procedures are included. So far, they have not bitten the bullet and dealt with what is covered, so they necessarily limit the *who*. Oregon is the first and only state to directly confront the trade-off between the *who* and the *what*.

If medical ethics and practice allow every health provider to deliver all "beneficial" medicine to each patient and charge commonly collected funds no matter how marginally beneficial, then we have an unsustainable model: a delivery vehicle that is all accelerator and no brake. In a pool of common resources, you cannot deliver maximalist medicine to every patient. Allocating commonly collected funds needs a broader vision, a new way of thinking, and evaluation of what is necessary and appropriate. We cannot avoid the reality of limiting in some way the demand for and supply of institutional resources.

Haavi Morreim brings together the trade-off between private need and collective funds in her concept of "contributive justice." Principles of equity and justice demand that we allocate commonly collected funds to maximize their effectiveness and recognize that spending resources on marginal procedures for *A* prevents us from doing justice to *B*, who pays into the same common pool and has a higher need. "Contributive justice protests when discretionary generosity for a few is bought at others' expense" (Morreim 1995, 250).

The new but painful obligation of modern medicine is to develop systems that set goals, limits, and priorities that are consistent with total societal reform. Whoever distributes limited funds must decide generally what is worth paying for and what is not worth paying for in light of total need. Limited funds should usually be budgeted according to relative need, and it is the duty of those allocating the pooled resources to set up a system of priorities that will maximize the health of the total group.

Both public policy and health plans have the obligation to look at the "opportunity costs" of pooled money. They must, for instance, compare the costs of using more expensive contrasting dyes (and avoiding a small risk) with the possibility of saving lives in other areas such as mammography, Pap smears, or improved cardiac care. All options to maximize limited funds should be weighed and considered. Southern California Kaiser has shown that it can save twice as many women for two-thirds of the money by concentrating mammography on women in the age group of the greatest risk (Eddy 1994b). It recognizes that to optimize the health of the group, you must occasionally suboptimize what is available to the individual.

This bites deeply into existing practice and culture. But it must be done. We must recognize that the price of modern medicine is to see the inevitability and desirability of forming procedures and strategies that fit infinite demands into finite resources.

The challenge of health care in an aging society is a particularly difficult one because it requires downsizing citizens' expectations of what is to be delivered, but more importantly because it involves moral and ethical issues relating to life and death on which there is no national agreement. In fact, even discussion on these issues has hardly begun (Klein 1998).

It is important to understand that confronting these policy and ethical issues was inevitable even before the age structure started to change. Ultimately, it is the proliferation of expensive medical technology and treatments that forces us to adopt a new moral vision. The aging of America merely accelerates this problem. Maturity, as I was once told, is the graceful acceptance of the inevitable. With that in mind, I would suggest the following new moral vision for the coming health care debate.

    1. A nation's health goal can never be, nor should it be, to fund the

sum total of all its citizen's individual needs. Public policy should seek a healthy public and recognize that medical care is an important part of that search, but only a part. It must find polices that maximize the health of the public, not merely respond to the medical need of its individuals. Thus, the legislature should not be limited to or controlled by the ethics of the physician-patient relationship. That relationship is important but not exclusive.

2. No funding system in health care will ever be able to fund all stakeholders' ailments and anxieties. Not only is it not in the public interest to fund everything "beneficial" to the patient, but, correctly analyzed, it is not always in the patient's best interest. The question for all health care funders will not be, What do we "need"? but, What can we reasonably afford? To the extent that health care and medical ethics do not incorporate fiscal realities, they will have to be rethought.

3. We do not maximize health by maximizing health care. Society must better analyze and study the determinants of health for a state and a nation. How do we keep a nation healthy? What factors produce health? In this we have the benefit of a number of other countries having considered the subject.

4. Public policy should concern itself more with extending the health care floor (i.e., maximize coverage) than raising the research ceiling. Public policymakers must care about the health of the total society as passionately as health providers care about an individual's health. When these conflict, it is the public health, not individual need, that must be controlled.

5. A "two-level" health care system is inevitable. Individuals have the right to spend their own money as they see fit. Thus, whatever "basic" level of health care is constructed by government or health plan, some will be able to enrich that benefit with their own funds.

6. We must recognize that more than 80 percent of health care is paid out of commonly collected funds, not individually out of pocket. Group funds, public or private, should maximize the health of the group. It is the duty of those distributing pooled money to optimize the health of all those in the pool. The doctor-patient relationship may be the most important relationship in health care, but it is not the only relationship. Doctors are patient advocates, but they are imperfect agents to maximize the health of a group of patients.

7. When people pool funds, they cannot maximize the amount of beneficial treatment to each member of that pool, and cost has to be a consideration when distributing those funds. The tort system must be amended to recognize these realities.

8. Not only is the Oregon health plan ethical; it is unethical for a state *not* to have a system of priorities. Likewise, those in health plans who distribute pooled resources have an independent ethical duty to prioritize and budget those funds to maximize the total health of the group. Governor Kitzhaber demands that we give our attention to the "hydraulic relationship" between coverage, benefits, and cost. All are important; all are interrelated. Public policy must find a way to prioritize *what benefits* are covered instead of *which citizen* is covered. We must recognize that because of that "hydraulic relationship," the problems of the uninsured and the problems of cost containment are not separate problems but are inextricably intertwined and must be solved together.

9. What may have been unethical under assumptions of infinite resources becomes ethical in the trade-off world of finite resources. Many concepts must be reconsidered and redebated. Does not a society owe a greater moral duty to a 10-year-old than a 90-year-old? Shouldn't a patient's smoking and drinking habits be laid on the scale for high-cost rescue procedures?

10. Life is precious but cannot be priceless. Death is always a loss, but now it is often a publicly subsidized event. There will always be "ten leading causes of death," no matter how brilliant our medicine. The threat to biological life cannot highjack a disproportionate share of finite resources needed elsewhere for the quality of life. People have a "right to die," but it is a negative right against interference, not a positive right to a state-subsidized death regardless of cost. The postponement of death is an important value but must take its place among other health values.

SUMMARY

Goethe warned, "If you are going to live in your father's house, you must rebuild it." We have not adequately structured the house of health policy or ethics to prepare ourselves for our increasingly aging society. We have overbuilt and overfurnished the first floor (the doctor-patient relationship), but most of the rest of the structure remains not only unfinished but also unframed. There is more than one level of ethical analysis in health policy; there are multiple levels. A legislator, a health plan, and a family member have different moral duties than a doctor has, and we need different levels of ethical analysis—corresponding to the various levels of moral obligation.

Health policy is not an island, complete in itself, but is instead part of the landscape of many needs. Our aging society has three overriding public policy obligations to meet if it is to have a just and adequate system. It must provide health care, income security, and long-term care, and we must be wise enough not only to balance the spending between these needs but also to do it while meeting the full spectrum of other governmental demands.

We are not alone in this challenge. Virtually all the world is growing older as birthrates drop, life expectancy increases, and technology advances. As Rudolf Klein (1998) states succinctly, "all countries, not just Britain, must decide how to allocate scarce health care resources at a time of rising patient demand and the proliferation of medical technology." This is politically difficult but conceptually possible, and it is economically necessary. Americans must rethink and rebuild their health policy. We must bring to America the wise words of President Jacques Chirac, who said when running for reelection as the president of France, "Politics is not the art of the possible, it is the art of making possible what is necessary." To which I say: Amen.

ACKNOWLEDGMENTS
I have been immensely influenced, in ways I cannot fully acknowledge, by Victor Fuchs, Garrett Hardin, and Herschel Elliott.

REFERENCES
Attinger, E. O. 1987. High Technology: The Pendulum Must Swing Back. *World Health Forum* 8:309.
Eddy, D. 1994a. Principles for Making Difficult Decisions in Difficult Times. *Journal of the American Medical Association* 271, no. 22 (June 8): 1792–93.
———. 1994b. Rationing Resources While Improving Quality. *Journal of the American Medical Association* 272, no. 10 (September 14): 817–24.
Klein, R. 1998. Rationing of Health Care Should Be an Incremental Process. *British Medical Journal* 317:959–60.

Lippman, W. 1925. *The Phantom Public*. New York: Harcourt Brace.

Morreim, H. 1995. Immoral Justice and Legal Justice in Managed Care: The Ascent of Contributive Justice. *Journal of Law, Medicine and Ethics* 23:247–65.

Murdoch, I. 1970. *The Sovereignty of Good*. Art. Ed. 1985. New York: Routledge Classics.

Olshansky, J. 1994. *Rocky Mountain News*, October 4, 23A.

Peterson, P. G. 1993. *Facing Up*. New York: Simon and Schuster.

Phifer, A., and L. Bronte, eds. 1986. *Our Aging Society*. New York: Norton.

Preston, S. 1976. *Mortality Patterns in National Populations*. New York: Academic Press.

Rice, D. P. 1989. Demographic Realities and Projections of an Aging Population. In S. Andreopoulos, ed., *Health Care for an Aging Society*. New York: Churchill Livingstone.

Rocky Mountain News, October 4, 1994, 23A.

Smith, S., S. Heffler, M. Freeland, and the National Health Expenditures Projection Team. 1999. The Next Decade of Health Spending: A New Outlook. *Health Affairs* 18, no. 4: 86–95.

U.S. Bureau of the Census. 1994. *Statistical Handbook on Aging America*. Washington, D.C.: U.S. Government Printing Office.

Usdansk, M. 1992. As People Live Longer, Choices Get Tougher. *USA Today*, July 23, 7A.

10

The Merits of Changing to Defined Contribution Programs

Mark V. Pauly, Ph.D.

Any public program that pays subsidies to households in general, conditional on the occurrence of unpredictable events, provides a kind of social insurance. Any subsidy program must define to some extent what the subsidized expenditures are to be used for. In the most fundamental sense, there are therefore many social insurance programs with some element of defined benefits. However, it is clear that both the proportion of the population eligible for a subsidy and the completeness with which benefits are defined can vary greatly. All or almost all persons who share a broad set of characteristics might be eligible for the subsidy, and the benefits may be defined very tightly; this plan is classic social insurance. Alternatively, the set of people eligible may be limited by a means test or other device, and the restrictions on how subsidized funds can be used may be loose. As one moves through this multidimensional spectrum, there are advantages and disadvantages to be realized. In this chapter I outline the advantages and disadvantages of moving two prominent American social insurance programs—Social Security and Medicare—from their current position on the spectrum, which approximates (though not perfectly) classic social insurance, to a new position involving both less definition of the benefits to be provided and more varied (and less extensive) terms for eligibility.

The reason for considering such changes is based on the hypothesis

218 Mark V. Pauly

that some structural alterations in current Medicare and Social Security are inevitable. The reason why things have to be changed is that the failure to do so would result in future tax rates so high as to generate unacceptable levels of excess burden or distortion on the economy. I argue that there may be substantial advantages, and what I judge to be relatively modest disadvantages, to moving both of these programs more toward an income-conditioned defined contribution framework. Along the way, I also emphasize some very important differences between Medicare and Social Security in how these general concepts might be applied. My own judgment is that bigger changes are both necessary and desirable for Medicare than for Social Security.

There has been some policy interest in means testing Medicare (Pauly 1999a, 1999b; Wilensky and Newhouse 1999). Some very modest steps in that direction were present in the Medicare Commission's proposal until the final (political) revisions were made (National Bipartisan Commission 1999). A defined contribution or "premium support" approach was also at the heart of that proposal.

SOME DEFINITIONS AND SOME DISTINCTIONS

Current policy with regard to Social Security and Medicare is somewhat ambiguous. Both plans have some elements of defined contribution and some elements of defined benefit. This is not unexpected, since the two concepts do not represent polar opposites. Instead, social insurance plan types can take a position along a continuum from pure defined contribution to pure defined benefit.

Social insurance is a program for older citizens in which contributions or premiums are not collected and disbursed on an individual-specific basis. That is, as at present, there is no *necessary* dollar-for-dollar linkage between what people pay in taxes or "premiums," and when, and the benefits they are eligible to receive.

The terminology of *defined contribution* and *defined benefit* was coined for private pension plans, and one interesting question is how well the terms carry over to public pensions or to health insurance for retirees, public or private. The textbook says that a defined benefit pension plan is one in which "the retirement benefit is known in advance but the contributions vary depending on the amount needed to fund the desired benefit." In contrast, a defined contribution plan is one "in which the contribution rate is fixed but the retirement benefit is variable" (Rejda 1995, G-4).

In this chapter I take a somewhat more general approach to definition. By *defined benefit* I mean that, for a given amount of revenue, all aspects of a social insurance program are prespecified and chosen collectively or politically. No decisions are left to the individual beneficiary. Key elements to be defined include

- How contributions or revenues are to be transformed into expenditures or outlays per beneficiary
- Under what conditions the beneficiary receives a payout or benefit
- What the beneficiary is allowed to do with the payout

By *defined contribution* I mean that the social insurance plan specifies only how much revenue is to be collected and divided among beneficiaries of a specific age group. In this case, what is to be done with the revenue—how much to spend now rather than later, and what to spend it on—is, within very broad limits, up to the individual.

Inevitably, Medicare has more defined benefit features than Social Security. Once the dollar amount of Social Security benefits is determined, the recipient can spend them on anything he desires; there are no "in kind" limits or requirements about spending on housing, food, entertainment, or knickknacks. The beneficiary also has some control over the age at which Social Security benefits are received. In contrast, Medicare benefits must be spent on medical care (and specific types of medical care at that), cannot be deferred or assigned to one's spouse or heirs, and can currently be claimed only by those over age 65 or by those who are eligible by reason of disability.

Thus, one distinguishing difference between the two types of plans is the amount of control the individual has over how funds are used. Economists would ordinarily think that people should prefer more choice to less, other things being equal, but insurance specialists do not always see things the same way. For example, "Another disadvantage [of a defined contribution pension] is that employees must make decisions on how the funds are invested" (Rejda 1995, 467). Defined contributions (at any level) *require* more choice and therefore are less paternalistic than defined benefits. For the present, we will remain agnostic on the value of choice.

Another feature usually mentioned as a distinction between the two types of plans is the degree of uncertainty. Benefits are specified in detail and guaranteed in defined benefit plans, whereas only the proceeds of a predetermined contribution policy are to be expected in a defined contribution plan. However, this difference only holds after the person has retired. Before that, as noted in the definition, workers may be required to contribute more to a defined benefit plan than they initially expected if the rate of return falls below that expected (or if aggregate wages fail to increase as expected). It is clearly possible that there could be more *lifetime* uncertainty with a defined benefit than with a defined contribution plan. Moreover, with regard to Medicare (but not Social Security), the only benefit guaranteed is insurance coverage, not insured services. If the reimbursement rate were set low, access to services and to new technology might prove difficult. If it were impossible to supplement the defined benefit (see the next section), a defined benefit plan could actually cause more uncertainty as and if the level of access fluctuated. However, here I will follow tradition and suppose that defined benefit gives the beneficiary real guarantees in return for rigidity.

Supplementability

An important characteristic of all public interventions to affect individual behavior, a characteristic that determines, most fundamentally, how much of an impact they will have, is something we may call *supplementability*. A plan that prohibits citizens from buying more or paying more for the services that are the subject of public expenditure is the quintessential nonsupplementable plan. Usually supplementability is not absolute but may vary in terms of ease. I can supplement the public primary school education my children receive by paying for tutoring or moving them back and forth between public and private schools; supplementation here is difficult. In contrast, under current policy, the government would actually help me buy a Medigap policy to supplement my government-run Medicare plan, both by helping to structure that market and by cross-subsidizing Medigap through community rated Medicare "premiums." But if I prefer a new-model hip joint that Medicare has not yet approved, I may not be able to get it at all. And if I want to pay my doctor more than 115 percent of Medicare's fee schedule in order to garner special attention, both of us could be in big trouble. It is sometimes even possible to have negative supplementation—people reduce some private activity that offsets an increase in public spending.

In the fully supplementable (positive and negative) world, the specificity of public spending becomes inconsequential, and all public programs become transformed into income transfer or "perfectly defined contribution" mechanisms only. More reasonably, if it is easy to add but hard to subtract, public spending does not affect resource allocation for those who do supplement (income effects aside); it only changes things for those who rely entirely on Social Security or Medicare. Trying to distinguish between allocative effects and income transfers will be an important issue in what follows.

What Are Our Social Objectives?

It is clear that social insurance programs have been created in part to satisfy citizens' desires to achieve some objectives that markets alone will not. (Realistically, they were also created to engineer various kinds of political transfers, not necessarily related to the highest aspirations of mankind, but we will temper cynicism with idealism here.) It would clearly help in evaluating alternative arrangements to have statements of those objectives that are both clear and politically supported and stable. Where does one go to find such statements?

Advocates of social insurance, usually a policy elite, provide many such statements, ranging from "the solidarity principle" to "guarantees of a decent old age." Two slogans (one slightly more elevated than the other) are descriptive: "We're all in this together" and "The big winner buys the drinks." The problem is that such statements are often unclear, usually inconsistent, and not uniformly agreed to.

The other strategy is to suppose that the objectives are the *result* of a decision in the political process that a community has chosen to make (and seems inclined to leave in place rather than tinker with). Objectives then become the preference of the person or group that is decisive in that political process (even though many others in society will disagree). In a very simplified model, this decisive person is the "median voter"; in other settings, identification of the person or group that makes decisions will be more complex. In what follows I will try to pay attention to both supporters' rhetoric and political reality, but the reader should be forewarned of two things: (1) some confusion is inevitable, and (2) when in doubt, I will opt for the democratic choice rather than the preferences of influential elites. There is an issue, even so, of which democratic choice at which time; there clearly are quasi-constitutional aspects of social insurance that can be changed but which may (and should) change slowly and deliberately.

The Classical Social Insurance Benchmark

Classical social insurance programs are government or government-regulated programs with the following characteristics:

- Compulsory
- Funded through income or wage-related earmarked taxes paid into separate funds, to provide partial self-support
- No means testing for benefits (beyond any statutory relationship with earnings); benefits paid as a matter of right
- Designed to achieve social goals
- Qualifying conditions and benefit rights prescribed by statute
- Additional redistribution in favor of lower income groups, though eligibility is linked to past behavior
- Intended to provide benefits

If the external circumstances were those happy ones that permit social insurance to pay high returns, we would not be considering restructuring of these programs. The falloff in population growth and the aging of the population (along with the secular increase in the relative cost of medical services) have made it much more difficult for classical social insurance programs to achieve the objectives postulated above and still levy compulsory payments that are moderate enough to be relatively nondistortive and politically stable. Opinions may differ on how serious "the problem" needs to be; other chapters in this volume address that issue. The main assumption here, however, is that if compulsory payments or taxes are to be kept below some unspecified but undeniable target level, at least some of the design features of classical social insurance will need to be modified. The question to be addressed in the remainder of this chapter, then, is which modifications do the least harm (or, in some cases, the most good) with regard to equity and efficiency.

Some Environmental Changes

There have also been some major changes in the circumstances and characteristics of the present (and future) elderly population that should be taken into account in planning reform. The following three trends are expected to continue:

- As the time since the Great Depression lengthens, the population over 65 has less fear of economic catastrophe (Bernstein 1999). Being old is no longer synonymous with being fearful.
- The distribution of income has shifted strongly in favor of people over age 65 (even without including the value of Medicare benefits). Being old is no longer synonymous with being poor.
- The education level and the economic sophistication of people over age 65 is growing. Being old is no longer synonymous with being ignorant and confused.

I do not want to overstate these arguments. Although the change has been in the directions noted, it is probably still true that there are large numbers of persons over age 65 who are fearful, poor, ignorant, and confused. But surely the proportion has declined significantly, and probably it is less than (or little different from) that of the under-65 population.

Defining with Money or Regulation?

Money, as all economists know, is fungible. It can be transformed nearly costlessly from one commodity to another, from one investment vehicle to another, and from one time period to another. The first assertion that justifies a shift from a defined benefit approach to a defined contribution approach for Medicare or Social Security is that people are now more capable of making such decisions themselves than formerly. However, there is also a need to preserve some kind of safety net. Perhaps what is called for, in both Social Security and Medicare, is a kind of hybrid in which people can choose at various points in time between a defined contribution and a defined benefit approach, once a basic level of benefits has been obtained. More options can surely be created, and eligibility for them could be limited to the nonpoor if low-income people were thought incapable of choosing or unable to bear the risk of a mistake that inevitably accompanies the power to choose.

The kinds of choices that people might be permitted to make differ between Social Security and Medicare. For Social Security, the main choices that might be made are (1) how to invest contributions made during one's working lifetime and (2) how to choose the pattern of payouts over the retirement period. An example of the first kind of choice would be a switch from the current pay-as-you-go system to a funded system supported by private sector investments. An example of the second choice would be for the person to be given greater opportunity to select the patterns of payment conditioned on retirement age. For example, the person could choose to take the high payments initially, or other annuity plans, as long as they have the same actuarial value. To prevent adverse selection, these choices would have to be made well in advance of retirement.

For Medicare, both of these kinds of choices are possible, but there are some additional ones as well. One could fund postretirement health insurance with a private investment fund (with contributions still compulsory); this is the kind of scheme suggested by Gramm, Retenmeyer, and Saving (1998). One could choose an earlier or later date for eligibility for Medicare, with offsetting adjustments in the level of Medicare benefits.

However, Medicare goes much further in defining benefits than Social Security does. Annuitants are free to spend their Social Security checks on whatever they want (including silly things); once a person is at the point of retirement, Social Security in effect switches from a defined benefit retirement plan to a defined contribution consumption-financing plan. In contrast, Medicare classically provided only one kind of medical insurance, with quite specific provisions about what services would be covered and what payments would be permitted to be paid to and received by providers. For example, a person could not accept a larger Part B deductible in return for catastrophic drug coverage, nor could one agree to pay doctors more than the Medicare fee schedule and reduce the Part A upper limit.

An interesting question is whether social insurance for medical care could ever have the same kind of defined working-life contribution that some now advocate for Social Security. Could the program consist solely of a requirement to set aside some proportion of wages into a fund that would be used to pay for health insurance premiums after retirement, but with the investment of the fund and the form of the insurance left up to the individual? One problem with this arrangement is not just that the private return on investment might in the future be lower than its long term average but also that the value of the fund on retirement might still be outdistanced by health care costs. Of course, a person could hedge against rising medical care costs by investing in medical firms' stocks; the value of these investments would presumably rise with health care costs. However, in what follows I rule out this kind of *really* defined contribution for Medicare.

It is important to note, however, that in recent years Medicare has in a de facto sense become virtually equivalent to a postretirement defined contribution plan. Specifically, beginning with the availability of the HMO option and continuing through the Balanced Budget Act modifications, beneficiaries have been able in effect to take the payment that would have been made to traditional Medicare on their behalf and transfer it to other organizations providing other kinds of benefits. The "contribution" available to beneficiaries each year for any of a large variety of different kinds of health benefits is the Average Adjusted per Capita Cost in the fee-for-service Medicare option.

Traditionally, the only limitation on how this contribution could be used was the requirement that alternative plans must cover the basic benefits that conventional Medicare covered. However, especially in the managed care setting, nominal coverage does not determine what benefits will actually be paid. The one limit is that a person who selects an alternative plan that is less costly than Medicare cannot receive the refund as an addition to their Social Security check or as a refund, but this provision may be changed. One could say that the "contribution" is still tied to an explicit benefit, since it needs to be enough to cover the cost of the basic benefits under conventional Medicare. However, since Congress fully controls the annual update, it can, within broad limits, define this "cost growth rate" however it wishes. Thus, for all practical purposes, Congress chooses a defined contribution. The link to conventional Medicare only serves to show how far that contribution can go when stretched to fund basic benefits through the fee-for-service Medicare plan. Note also that this plan provides a fallback option for all beneficiaries.

Efficiency and Equity Characteristics of a Reformed Plan

My judgment is that many senior citizens are capable of dealing with defined contribution plans for health and for pensions and that some of them are well enough off to avoid dealing with Medicare entirely. I am less certain about the need for further means of testing Social Security, but I think the idea deserves consideration. Choice and means testing are both feasible.

The level of benefits an average-income worker can expect to receive either from Medicare or from Social Security ordinarily exceeds the equivalent value of the taxes he paid over his lifetime; there is presently redistribution from the working generation to those who are retired or near retirement. What is the pattern of the redistribution?

Social Security has adopted a nominally more complex and conflicted approach to such redistribution. On the one hand, there is a positive correlation between the person's lifetime wages and his or her Social Security benefits, since the size of the benefit is based to some extent on the size of covered wages and the extent of participation in the program. Higher wages when working are highly correlated with higher income when retired, above and beyond the effect of Social Security. However, the benefits rise less than proportionately with wages, there is a minimum level of benefits, and high earnings have sometimes been taxed. For these reasons, the *net* benefit in Social Security is already means tested to some extent; lower-income people receive net transfers and higher-income people pay them. This effect is modestly offset by positive effects of additional earnings (for someone who chooses not to retire until age 70) on future pension levels. Moreover, benefits are subject to income taxes to some extent.

Medicare, in contrast, makes the same nominal amount available for the insurance of every covered person. Since Medicare taxes rise with income (especially because there is no upper limit on taxable income for Medicare as there is for Social Security), there is a possibility of redistribution within each generation as well as across generations.

Nominal Medicare benefits are uniform across income levels, whereas lifetime tax payments increase with income. However, McClellan and Skinner (1999) find evidence that actual lifetime benefits increase with income, because higher-income beneficiaries live longer and use more costly services. They suggest that Medicare may even have made a net lifetime transfer from lower-income people to higher-income people.

Whatever the current distributional pattern, means-testing approaches would in effect make that redistribution more progressive (or less regressive). Why might such a change be desirable? Somewhat surprisingly, greater equity alone is not a very persuasive reason. Using Social Security or Medicare is both a more complex and a less consistent way to redistribute than simply adjusting general revenue taxes (with refundable tax credits) to transfer more from the rich to the poor.

However, if we view redistribution from a short-term perspective, it seems obviously inequitable to fund generous Medicare or Social Security benefits for the well off with taxes levied on workers who are on average less well off. More specifically, if the baby boom generation, under current law, would receive a large net transfer from the succeeding generation, larger than the transfer that generation will receive from the one following it, and if this "one time" transfer is judged to be unfair, reducing it may be desirable.

The efficiency calculus for this case (as opposed to the distributional calculus) is more complex. Choosing insurance that pays lower benefits to well-off seniors obviously reduces the level of wage or income taxes under pay-as-you-go financing and therefore reduces tax related work disincentives. However, if workers expect to have benefits reduced if they have high postretirement income, that implicit lifetime net tax may discourage work effort, shift the pattern of lifetime consumption to preretirement years (or early retirement years), and skew savings and investment toward assets that yield unmeasured income (such as owner-occupied housing). One set of distortions is improved, relative to non-means-tested benefits, but another set is worsened; at this level of abstraction, it is not possible to determine what the net effect will be. (Of course, if Medicare actually pays more the higher a person's income, people might respond by making more [perhaps even excessive] efforts to earn income. It is unclear whether I would decide to work harder to earn more income so that I would live longer and therefore collect more benefits from Medicare [and Social Security], but anything is possible.)

There are, however, some conjectures that may lead to more authoritative speculation. First, if the upcoming generation of retirees have higher average incomes than worker-taxpayers have, and if this also reflects higher lifetime income, the intergenerational transfer to them—which will surely be positive—may be thought to be inequitably high.

Second, suppose there is no transfer across generations, but current workers do plan to make a given transfer to members of their cohort with low lifetime incomes. In an idealized (and interest-free) world, it would not matter when and how the transfer is made if the relevant persons could be identified. Those with high lifetime incomes could either pay high taxes when working and then receive benefits independent of income when they retire, or they could pay lower working-age taxes (enough to cover the intergenerational transfer only) but receive no benefit on retirement.

In a more realistic model, the two schemes may have different effects. For one thing, if social insurance benefits are expected to be lower, persons with high lifetime wealth may save more privately, to replace those lost benefits. Second, there is sure to be some uncertainty that will diminish as the person ages and has lived more of her or his life. One can guess more accurately about one's own lifetime income after retirement than before. Both the progressivity of the income tax (which funds Medicare) and the absence of full offsets for losses mean that a person could risk paying a high lifetime tax because of a few years of high income, followed by years of low or negative income. In contrast, by waiting until after retirement and then making the transfers, the identification of who should pay what is more certain. Waiting until the end of the evening to decide who is a big enough winner to buy drinks for the losers is sensible. Moreover, although the argument is less certain, it may be that the value of sacrificed consumption or wealth is lower in postretirement years. (It is probably lowest of all after death.)

Beyond these kinds of preferences for the form of distributional transfers, are there efficiency effects of the provision of high social insurance benefits to the nonpoor? Perhaps, yes. At least some of these persons will optimally prefer less insurance coverage than Medicare requires. Such forced overconsumption is inefficient. For people who would have preferred more coverage than Medicare furnishes, the important allocative issue is whether public coverage can be supplemented efficiently. There are two reasons for inefficiency. There are administrative costs to supplementation, principally associated with choosing and paying for Medigap coverage. The other reason is that the community rated structure of current Medicare encourages excessive Medigap coverage (and actually discriminates against Medicare managed care). Finally, there is a practical argument. If Medicare did not provide coverage to well-off seniors, they could and would choose private coverage that matches their preferences. Although traditional Medicare has not thus far managed its benefits to any great extent, such policies as the ban on payments to high-priced physicians and the increasing set of rules on covered services suggest that more limitation is in store. If this is true, having the better-off opt out of Medicare at least gets them out from under the perceived heavy hand of government regulation (for a price).

These arguments are much stronger for Medicare than for Social Security. The level of the Social Security annuity is virtually certain to be less than the private pension the person would have chosen. There is little moral hazard, and administrative costs are likely to be low.

TOWARD A SOLUTION

How might a defined contribution approach be blended with introduction of means testing in ways that are synergistic and help to solve Medicare or Social Security's long-term financing problem? I first outline the contours of a proposal for Medicare and then turn to Social Security. In these cases, the seriousness of the long-term financing problem requires bold, not timid changes; these changes in turn are not advanced as the ideal proposal to improve either program relative to its current unsustainable form but rather as among the least painful solutions to what would otherwise be program degradation. I then close by outlining the contributions that means-tested defined contributions can make to solving the financing problem, relative to the alternative solution of raising tax rates or imposing regulation.

Means-Tested, Defined Contribution Medicare

The most fundamental part of this reform would be a definition, for those not yet retired, of the dollar value of the Medicare contribution, voucher, or credit at alternative levels of postretirement income or (ideally) wealth at some future date. It might be easiest to administer (and to describe) the program if we think of income or wealth categories rather than continuous variation. The choice of which categories should be used is a political one; here I describe things in qualitative terms.

Below some minimum income level, the contribution or credit would be enough to buy approximately the current Medicare benefit package. It would define that package in at least as much detail as conventional Medicare now does. The value of this credit would increase over time at the politically chosen sustainable growth rate. The structure of multiple approved plans, set in place by the Balanced Budget Act, would remain. If a plan that met the minimum benefit characteristics could be offered for less than the credit, those who chose it could take the difference in cash. Thus, at this income level, there would still be some elements of defined benefit, but they would be minimal. At the other extreme, perhaps for the top 5 percent of the income or wealth distribution, no credit would be offered, although this population could choose to belong to one of the Medicare plans (at a premium that would cover the cost) or any other insurance. In this case there would be nothing to define. For the other people in the top part of the income distribution (perhaps the top quarter), there would be a credit linked to a catastrophic low coverage plan. The size of the maximum permitted deductible would increase with income. It might be possible to make the credit reasonably close to (but less than) the premium for catastrophic coverage; a 50 to 75 percent subsidy rate would probably be appropriate.

The credit would be set above average for people with high-risk chronic conditions; certification of those conditions could be performed by one of the Medicare certified plans, which would then receive the larger credit as a risk-adjusted contribution. It is less clear that it is necessary for the credit to increase with age for those without chronic conditions, since this increase would be perfectly predictable.

The rate at which the value of the partial credit would increase over time is a matter of political choice—the choice of the amount of new technology that needs to be subsidized. If the credit grew at only the economy-wide inflation rate, beneficiaries who are not poor could still buy the same old technology at the same price as before, but they clearly would have to pay more themselves for new technology. The key question is the social devices (or obligation) to subsidize new technology for those who are not poor. My personal preference would be to subsidize such technology partially (by paying the subsidy to private premiums) but to reduce the subsidy as income grows and as time goes on.

Such a reduction in benefits for the better-off should be phased in gradually. Doing so would be expected to increase the level of savings in order to be able to cover the deductibles (for the more risk averse) or to purchase private supplemental coverage.

Panacea or Palliative?

How much good would it do to income-test Medicare in this fashion? The answer obviously depends on the extent to which benefits would be reduced. Modest means testing of the Part B premium would not appreciatively affect Medicare's total budgetary cost (Bernstein 1999). However, if these income reductions were targeted to the top 25 percent of beneficiaries, it is plausible that costs might be reduced by 10 percent or so (Pauly 1999a).

Would this help to "save" Medicare? There is no doubt that anything would help. It would postpone the date at which the Medicare trust fund would finally be exhausted. But the key driver of future cost will not be current cost per beneficiary. Rather, the future tax rate is driven by the rate of growth in the Medicare population relative to the rate of growth in the tax base and by the rate of growth in spending per beneficiary. The tax base in turn grows at a rate that reflects the growth in number of workers and the growth in tax base per worker. The difference between the growth rates for the elderly population and for workers, given current birthrates and immigration policy, is a little less than 1 percent, but this difference could balloon to nearly 2 percent at some point in time. Could growth in the tax base for workers make this up?

The real growth in the payroll tax base has historically been a little less than 1 percent, but because the Medicare tax applies to all wages and supplemented income, its growth is plausibly in excess of 1 percent. Even so, calculations of future GDP shares of tax rates twenty or thirty years hence can be affected by small differences between the "excess" growth in the number of elderly and the growth in the tax base (NASI 1999).

Limiting growth in expense per beneficiary to a rate of growth no greater than that which taxes are likely to be able to cover would prevent "inflation" but appears to be quite sensitive to small and unpredictable variations in rates.

Growth in expenses per beneficiary can be constrained by the defined contribution approach of the nonpoor. For the poor and the nonpoor, the permitted growth in the contribution will largely determine the cost of the technological change that can be covered. Even with the strong cost containment efforts and good luck, the GDP share will probably increase modestly over this period.

This model of defined benefit plans for the poor gradually changing, as wealth rises, to defined contribution plans for the nonpoor has both programmatic and political advantages. The programmatic advantage is that the tight level of the safety net under the poor can prevent the consequences of opportunistic behavior. For instance, allowing a poor person to choose a high- deductible policy with a Medical Savings Account (e.g., in order to obtain funds for some lifestyle-enhancing treatment) raises the issue of denying medical care in a serious illness if the person cannot afford the deductible. It may be better to forbid what we cannot tolerate (an idea that extends to Medicare Medical Savings Accounts themselves, should they ever become operable). In contrast, the wealth cushion available to the nonpoor paradoxically allows deductibles and other incentive-improving but risk-expanding choices to be more effective.

In addition, the opportunity for private, marketlike choices among the nonpoor has merits of its own. A nonpoor retiree can substitute drug coverage for a higher outpatient deductible in a private Medicare plan without raising the issues of monopsony that are central to the current controversy. Requiring pharmaceutical firms to discount prices to the government may be acceptable if only the poor are eligible for coverage benefiting from such discounts. The political issue here is the likelihood of contrast between the "safe" coverage the poor would be required to take and the opportunity to choose an alternative available to the nonpoor. The best evidence that the safe coverage is excessively restrictive would be if the nonpoor reject it. Advocates for the poor may then find it less attractive to maintain a strongly paternalistic position.

Means-Tested Social Security

Means-tested Medicare could limit the increase in the Medicare tax rate to another percentage point or so. This remaining modest increase alone would not result in macroeconomic Armageddon. However, the behavior of the much larger payroll tax for Social Security is likely to be more important than the smaller Medicare tax. In the near future, since current Social Security taxes exceed current benefits, Social Security's fiscal problems are less pressing. There would be time to phase in a process of gradual reduction in real benefits for the well off (perhaps simply by leaving their benefits unadjusted for inflation). By the time the Social Security trust fund would have reached a crisis phase twenty or so years hence, reforms may be in place. Of course, if Medicare benefits are converted to defined contribution and then cut back, it could be desirable to increase Social Security benefits for a time to cushion and facilitate the phase-in of means-tested Medicare.

CONCLUSION

The emergence of a sizable, well-educated, high-income segment of the over-65 population is a sociodemographic fact that the Medicare policy world should recognize. Although even dramatic steps probably cannot save Medicare from some kind of eventual tax increase, the increase can be held to manageable levels. Benefits could be maintained for the needy among the elderly, if there was a process to make that choice.

However, some fear not the economic consequences of converting to defined contributions and means testing but the supposed political outcomes. The fear is that political support for a redistributive system will erode if benefits decrease for the better-off, if Medicare becomes a "welfare" program. This need not happen, of course, if the proportion of the population with reduced benefits is less than a majority. The remaining individuals may still favor high benefits. (Because upper-middle-class people may have disproportionate political influence, it is possible that means testing could lead to lower political support for generous benefits for the poor.)

In democratic political philosophy, there is no justification for preventing such a political choice. That is, if voters would choose to reduce the level of transfers when the program was redesigned, there is no obvious analytic basis that could judge that choice to be inappropriate. Those of us who favor generous support of the poor would have to work harder to resist cuts, and we might be disappointed, of course, but the rules of democratic process that we have chosen should be allowed to work.

My own belief is that, relative to the alternative scenario of microeconomic and macroeconomic dislocation from high tax rates and their attendant excess burden and political confusion, the prospects of preserving the sensible transfers embodied in social insurance are greater if that insurance is converted to a means-tested form using defined contributions as the vehicle. No one can claim to forecast politics accurately, so in this essentially political choice there can be no guarantees. There can, however, be ways of increasing the odds of the best outcome.

REFERENCES
Bernstein, J. 1999. Should Higher Income Beneficiaries Pay More for Medicare? Medicare Brief no 2, National Academy of Social Insurance, Washington, D.C.
Gramm, P., A. Rettenmaier, and T. Saving. 1998. Medicare Policy for Future Generations: Search for a Permanent Solution. *New England Journal of Medicine* 338 (April 30): 1307–10.
McClellan, M., and J. Skinner. 1999. Medicare Reform: Who Pays and Who Benefits? *Health Affairs* 18, no. 1: 48–62.
National Academy of Social Insurance (NASI), Study Panel. 1999. The Financing Needs of a Restructured Medicare Program. Medicare Brief no. 5, September, National Academy of Social Insurance.

National Bipartisan Commission on the Future of Medicare. 1999. *Medicare Financing Sources.* Washington, D.C.: U.S. Government Printing Office.

Pauly, M. V. 1999a. Can Beneficiaries Help Save Medicare? In R. B. Helms, ed., *Medicine in the Twenty-First Century: Seeking Fair and Efficient Reform,* chap. 4. Washington, D.C.: AEI Press.

———. 1999b. Should Medicare Be Less Generous to Higher-Income Beneficiaries? In A. Rettenmaier and T. Saving, eds., *Medicare Reform: Issues and Answers,* chap. 3. Chicago: University of Chicago Press.

Rejda, J. 1995. *Principles of Risk Management and Insurance.* 5th ed. New York: HarperCollins.

Wilensky, G., and J. Newhouse. 1999. Medicare Reform: What's Right? What's Wrong? What's Next? *Health Affairs* 18, no. 1: 92–106.

11

The Case for Retaining
Defined Benefit Programs

Alicia H. Munnell, Ph.D.

Proposals abound to transform some or all of the Social Security system from a defined benefit (DB) plan, with benefits based on lifetime earnings, to a defined contribution (DC) plan, in which benefits depend on contributions and investment returns. Similar proposals would transform Medicare's commitment from reimbursement for a bundle of services to a dollar payment to purchase insurance. What is behind these proposals, and what impact would they have on the respective programs and participants?

Before answering these questions, it is important to narrow the issue under debate. First, the debate is not about the general merits of defined contribution versus defined benefit plans. Neither defined contribution nor defined benefit plans are intrinsically superior; they involve a number of trade-offs. The question is which is most appropriate for the basic level of income and health care support. Once basic benefits are ensured, most observers support defined contribution accounts to supplement public programs.

Second, the debate is not about prefunding—that is, building up reserves in advance of benefit payments. There is considerable support for using social insurance programs to increase national saving. The desire to accumulate reserves does not argue for either defined benefit or defined contribution, however, since prefunding can be accomplished under either arrangement.

Third, the debate is not about broadening investment options. Most observers would like to see Social Security participants—particularly those with no other assets—have access to the higher returns associated with equities. But individuals can reap the benefits of investing in equities under either a defined benefit or a defined contribution arrangement.

Thus, the debate is—given the desires to ensure basic protection in retirement, to increase national saving through prefunding, and to broaden investment options—whether providing basic retirement income and health care is better done through a defined benefit or a defined contribution arrangement.[1]

The chapter begins by describing the role that defined benefits have played in the U.S. social insurance system and then explores the factors behind the enthusiasm for DC plans. Later sections look at the potential impact on individuals and on society of shifting from DB to DC arrangements in the public sector.

The conclusions of this analysis differ somewhat for the two programs. In the case of Social Security, any potential gains from increased control and self-reliance are outweighed by the higher administrative costs, increased risk to participants, and potential harm to low-wage individuals. For Medicare, the story is more complicated: although a DC approach is likely to put low-income individuals at great risk, it might be an effective mechanism for reforming a complex system.

THE ROLE OF DEFINED BENEFITS IN U.S. SOCIAL INSURANCE

Both Social Security and Medicare provide a defined benefit—in one case, cash, and in the other case, reimbursement for a package of medical services.

Social Security

The 1935 Social Security Act set up a defined benefit system that had a much stronger resemblance to private insurance than to Social

Security as we know it today. The initial legislation planned for the accumulation of reserves and stressed the principal of a fair return for each worker. By 1939, however, it was evident that the states' old age assistance programs were not meeting the needs of those near retirement whose lives had been disrupted by the Great Depression. At the same time, these older workers had not had the chance to build up credits under the new Social Security system. To pay Social Security benefits to individuals without a lifetime of contributions, the 1939 amendments to the Social Security Act shifted to a radically different defined benefit arrangement that based benefits on a shorter period of coverage. The new formula also provided proportionally much greater benefits to low-income workers than to the higher-paid. The legislation also added monthly benefits for the dependents and survivors of insured workers. Thus, a defined benefit approach made it possible to pay benefits to people about to retire, to provide income redistribution, and to add dependent support.

Because income redistribution has been an integral part of America's social insurance program, Social Security has been successful not only in providing basic retirement income to working Americans but also in reducing poverty among the elderly. It has served as insurance not only in the event of the retirement, disability, or death of a breadwinner but also against the risk of a lifetime of low earnings. Income redistribution through a social insurance program with broad-based middle-class support is also more secure and predictable than that provided through a means-tested program. The mere fact that Social Security has been financed by an earmarked payroll tax has meant that it has not been subjected to the annual appropriations battles faced by programs financed through general revenues.

Despite Social Security's successes, a confluence of events has led to numerous proposals to introduce defined contribution individual accounts for Social Security. Indeed, a shift toward individual accounts has occurred in the private sector. There, however, a legitimate and important argument in favor of the defined contribution approach is that it is superior for mobile employees who often are shortchanged under defined benefit plans as they move from one job to another. No such rationale exists, of course, in the case of Social Security, since virtually all employment is covered, so workers do not forfeit benefits as they change jobs. Similarly, the regulatory compliance costs in the private sector are higher for defined benefit plans than for defined contribution plans, but again this factor is not relevant for the Social Security debate. What, then, is behind the enthusiasm for DC plans in the public sector? We will consider this question below.

Medicare

When Medicare was established in 1965, the government was not dealing with an economic catastrophe like the Great Depression but rather with inadequate provision of private sector services. Relatively few retired and disabled persons had health insurance; the private health insurance for these groups was very expensive, offered inadequate coverage, and was not automatically renewable. As a result, many elderly faced bankruptcy in the event of a serious illness or the possibility of receiving inadequate care.

After extended debate, Congress decided to provide the elderly with insurance similar to that offered to working-age individuals and their families.[2] Like private health insurance, it was a system of fee-for-service reimbursement. That is, the elderly could seek services from an unrestricted choice of providers, and then Medicare would pay doctors and hospitals for the services they provided to Medicare beneficiaries. The current Medicare system is a defined benefit arrangement because the Medicare program is committed to paying for a given basket of medical services.

Medicare has been enormously successful. Today nearly all elderly and disabled persons have coverage for acute medical needs, and the risk of impoverishment from uninsured medical costs has been greatly reduced. Medicare operates with relatively low administrative costs and enjoys widespread public support. But Medicare today also faces formidable challenges, including a long-term budget gap, an inadequate benefit package, and an inefficient delivery system.

In short, both Social Security and Medicare have provided defined benefit packages; participants know what they can expect to receive, and the risks of providing those packages have been borne by the taxpayer. A shift from DB to DC arrangements for Social Security and Medicare would transfer risks to the beneficiary. Why the enthusiasm for the DC approach, and what impact would such an approach have on individuals and society?

WHAT'S DRIVING THE ENTHUSIASM FOR DC PLANS?

The impetuses for change in Social Security and Medicare are somewhat different, although in both cases rising program costs associated with an aging population is an important factor. In the case of Social Security, the enthusiasm for DC plans comes primarily from the conservative side of the political spectrum and reflects a basic distrust of government and confidence in individual initiatives. With regard to Medicare, both liberal and conservative observers appear willing to explore the notion of moving from a DB to a DC arrangement.

Social Security

With regard to Social Security, five factors have been driving the enthusiasm for the DC approach: the emergence of a long-term deficit, the decline in returns, demographics, growing inequality, and Wall Street.

The Emergence of a Deficit. Social Security would in all probability not be on the national agenda if the system were not facing a projected long-term deficit. The intermediate projection from the most recent Annual Report of the Social Security Trustees (Board of Trustees 2000) shows that between now and 2015 the Social Security system will bring in more tax revenues than it pays out. From 2015 to 2025, adding interest on trust fund assets to tax receipts will produce enough revenues to cover benefit payments. After 2025, annual income will fall short of annual benefit payments, but the government can meet the benefit commitments by drawing down trust fund assets until the funds are exhausted in 2037.[3] From this point on, if no tax or benefit changes were made, current payroll tax rates and benefit taxation would provide enough money to cover about 70 percent of benefits. It is this long-run gap between 70 and 100 percent that needs to be filled.

Over the next seventy-five years, Social Security's long-run deficit is projected to equal 1.89 percent of covered payroll earnings. That figure means that if the payroll tax rate were raised immediately by 1.89 percentage points—less than 1 percentage point each for the employee and the employer—the government would be able to pay the current package of benefits for everyone who reaches retirement age at least through 2075.[4] Although such a tax increase is neither necessary nor desirable, it provides a useful way to gauge the size of the problem.

The reemergence of a long-term deficit was particularly disconcerting given the general belief that Congress had fixed Social Security in 1983. The legislation enacted in 1983, based on the recommendations of a commission chaired by Alan Greenspan, was supposed to keep the Social Security system solvent for seventy-five years and produce positive trust fund balances through 2060. Only a year after Congress enacted the legislation, however, the trustees began to project a small deficit. The deficit grew more or less steadily for the next decade. Even though it is easy to explain what happened,[5] the fact that the fix did not solve the problem created more uneasiness about the long-run financial security of the program.

The reemergence of a deficit made Social Security vulnerable to critics' attacks, and the critics greatly exaggerated the problems in order to justify dramatic solutions. One of the most persistent voices has been that of Peter Peterson, an investment banker who was secretary of commerce during the Nixon administration. His first essay on the perils posed by Social Security appeared in the *New York Review of Books* in 1982, and he has published numerous books and articles over the last eighteen years. Peterson paints a dire financial picture by lumping together the costs of Social Security and Medicare and treating them as a single, overwhelming crisis. A 1997 *New Yorker* article, "Spooking the Boomers," summarized his efforts as follows: "The Social Security critic Pete Peterson has whole segments of America fearing an impoverished old age" (Cassidy 1997). Peterson is not alone, of course; all the advocates of privatization claim that the system is not viable and demands dramatic restructuring.

The Decline in Returns. A deficit by itself would probably not have been enough to stimulate a major movement to restructure Social Security, since the program's financing shortfall does not require radical changes in the system. The deficit emerged, however, just as the system matured, making apparent the full cost of the program and the low expected returns on Social Security contributions—the so-called money's worth issue. Unlike earlier generations, who received large benefits relative to the taxes they paid, today's workers can expect to receive relatively low returns on their payroll tax contributions. Since raising taxes or reducing benefits will only worsen returns, almost all reform plans involve trying to increase returns through equity investment in one form or another.[6] Given that equity investment is viewed as desirable, those who do not trust the government conclude that individual accounts are the only mechanism through which this form of financial diversification could be achieved. Supporters of the existing defined benefit structure agree on the need for safeguards but think it is relatively easy to create a process that would enable the government to accumulate reserves in the trust funds and hire private sector managers to invest part of those reserves in private stocks and bonds without political interference (Advisory Council on Social Security 1997; Munnell and Balduzzi 1998; Aaron and Reischauer 1998).

The opponents of trust fund investments have some powerful allies—most notably Alan Greenspan (1999)—who characterize trust fund investment as the first step toward socialism. These opponents typically point to state and local pensions and claim that these funds often undertake investments that achieve political or social goals, divest stocks to demonstrate that they do not support some perceived immoral or unethical behavior, and interfere with corporate activity by voting proxies and other activities. They charge that if the investment options are broadened at the federal level, Congress is likely to use trust fund money for similar unproductive activities. The critics are wrong; recent research documents that political considerations have had almost no effect on investment decisions at the state and local level (Munnell and Sundén 1999).[7] Nevertheless, the desire to broaden Social Security's portfolio combined with ideological opposition to the government's investing in the private sector securities is a major impetus for individual accounts.

Demographics. The third factor influencing the Social Security reform debate is demographics. Longer life expectancies and a rapidly aging population will greatly increase the cost of supporting the aged, and almost everyone agrees that it is prudent to save in anticipation of such an event. Increased national saving will produce more national output so that supporting the elderly will be less burdensome on workers and will also avoid the high payroll tax rates (19.5% by 2075 under the intermediate assumptions) that are projected under the current pay-as-you-go system. Like the debate about government's investing in equities, the issue is whether saving can be done at the government level.

Some of those who oppose the accumulation of reserves at the federal level base their conclusion on faulty analysis. They claim that because the trust funds loaned money to the federal government and the federal government spent that money on submarines, the accumulation of trust fund reserves had no effect on the economy. That is incorrect; Social Security surpluses reduced the unified budget deficit and thereby lowered government dissaving. More sophisticated opponents contend that the existence of Social Security surpluses encouraged either taxes to be lower or non–Social Security spending to be higher than they would have been otherwise. Although little evidence exists to support this contention, a unified budget and large deficits during the 1980s and most of the 1990s blurred the picture. In the view of those who support individual accounts, the attempt to save at the federal level has been a failure, and the only way to increase national saving is for each individual to contribute to his own account.

These proponents of individual accounts fail to acknowledge that the changed federal budget picture—the non–Social Security portion of the budget is now in balance—alters the likelihood of success. It should now be much easier to revise the presentation of government accounts to separate Social Security completely from the rest of the budget, which would clarify the extent to which the system adds to national capital accumulation. Current congressional efforts to create a "lockbox" for Social Security, which would ensure that Congress does not use surpluses in Social Security to cover deficits in the non–Social Security part of the budget, are aimed at precisely the problems that arise from focusing on the unified budget.[8] These budgetary restrictions should be useful in enabling the federal government to accumulate reserves and add to national saving.[9] Nevertheless, the need to save in anticipation of the rapidly rising pay-as-you-go costs associated with the aging of the population is another factor in the enthusiasm for individual accounts.

Growing Inequality. Another development that could have influenced attitudes about redistributive defined benefit social insurance is the growing inequality in income and wealth. The facts are well known. Between 1980 and 1999, the share of the income going to the highest quintile has increased from 43.7 percent to 49.4 percent. Over the same period, the share going to the bottom two quintiles has declined from 14.6 percent to 12.5 percent (U.S. Bureau of the Census 2000). The statistics for the distribution of wealth are even more startling. Data from the Federal Reserve Board's Survey of Consumer Finances show that the net worth of the top quintile of the wealth distribution increased from 81.8 percent in 1983 to 83.4 percent in 1998, while the net worth of the bottom 40 percent fell from 0.9 percent to 0.2 percent (Wolff 2000). In fact, Bill Gates alone in 1995 was worth as much as all the 40 million households at the bottom of the wealth distribution (Wolff 1998).

The mechanism through which inequality might affect the DC-DB debate is twofold. First, the successful could view the continuation of these programs as a continued drag on their well-being, especially as the population ages. The second, and more likely, mechanism is that the successful believe that they could do much better investing in their own accounts and do not see the need to be part of any collective arrangement. This second factor reflects a shift in public attitudes over the 1980s and 1990s toward individual responsibility and self-reliance.

Wall Street. The potential for "taking the system private" quickly caught the attention of the nation's financial institutions, and they have been very supportive of conservative think tanks leading the charge toward privatization. The Cato Institute, which is the point for a phalanx of organizations in favor of privatization, was reported as of 1997 to have raised $2 million for its project on Social Security Privatization, one-fourth of it from Wall Street firms. Cato presented numerous seminars in New York to potential supporters in an effort to raise money for its projects. A key speaker at these seminars has often been Jose Piñera, Chile's ex–labor minister, extolling the successes of the Chilean pension system and saying, "I'm a firm believer that this can be done in the United States" (Lieberman 1997).

Cochair of Cato's privatization project along with Piñera is William Shipman, a principal of State Street Global Advisors, a division of State Street Bank. Although State Street has now carefully separated itself from the privatization effort, Shipman's efforts in behalf of the cause have been prodigious. He coauthored a book on Social Security privatization, wrote a long article in *Foreign Affairs*, and gave scores of speeches both here and abroad on how to reform the system. His presence plus financial support from State Street has greatly helped the Cato initiative.

On the low-budget end of the phalanx has been the Third Millennium, famous for its whimsical poll results showing that more young people believed in UFOs than in Social Security's viability. Although the group is small and has a relatively small budget, it has repeatedly been called to testify before Congress. Third Millennium's message is that the system is in dire shape and "Band-Aids" will not fix it. As of 1997, it was reported that Third Millennium's second largest funder was Pete Peterson, the New York investment banker discussed above.

Financial institutions, which once thought that individual defined contribution accounts would be a gold mine, now seem to have backed away from wholehearted endorsement of efforts to privatize Social Security. Their reversal appears to reflect the recognition that setting up and maintaining accounts for millions of low-wage workers would be very expensive and that the profit potential is much less than originally envisioned. Moreover, such an effort would likely bring scrutiny and regulation from the federal government that could harm other aspects of their business. Nevertheless, their initial excitement and the financial support they provided for conservative think tanks was a major factor behind the enthusiasm for individual accounts.

In summary, the emergence of deficit, interest in improving Social Security returns, the desire to save in advance of the retirement of the baby boom, the self-confidence of a growing number of higher-income individuals, and profit motivation from financial institutions have all contributed toward the enthusiasm for the DC approach. This list is in no way exhaustive, however, in that political calculations have also entered into proposals. For example, several proponents of introducing a small individual account into the current Social Security program concluded that a tax increase to support the current system was impossible and introducing a small individual account was the only way to get more money in the program. Thus, political assessments as well as value judgments and economics have all played roles in bringing the DC-DB debate to the fore. The question is what such a shift would mean for individuals and for society as a whole.

Medicare

The sources of enthusiasm for a DC arrangement for Medicare seem somewhat less complicated. Even after significant spending cuts made by the Balanced Budget Act of 1997, Medicare faces a long-term budget crunch. The most recent trustees' reports project exhaustion of the Hospital Insurance trust fund in 2023 and spending under the Supplementary Medical Insurance portion of Medicare to increase even faster. This crunch reflects both the aging of the population and the growth in per capita health care spending. The population 65 and over will double by 2030, and medical outlays for older people are four times those for the working age population. More importantly, however, per capita Medicare spending is projected to increase significantly, driven by technological breakthroughs in medicine and their increasing utilization.

While Medicare's projected long-run deficit is spurring calls for reform, the program's benefits, in fact, are less comprehensive than much private sector insurance. For example, Medicare does not cover prescription drugs and provides only very limited mental health benefits. Moreover, Medicare does not place an upper bound on cost sharing responsibilities for hospital stays, skilled nursing facility care, or physician costs. As a result, people with long and complicated illnesses and no supplementary private insurance could incur tens of thousands of dollars of out-of-pocket expenses. The challenge, then, is not only to control the costs of the benefits currently provided by Medicare but also to create some room for improvement in the benefit package.

Despite its success and popularity, almost everyone agrees that the current system is inefficient, not because it spends excessive money for administration but rather because it pays for some health care that may not be worthwhile and because it does not act as a prudent purchaser on behalf of the nation's elderly (Reinhardt 1999). The tendency to cover unnecessary care is reflected in the large and persistent regional differences in the level of Medicare spending that appear to have no demonstrable effects on health care outcomes. In its role as purchaser of goods and services, current law prevents the government from using such efficiency-enhancing measures as competitive bidding, selective contracting with preferred providers, and disease and case management techniques common in the private sector.

The obvious inefficiencies and the projected long-term deficit have spurred calls for reform. Because Medicare currently offers a defined package of services to all enrollees, the government faces significant risk for any rise in the cost of services, whether it is related to changes in technology, prices, or volumes. Some have suggested that the government could limit future expenses, spur competition and efficiency, and increase beneficiary choice, by guaranteeing a specified contribution toward health insurance expenses for the elderly and leaving the choice of the specific insurance plan to the individual. In short, enthusiasm for the DC-type approach appears to stem from a desire to hold down costs and the belief that competition among private plans will hold down costs better than reform of the traditional Medicare program. Proposals for major restructuring of Medicare, unlike those pertaining to Social Security, come as much from traditional supporters of the program as from critics. The proposals for defined contribution plans under Medicare fall into two major categories, pure defined contribution (the voucher approach) and premium support.

THE IMPACT ON INDIVIDUALS OF A SHIFT FROM DB TO DC

Neither DC nor DB plans are intrinsically superior; they involve a number of trade-offs (Bodie, Marcus, and Merton 1988). The question is which is most appropriate in terms of basic income support and political implications.

Social Security

Social Security benefits are currently based on career earnings, indexed to reflect the growth in average wages over time. The benefit structure is progressive in the sense that it replaces a higher percentage of the preretirement earnings of a low-wage earner than of a high earner. In 2000 the replacement rate for an individual retiring at age 65 with a history of average earnings was 43.0 percent; for the low earner,

57.8 percent; and for the person earning at the taxable maximum, 25.4 percent (U.S. House 1998). Benefits are adjusted fully for changes in the cost of living after retirement. Social Security provides additional benefits for spouses and for survivors, who are usually women. Proponents of privatization would replace some of this defined benefit arrangement with defined contribution accounts so that benefits would depend on contributions and investment returns.

The arguments for the defined contribution approach rest more on value judgments and political assessments than on economics. As discussed by Geanakoplos, Mitchell, and Zeldes in chapter 12 of this book, a defined contribution approach alone—without prefunding—will not raise returns. Not all proponents of a DC approach understand this point; some suggest that simply sending payroll taxes to Fidelity or Merrill Lynch instead of the Treasury will enable participants to enjoy higher returns, but such assertions completely ignore the burden of transition costs. Prefunding would eventually raise returns, but higher returns to future generations would be gained at the expense of lower returns to current generations who have to pay twice, first to cover promised benefits for others and second to build up reserves in their own accounts. The question of how much to prefund requires weighing the welfare of one generation against that of another. Moreover, prefunding can be accomplished either in the trust funds or individual accounts.

The legitimate arguments for a defined contribution component for Social Security rest more on the merits of individual control and the ability to match risks to tastes. Many proponents also think that a combined defined benefit–defined contribution approach is more politically stable in the long run than the current system. Others believe that avoiding social investing issues associated with trust fund purchases of equities more than outweighs the additional costs of setting up individual accounts and regulating their activities.

The basic argument against shifting from a defined benefit to a defined contribution plan for Social Security is that it would put people's benefits at risk and make them unpredictable. As argued by the late Herbert Stein (1997), an uncertain amount is fundamentally inconsistent with the philosophy behind the program. "If there is no social interest in the income people have at retirement, there is no justification for the Social Security tax. If there is such an interest, there is a need for policies that will assure that the intended amount of income is *always* forthcoming. It is not sufficient to say that some people who are very smart or very lucky in the management of their funds will have high incomes and those who are not will have low incomes and that everything averages out."

In other words, retirement income that depends on one's skills as an investor is not consistent with the goals of a mandatory Social Security program. Remember that Social Security is the major source of income for two-thirds of the 65-and-over population and virtually the only source for the poorest 30 percent. The whole point of having a Social Security system is to provide workers with a predictable retirement benefit. Social Security benefits are quite modest; the average worker retiring at age 62 in 2001 got $892 per month (Social Security Administration 2001). That modest benefit should be an amount that people can count on and supplement with income from private pensions and other sources. It should not depend on investment decisions in a volatile stock market.

In addition to the philosophical argument, individual accounts raise a host of practical problems such as potential access before retirement, lack of automatic annuitization, and cost.

Access before Retirement. Individual accounts create a very real political risk that account holders would pressure Congress for access to these accounts, albeit for worthy purposes such as medical expenses, education, or home purchase. Although most proposals prohibit such withdrawals, experience with existing IRAs and 401(k)'s suggests that holding the line is unlikely. To the extent that Congress acquiesces and allows early access—no matter how worthy the purpose—retirees will end up with inadequate retirement income.

Lack of Automatic Annuitization. Another risk is that individuals stand a good chance of outliving their savings, unless the money accumulated in their individual accounts is transformed into annuities. But few people purchase private annuities, and costs are high in the private annuity market.[10] Even if costs were not high, the necessity of purchasing an annuity at retirement exposes individuals to interest rate risk; if rates are high, they will receive a large monthly amount, if rates are low, the amount will be much smaller. Moreover, the private annuity market does not offer inflation-adjusted benefits. In contrast, by keeping participants together and forcing them to convert their funds into annuities, Social Security avoids adverse selection and provides a good vehicle for inflation-adjusted benefits.

Cost. The 1994–96 Social Security Advisory Council estimated that the administrative costs of an IRA-type individual account would be 100 basis points per year.[11] A 100-basis-point annual charge sounds benign, but it would reduce total accumulations by roughly 20 percent over a forty-year work life. Moreover, although the 100-basis-point estimate includes the cost of marketing, tracking, and maintaining the account, it does not include brokerage fees. If the individual did not select an index fund, then transaction costs could be twice as high. Indeed, the United Kingdom, which has a system of personal saving accounts, has experienced considerably higher costs (Murthi, Orszag, and Orszag 2001). Finally, because these transaction costs would involve a large flat charge per account, they would be considerably more burdensome for low-income participants than for those with higher incomes.

Many advocates of individual accounts have now recognized the very high administrative costs of the IRA approach and have fallen back to recommending a 401(k) or federal Thrift Savings Plan (TSP) mechanism. Costs would be substantially less under this alternative, although it would still double the costs of the current Social Security program. Moreover, for those concerned about government involvement, this approach has the government picking the appropriate equity funds and retaining control of the money. This is not a particular problem in my view, but for those who are concerned about government investment in private sector activities, the TSP approach raises all the same issues as investment by the central trust funds.

In addition to all the economic arguments advanced above against shifting from a DB to a DC arrangement for Social Security, the most serious concern is that even a small individual account component contains the seeds of dissolution for the entire Social Security program.[12] The fear is that as the mixed DC-DB system develops over time, moderate and high earners will think that they are getting a much better return in their individual account than in the reduced Social Security plan. Of course, the comparison is unfair since Social Security must pay benefits to earlier generations of retirees, finance disability and survivor insurance, and provide adequate benefits to low-income workers and women who spend time out of the labor force. Nevertheless, these higher earners will press for further reductions in the traditional defined benefit in order to have more money directed to individual accounts. The fundamental concern is that in the end, under this scenario, Social Security will dissolve into a system of defined contribution accounts plus some form of safety net for the lowest earners. In the process, low earners will lose the redistributional provisions that are an integral part of Social Security and instead become dependent on some targeted program, subject to all the uncertainties associated with the annual appropriation procedures of Congress. Thus, whereas individual accounts are merely risky and costly for the average and above average worker, they could end up being disastrous for vulnerable workers in the future.[13]

Furthermore, it is not clear that switching from a defined benefit plan to a two-tier system with a defined contribution component will improve efficiency. Many proponents of a two-tier approach for Social Security argue that strengthening the link between benefits and contributions in the top tier will reduce the extent to which the payroll tax distorts labor supply decisions. But it is impossible to evaluate the merits of that hypothesis by looking simply at the defined contribution component. The extent to which the payroll tax distorts labor supply decisions depends on the whole Social Security system, not just one part of it.

The two-tier approach trades a complicated and varying relationship between taxes and benefits under the existing system for two benefit programs—one in which the benefit is more linked to taxes and one in which it is less linked. In the extreme, some have proposed a flat benefit for the bottom tier, which would make the payroll tax for that portion of the program purely distortionary. With one tier more linked and the other tier less linked, the two-tier approach would have the same amount of linkage on average as the current system, although the pattern would be different for different workers. Thus, there is no reason to think that the two-tier approach, considered as a whole, would be less distortionary than the current system.

An issue also arises as to how people might respond with respect to total saving under the two approaches. The DC arrangement makes very transparent the level of individual contributions but obscures how adequate benefits will be compared to preretirement income. The DB approach makes future replacement rates apparent but obscures how benefits are related to contributions (Diamond 1999). In addition, individuals bear more investment risk under a DC than under a DB arrangement. People could respond to these different environments in one of two ways. On the one hand, since individuals bear more risk under the DC formulation, they might save more than they would under Social Security's DB commitment. Alternatively, individuals could suffer from "wealth illusion" in that the accumulation of a large pile of assets makes them feel rich, and they save less than they would under a Social Security defined benefit plan. In other words, the form in which retirement income is provided could affect how much people save.

In summary, although individuals would have more control over their investments if Social Security moved from a DB to a DC arrangement, this increased control would come at a steep price.

Medicare

The impact on individuals of a DC approach for Medicare depends on whether the restructuring takes the form of a pure DC payment or a premium support formulation. Under the most extreme form of the DC payment, the initial amount could be unrelated to health care costs; it could be set simply to achieve a targeted level of health care spending. Similarly, increases in the DC payment over time could be tied not to increases in health care costs but rather to the Consumer Price Index or the gross domestic product (GDP). This approach would shift all the risks for high health care spending from the government to individuals.

Under the premium support approach, the initial payment is more closely linked to the actual costs of care. Insurance providers in a given geographical market could be asked to bid on the cost of insuring a minimum package of services, and the average of those bids could then be used to set the dollar payment to each Medicare beneficiary in that market. The government would be responsible for paying a percentage of the required premium. The level of premium support would increase in line with the costs of insurance. As a result, both the government and the individual would share the risks of higher health care costs.

Both the DC and premium support approaches differ from the current DB arrangement in that the premiums paid by different individuals will vary. Under the current system, beneficiaries pay their Part B premium as well as any required cost sharing, and they are guaranteed the basic insurance package. But under either of the restructuring options, beneficiaries who wanted lower deductibles or copayments or more doctor or hospital options could use their own money to buy more expensive policies. Beneficiaries who wanted to save money could join cheaper plans and receive the difference between the amount of the fixed payment and their premium contribution. The whole purpose of the exercise is to make beneficiaries sensitive to the variation in costs among plans, so that individuals have the incentive to get the best deal for their money.

The question is, What would happen to Medicare costs, and particularly Medicare beneficiaries' out-of-pocket expenses, under either a pure defined contribution (voucher) or a premium sharing arrangement? The importance of that question is highlighted by the fact that health care costs are already a significant financial burden for the elderly. As a percent of family income, health spending in 1996 amounted to 21 percent for all elderly but ranged from 11 percent for those with higher incomes to 30 percent for the poor and near-poor (Reinhardt 1999).[14]

A recent study compared beneficiaries' out-of-pocket expenses as projected under the existing Medicare plan with those estimated under both a pure defined contribution (voucher) and a premium support option (Moon 1999). Without cost savings, the voucher approach would raise out-of-pocket expenses of Medicare beneficiaries in 2025 by between $835 and $2,011 (1998 dollars), depending on whether the initial voucher amount was adjusted over time by the growth in GDP or the growth in per capita GDP.[15] These increases should be compared with projected baseline out-of-pocket spending per beneficiary in 2025 of $3,074 (compared to $1,472 in 1998). Advocates of the voucher approach claim, however, that costs will be lower than the baseline because of the competition that comes from the restructuring. Assuming that per capita spending grew 0.5 percent less each year than projected in the baseline, vouchers could reduce beneficiary out-of-pocket expenses in 2025 by $324 or raise them by $889, again depending on how the initial amount was adjusted over time.

In contrast to the voucher option, where the Medicare beneficiary bears all the risks associated with higher health care costs, the premium support approach allows the government and the beneficiary to share in these risks. Thus, the burden for the typical beneficiary would be less under the premium approach than under the voucher mechanism. For example, in the study cited above, if the government paid an amount equal to 85 percent of the median premium (and even if the reform achieved no cost savings), out-of-pocket expenses would rise by only $137 (1998 dollars) by 2025.[16]

Although the premium support approach has the desirable feature of sharing the burden of higher health care costs between the government and beneficiaries, it still has some downside risks. The most serious is the possibility that differential cost savings could ultimately price low-income individuals out of the traditional fee-for-service Medicare plan. Assume that private plans saw a 0.5 percent reduction in their projected rate of future growth per year and the traditional Medicare plan saw no reduction. Both the out-of-pocket payment for the person choosing the median-priced private plan and the government's payment, which is set at 85 percent of the median-priced private plan, would decline relative to the baseline. At the same time, the reduced government payment would sharply raise the cost of choosing the traditional Medicare plan, which did not see any reduction in program costs. For example, in the study cited above, whereas the 2025 out-of-pocket cost of those choosing the median plan would decline by $25, the cost of those choosing the traditional Medicare plan would rise by $1,199. If those going into the high-priced Medicare plan were only the wealthy, such an outcome might not be a problem. But if those wanting the traditional plan were the very old, who were afraid to switch plans, or the very ill, the outcome would be less acceptable.[17] Given that the older and sicker—and therefore the poorer—are the most reluctant to change plans, the erosion of Medicare's entitlement to an affordable fee-for-service option would fall on the most vulnerable.

THE IMPACT ON SOCIETY OF A SHIFT FROM DB TO DC

Shifting from DB to DC arrangements for the nation's health and retirement systems would have a profound affect on society. Although the precise impacts differ for Social Security and Medicare, the overall effect would be more unequal outcomes, worsening the distribution of income and wealth.

Social Security

Shifting funds to individual accounts reduces the ability to redistribute income. The whole point of such a shift is to emphasize individual equity, that is, a fair return for the individual saver, rather than adequacy for all. Taking part of what the high earner makes to improve the return for the low earner would be contrary to the spirit of such a plan. To meet this objection, many advocates of the DC approach provide either a flat benefit amount or a healthy minimum benefit for low-wage workers. In either case, maintaining redistribution within the program is unlikely to be sustainable.

A mixed DB-DC system with a flat benefit and a DC account is likely to respond very differently to change over time than the existing DB arrangement. For example, suppose that the overall size of Social Security was viewed as too large as the retirement of the baby boom neared. Benefit cuts under the existing program would likely affect all people at all points in the income distribution proportionately; for example, the extension of the normal retirement age in 1983 was a form of across-the-board cut. Congress might even make some attempt to protect the benefits of workers with low incomes. Cuts under a mixed DB-DC system are likely to be very different. Congress would likely view the DC component as individual saving and see little gain from cutting it back. The more likely target would be the flat minimum benefit, which goes to both those who need it and those who do not. Higher-wage workers would find that they got very little for their payroll tax dollar from such a residual Social Security program and would withdraw their support. As the minimum was cut repeatedly, it would become inadequate for low-wage workers. In response, Congress would be likely to replace the flat benefit with a means-tested program.

Observers sometimes argue that the same economic outcome can be achieved either through means-tested benefits or through universal payments that are then taxed back. The thrust of this argument is that, in economic terms, little difference exists between means-tested public assistance and more general programs that usually fall under the heading of social insurance. This conclusion ignores psychological, social, and institutional factors. In fact, the two approaches differ dramatically: they grow out of different historical traditions, they have different impacts on their recipients, and they are viewed very differently by the public.

Social insurance reflects a long history of people getting together to help themselves.[18] The origins and tradition of social insurance are the nearly universal response of wage economies to the fact that most of the people are dependent on earnings; they grow out of efforts of workers to protect themselves and their families from the loss of those earnings. This self-help approach means that individuals have an earned right to benefits; they receive payments based on their past earnings from funds to which they have contributed. The programs involve no test of need, other than the reduction or loss of earnings, and program benefits can be supplemented with income from saving or other sources.

Public assistance, in contrast, grows out of the punitive and paternalistic poor-law tradition.[19] This tradition is based on individual self-reliance and recognizes only begrudgingly a public responsibility for providing for the impoverished. The association between poverty and moral failing has produced systems that distinguish between the "deserving poor" and others, and the elderly are certainly viewed as more deserving than the nonelderly poor. As a result, programs aimed at the elderly, such as Supplementary Security Income (SSI), were better structured and more stable than Aid to Families with Dependent Children and other programs for the nonelderly poor. SSI is based on national standards, benefits are adjusted for inflation, and Congress does not make abrupt changes in the program. In contrast, means-tested programs for the nonelderly have always varied from one state to another, benefits have never been indexed for inflation, and Congress has felt perfectly justified in making abrupt changes.

The fact that means-tested programs for the elderly are better than means-tested programs for the nonelderly does not mean that they are desirable. They suffer from two major flaws. First, benefit levels are inadequate. SSI benefits alone fall significantly below the poverty line, although the $20 disregard ($30 for a couple) of some Social Security or other non-means-tested income and the value of food stamps eliminate some of the gap.[20] Couples fare somewhat better than single individuals, as do people who live in states that provide supplemental benefits. But on balance, benefits are inadequate judged by standards of poverty. Moreover, unlike Social Security benefits, SSI benefits are not adjusted to reflect the increase in society's standard of living. The program and the government's whole concept of what constitutes poverty make no adjustment for the increase in economic well-being that working people enjoy as a result of productivity growth.

The second major problem is the stigma attached to the receipt of SSI; no stigma is associated with Social Security benefits, which are viewed as an earned right. As a result, many who are eligible for SSI never claim their benefits. Studies done in the 1980s suggest that only 50 percent of the aged and 55 percent of the disabled who are eligible for benefits actually participate in the program (Zedlewski and Meyer 1989). Although those with the greatest need have higher probability of claiming benefits, even among the most needy participation hovers at 70 percent. For recent years, the only information is for participation among the elderly poor; this figure, which averaged 57 percent in the 1980s, also was 57 percent for the period 1990–95 (*Greenbook* 1998, table 3-18, p. 307). Thus, it appears that many who are eligible continue not to claim benefits.

The point is that income support provided outside of Social Security is likely to be far less adequate than that provided within the program. As a result, people at the low end of the income distribution are likely to be worse off than they would be under the existing DB Social Security system. This means that moving from a DB to a DC arrangement is likely to produce a society with even more unequal distribution of income and wealth than we have already experienced and with the decline in social cohesion that accompanies such inequality.

Medicare

The rationale for moving to a DC or premium support approach for Medicare is that competition among plans would be more successful at holding down the growth in health care costs than the traditional Medicare program. To the extent that it would simplify the government's obligations and permit better control of health care costs, such a dramatic restructuring would be the key to reforming a relatively inefficient Medicare system.

If the savings did not materialize, then future Medicare beneficiaries would see a big rise in out-of-pocket expenditures. And even if the savings were achieved, serious problems could emerge (Moon 1999). For example, even with the cost savings, a DC plan indexed to per capita GDP would produce roughly a 20 percent increase in beneficiary liability by 2025. Similarly, in the case of a premium support option, even if the premium for the average individual did not increase, variations in plan premiums could place vulnerable beneficiaries at risk.

The second problem, which is shared by both the voucher and the premium support approach, is that any system based on choice in insurance markets has the potential to isolate the sickest population into small high-cost pools. Unless sophisticated risk-adjustment methods (which do not currently exist) could be used to vary the government payment rate with the level of expected medical expenses, market forces would put those in poor health at particular risk. Healthy individuals would have incentives to take policies with low premiums and limited coverage, which would drive up costs in the more comprehensive plans favored by less healthy persons. The result would be a system segmented not only by rich and poor but also by healthy and unhealthy.

The question is whether the potential gains from shifting to a premium support approach outweigh the potential risks to a vulnerable population. Some advocates clearly think it is the only way to solve the problem of rapidly rising Medicare costs (Aaron and Reischauer 1995); other experts disagree (Moon 1999). Skeptics of the cost saving argument point to the fact that although private plan performance has been good in the 1990s, over longer periods of time Medicare per capita spending has grown more slowly than private sector spending (Moon and Segal 1999). If the savings did not materialize, then future Medicare beneficiaries would see a big rise in out- of-pocket expenditures. And, as discussed above, even if the savings were achieved, serious problems could emerge. In short, movement to a defined contribution or premium support arrangement has the potential of putting low-income and sickly people at risk.

CONCLUSION

The conclusion that emerges from this analysis is that moving the nation's social insurance arrangements from DB to DC arrangements would have a profound effect on individuals and on society. In both cases, risks would shift from society as a whole to the individual, and vulnerable people could suffer significantly. Such a shift would probably accelerate the trend toward increased economic inequality and social segmentation.

The question is whether the gains from the DC approach are worth the costs. In the case of Social Security, the answer seems clearly no. If it is appropriate for the government to interfere with private sector decisions to ensure a basic level of retirement income, it does not make sense for that basic amount to be uncertain, depending on one's investment skills. Defined contribution plans also are costly and expose participants to the risks of early withdrawal and the risks associated with private annuitization at retirement. More fundamentally, separating income support from social insurance will almost certainly produce less redistribution, which will harm future generations of low-wage workers.

The answer is more difficult for Medicare, primarily because it is a more complicated problem. The current system is clearly inefficient in that it provides some care that is not needed and overpays for many services. The question is how best to reform the system. Can it be done within the current program, or is a major restructuring the only answer? The risks associated with a DC or premium support approach are clear: vulnerable people who already pay up to 30 percent of their income for health care face the prospect of even higher costs. The potential gains are less obvious, and the evidence that the new approach would be successful is sketchy. Thus, the answer may be that change should wait for more compelling evidence about the success of private sector competition.

NOTES

1. Under a defined benefit plan, the employer or the government promises a specific benefit, and employers or, in the case of Social Security, employers and employees make the contributions necessary to fund such benefits. In the private sector, the benefit would be a certain percentage of pay (most often the highest average pay over a three- or five-year period) for each year of service. Social Security provides benefits based on workers' lifetime earnings (indexed by the growth in wages in the economy over time) and adjusts the benefit for inflation after retirement. In contrast, under defined contribution plans, individuals and their employers make contributions for the account of participating employees, and benefits are based on the contributions and accumulated earnings.

2. Medicare is composed of two programs. Part A covers inpatient hospital services, skilled nursing facilities, home health care, and hospice care. Part B covers primarily physician and outpatient hospital services. Part A is financed by a 2.9 percent payroll tax, shared equally by employers and employees. Medicare Part B is financed primarily from general revenues and enrollee premiums. By 1999 premiums contributed about 25 percent of the fund's income, with most of the remainder from general revenues.

3. Social Security financing will put increasing pressure on the unified federal budget before the trust fund balances are exhausted. Although shortfalls between 2015 and 2037 can be met in a technical sense from the program itself, first by drawing on the interest earned on the trust funds and then by drawing on the funds themselves, these actions will lead to a higher unified deficit unless the government raises taxes, reduces other spending, or increases federal borrowing.

4. Social Security's long-term financing problem is actually somewhat more complicated. Under current law, the tax rate is fixed while costs are rising, and this pattern produces surpluses now and large deficits in the future. As a result of this profile, under present law, each year the 75-year projection period moves forward, another year with a large deficit is added to the 75-year deficit. Assuming that nothing else changes, this phenomenon would increase the 75-year deficit slightly (0.08% of taxable payroll with today's deficits) each year. Many policymakers believe that the system should not be left with a huge deficit in the 76th year. Stabilizing the trust fund ratio—the ratio of assets to next year's outlays—would achieve this aim. A stable trust fund ratio means that the flows into and out of the trust fund are balanced, and therefore additional years do not increase the deficit as they are included in the projection period.

5. Interestingly enough, worsening economic and demographic assumptions have not—on balance—been responsible for the current deficit. Since 1983 the demographic developments have been positive—at least from the program's perspective. Life expectancy assumptions have been lowered slightly, thereby reducing long-run costs. The positive impact on long-run costs from changing demographic assumptions was roughly offset, however, by changing economic assump-

tions. In particular, the trustees lowered the assumed rate of real wage growth as it became clear that the productivity slowdown was more persistent than originally contemplated. On balance, the economic and demographic changes have roughly offset each other. About a third of the emerging deficit came from the fact that as time passes, the seventy-five-year valuation period ends in a later year, so more high-cost out-years are included in the projections. Including more deficit years raises the seventy-five-year deficit. Another third came from the disability caseload: disability cases grew much faster than anticipated, primarily because of legislative, regulatory, and judicial action that made it easier for individuals to qualify for disability benefits. The final third involved one-shot changes in the methodology used to project the future. For example, the large increase in the deficit from 1993 to 1994 was due mainly to new data suggesting that workers have more years of covered employment than previously had been thought and therefore were entitled to higher projected benefits.

6. For example, all three proposals emerging from the 1994–96 Advisory Council on Social Security (1997) advocated equity investment.

7. First, economically targeted investments (ETIs) account for no more than 2.5 percent of total state and local holdings. Although early studies showed plans sacrificing considerable return for targeting their investments to in-state activities, recent survey data reveal no adverse impact on returns as a result of the current small amount of ETI activity. Second, public plans in only three states have seriously engaged in shareholder activism, and this activism appears to have been motivated by a desire to improve the bottom line rather than to make a political statement. The literature suggests that this activity has had a negligible to positive impact on returns. Third, the only significant divestiture that has occurred was related to companies doing business in South Africa before 1994. This was a unique situation where worldwide consensus among industrial nations led to a global ban on investment in that country. With respect to tobacco, public plans have generally resisted divestiture, and only a few have actually sold their stock. Finally, state and local governments have borrowed occasionally from their pension funds or reduced their contributions in the wake of budget pressures, but this activity has been restrained by the courts and frequently reversed. Thus, the story at the state and local level is that although in the early 1980s some public plans sacrificed returns for social considerations, plan managers have become much more sophisticated. Today, public plans appear to be performing as well as private plans.

8. Although many lockbox proposals exist, they are all quite similar to that included in the Social Security and Medicare Safe Deposit Act of 1999, which the House of Representatives passed in May. This legislation changes the budget process so that Congress cannot use Social Security revenues to cover spending on non–Social Security programs unless there is a majority vote to do so. Theoretically, the vote requirement would have a chilling effect in that it would put on record those who supported such an action.

9. It is important to remember, however, that lockbox initiatives are designed to limit deficits in non–Social Security spending, not to restore balance to the Social Security program itself.

10. The reason for the high costs is adverse selection: people who think they will live for a long time purchase annuities, whereas those with, say, a serious illness keep their cash. Private insurers have to raise premiums to address the adverse selection problem, and this makes the purchase of annuities very expensive for the average person.

11. In addition to costs, a study by the Employee Benefit Research Institute (EBRI 1998) raised real questions about the ability, in anything like the near term, to administer a system of individual accounts in a satisfactory way. Unlike the current Social Security program, which deals with the reporting of wage credits, a system of personal accounts would involve the transfer of real money. It is only reasonable that participants would care about every dollar, and therefore employer errors in account names and numbers that arise under the current program would create enormous public relations problems under a system of individual accounts.

12. Most proposals that move toward DC arrangements also involve a cut in benefits for disabled workers. These proposals typically involve a reduction in Social Security benefit levels for both the disabled and retirees that, in theory, workers would make up through lifetime accumulations in their individual accounts. Thus, projections for the various reform proposals generally show for the average retired worker that the combined payment from the personal saving account and the reduced Social Security program would equal the benefit currently promised under Social Security. Unlike retirees, however, disabled workers would not have time before their disability to build up any significant reserves in their personal saving account to finance a full supplementary benefit. As a result, disabled workers would be likely to experience a substantial reduction in benefits.

13. Finally, women face the most risk from moving from a DB to a DC system. They could lose not only the progressive benefit formula, which is very important since women tend to be low earners, but also spouses' and widows' benefits, which help support women who spend time out of the labor force taking care of their families. Also, the inflation-indexed monthly benefits for life are particularly valuable to women, who on average live longer than men.

14. Poor is defined as less than 100 percent of the poverty line and near-poor as between 100 and 125 percent of the poverty threshold.

15. The key to the alternative outcomes is the mechanism used to establish the annual rate of growth for the vouchers. In the simulations, the voucher amounts were tied alternatively to total and per capita GDP growth. Since with a growing population, per capita GDP growth is slower than total GDP growth, it is a more stringent constraint on Medicare spending. The voucher amounts were calculated for 2025 and then compared to projected Medicare spending in that year for the typical beneficiary under the baseline scenario to calculate projected out-of-pocket costs.

16. Even if the government contribution were set at 80 percent of the median plan, beneficiaries' out-of-pocket expenses would rise by only $648.

17. Because the high costs would force many elderly persons out of the traditional plan, even though they are often fearful and skeptical of managed care, the Clinton administration proposed the "competitive defined benefit program." Instead of paying a fixed amount based on the average cost of competing plans, the government would pay based on the actual bids of the providers. If a person selected a plan costing less than Medicare's fee-for-service plan, he or she could keep 75 percent of the savings. This program would preserve entitlement not only to a specific set of benefits but also to fee-for-service medicine with unlimited choice among providers. The problem is that the administration's approach does not save much money.

18. As early as the Middle Ages, the guilds established formal benefit plans under which members made predetermined contributions while they were working and received specific benefits in the event of disability or death. The "customary funds" found in the mining districts of Austria and other central European countries as early as the sixteenth century were another forerunner of social insurance. Later, fraternal orders and friendly societies were organized by the hundreds for the central purpose of providing insurance protection for their members. Trade unions throughout the world developed protection plans against the risk of income loss.

19. The Elizabethan Poor Law of 1601, the first codification of social welfare policy in England, established the legal right of the poor to state-provided relief, which meant that they were no longer dependent on private charity. The 1601 legislation was deeply rooted, however, in the philosophy that individuals have moral responsibility for their own economic well-being. As a result, those capable of work but unwilling were given nothing; those able and willing to work but who were victims of economic circumstances were provided work; only those who were incapable of work, mainly the aged, the sick, and small children, were to be helped with public funds. Late in the eighteenth century, this was temporarily supplemented by the so-called Speenhamland system of providing allowances to workers who received wages below what was considered a subsistence level. The resulting increase in public expenditures was so great, however, that a new Poor Law was enacted in 1834. The new system, which once again stressed individual responsibility for one's own welfare, was considerably harsher than the one that preceded it.

20. In 1997 the federal SSI benefit for an individual was 77 percent of the $7,525 poverty line. Adding food stamps and the $20 disregard of income from Social Security or other (non-means-tested) sources brought that level to 88 percent. For couples, the basic benefit was 92 percent of the $9,491 poverty line, and food stamps and the $30 disregard brought the total to 104 percent of poverty (U.S. House 1998, tables 3-9 and 3-10, pp. 392–93).

REFERENCES

Aaron, H. J., and R. D. Reischauer. 1995. The Medicare Reform Debate: What Is the Next Step? *Health Affairs* 14, no. 4: 8–30.

————. 1998. *Countdown to Reform: The Great Social Security Debate.* New York: Century Foundation Press.

Advisory Council on Social Security. 1997. *Report of the 1994–1996 Advisory Council on Social Security.* Washington, D.C.: U.S. Government Printing Office.

Board of Trustees, Federal Old-Age and Survivors Insurance and Disability Insurance Trust Funds. 2000. *2000 Annual Report of the Board of Trustees of the Federal Old-Age and Survivors Insurance and Disability Insurance Trust Funds.* Washington, D.C.: U.S. Government Printing Office.

Bodie, Z., A. J. Marcus, and R. C. Merton. 1988. Defined Benefit versus Defined Contribution Plans: What Are the Real Trade-offs? In Z. Bodie, J. Shoven, and D. Wise, eds. *Pensions in the U.S. Economy,* chap. 5. Chicago: University of Chicago Press.

Cassidy, J. 1997. Spooking the Boomers. *New Yorker,* January 13.

Diamond, P. A. 1999b. The Transparency Myth. The World Bank (October). Mimeographed.

Employee Benefit Research Institute (EBRI). 1998. Individual Social Security Accounts: Issues in Assessing Administrative Feasibility. EBRI Issue Brief no. 203. EBRI, Washington, D.C.

Greenspan, A. 1999. *On Investing the Trust Fund in Equities.* Testimony before the Subcommittee on Finance and Hazardous Materials, Committee on Commerce, U.S. House of Representatives, 106th Cong., 1st sess., March 3.

Lieberman, T. 1997. Social Insecurity: The Campaign to Take the System Private. *Nation,* January 27.

Moon, M. 1999. Restructuring Medicare: Impact on Beneficiaries. Commonwealth Fund, New York, May.

Moon, M., and M. Segal. 1999. Beneath the Averages: An Analysis of Medicare and Private Expenditures. Henry J. Kaiser Family Foundation, Menlo Park, Calif.

Munnell, A. H., and P. Balduzzi. 1998. Investing the Social Security Trust Funds in Equities. No. 9802, March, Public Policy Institute, American Association of Retired Persons.

Munnell, A. H., and A. Sundén, with the assistance of C. Perry and R. Kling. 1999. Investment Practices of State and Local Pensions. In A. D. Arnold, M. J. Graetz, and A. H. Munnell, eds. *Pension in the Public Sector.* Pension Research Council Publication. Philadelphia: University of Pennsylvania Press.

Murthi, M., M. Orszag, and P. R. Orszag. 2001. Administrative Costs and Individual Accounts: Lessons from the U.K. Experience. In R. Holzmann and

J. Stigitz, eds., *New Ideas about Old Age Security*. Washington, D.C.: World Bank.

Reinhardt, U. E. 1999. Can America Afford Its Elderly Citizens? Thoughts on the Political Economy of Sharing. Policy Options for Reforming the Medicare Program, Washington, D.C.

Social Security Administration. 2001. *Fast Facts & Figures about Social Security*. Washington, D.C.: Office of Policy.

Stein, H. 1997. Social Security and the Single Investor. *Wall Street Journal,* February 5, 1997.

U.S. Bureau of the Census, Current Population Reports. 2000. *Money Income in the United States, 1999*. P60-206. Washington, D.C.: U.S. Government Printing Office.

U.S. House Committee on Ways and Means. 1998. *1998 Green Book*. Washington, D.C.: U.S. Government Printing Office.

Wolff, E. 1998. Recent Trends in the Size Distribution of Household Wealth. *Journal of Economic Perspectives* 12, no. 3: 131–50.

———. 2000. Recent Trends in Wealth Ownership. Working paper no. 300, Jerome Levy Institute, Annandale-on-Hudson, New York.

Zedlewski, S. R., and J. Meyer. 1989. *Toward Ending Poverty among the Elderly and Disabled through SSI Reform*. Urban Institute Report 89-1. Washington, D.C.: Urban Institute Press.

12

Private Accounts, Prefunding, and Equity Investment under Social Security

John Geanakoplos, Ph.D., Olivia S. Mitchell, Ph.D., and Stephen P. Zeldes, Ph.D.

As the U.S. Social Security system has matured, the rate of return received by participants has fallen. In the coming years, around the time the baby boom generation retires, the system will experience a budget shortfall. First, tax revenues will fall short of promised benefits, requiring spending the interest earnings, and then the principal, of the trust fund. Eventually, the trust fund will be depleted. This projected insolvency will necessitate benefit cuts or tax increases, leading to further declines in the rates of return individuals can expect.

Many advocates of reform suggest that an answer to this problem is to privatize Social Security. They argue that the creation of individual accounts invested in private capital markets, and especially in the stock market, will produce better rates of return for individuals than Social Security will. For example, Stephen Moore (1997) of the Cato Institute claimed that "privatization offers a much higher financial rate of return to young workers than the current system . . . if Congress were to allow a 25-year-old working woman today to invest her payroll tax contributions in private capital markets, her retirement benefit would be two to five times higher than what Social Security is offering." Presidential candidate Steve Forbes (1996) criticized Social Security because "the average worker retiring today receives a lifetime return of only about 2.2 percent on the taxes he has paid into the system. Contrast this with the historic 9–10 percent annual returns from stock market investments. . . . The advantages of an IRA-type approach are overpowering."

Our goal in this chapter is to challenge the following popular argument: projected returns to Social Security are low relative to expected returns on stocks and bonds, and therefore everyone would receive higher returns and be better off if the United States moved to a privatized system in which individuals could directly invest their contributions in stocks and bonds. We argue that for households with access to diversified capital markets, privatization without prefunding would not increase Social Security returns, when properly measured. Privatization together with prefunding would eventually raise the rate of return to future generations of participants, but at the cost of a lower rate of return to early generations.

The real economic benefit of privatization is the diversification that would be made available to constrained households that cannot participate on their own in diversified capital market investment portfolios. The improved-rate-of-return argument in favor of privatization thus has no force unless there are constrained households without access to diversified capital markets. However, this group of people is not generally recognized to be key to the popular argument just quoted. Indeed, in the presence of such constrained households, young market-savvy workers, who according to the popular argument should find privatization most appealing, will probably get lower returns as a result of privatization.

We begin by defining what privatization means and by distinguishing that concept from diversification and from prefunding. Next, we ask whether projected returns on Social Security are in fact below those anticipated from U.S. capital markets.[1] Finally, we ask whether low Social Security returns are a valid reason to support a privatization that does not involve prefunding. We conclude that several valid rationales can be offered to support privatization but that, taken by itself, the low rate of return on Social Security is not among them.

WHAT DO WE MEAN BY SOCIAL SECURITY PRIVATIZATION?

To begin, it is useful to draw a clear distinction between three terms that are often confused: *privatization* versus *diversification* versus *prefunding* of Social Security. By privatization we mean replacing the current, mostly unfunded, defined benefit Social Security old age program with a defined contribution system of individual accounts held in individual workers' names. By diversification we mean investing funds (either from the personal accounts or from the Social Security trust fund) into a broad range of assets. These assets might include U.S. private sector stocks and bonds and foreign securities, in addition to the government bonds now used exclusively by the Social Security trust fund. The focus is currently on diversifying into stocks. By prefunding we mean reducing the sum of the system's implicit and explicit debt (see Table 12.1).[2]

In the public debate, these terms are often linked, but they are conceptually different. It is easy to see why all three categories nevertheless appear together in the public mind. Suppose the Social Security system had begun as a forced saving plan in which all workers were obliged to set aside money for their retirement, which would be put into private accounts invested in a balanced portfolio of stocks and bonds. Then from the beginning the system would have been privatized, diversified, and completely prefunded.

The situation is quite different now from what it was in 1935 when the U.S. Social Security system began. Social security systems in the United States and in most other developed economies have amassed substantial unfunded liabilities; assets on hand are insufficient to pay for the present value of benefits that have been accrued and promised to workers and retirees based on contributions already made.[3] In the United States, for instance, the unfunded present value of Social Security promises totals about $9 trillion (Goss 1999). Although this Social Security debt is implicit rather than explicit, it is economically significant. The United States will surely not decide to eliminate this implicit debt by ignoring all of the promised benefits.

Our tripartite decomposition is intended to emphasize that Social Security reform could change any one of these three categories without changing the other two. For example, the trust fund could invest in

Table 12.1. Differentiating Privatization, Prefunding, and Diversification of Social Security

- **Privatization:** Replace existing social security system with a system of individual accounts held and managed by individuals.
- **Prefunding:** Raise contributions and/or cut benefits so as to lower the sum of explicit and implicit debt associated with the system.
- **Diversification:** Invest social security funds into a broad range of assets, including equities.

Privatization, prefunding, and diversification are distinct concepts. It is possible to have any one, without either of the other two.

		Privatization	
		NO	**YES**
Prefunding	**NO**	• Current system	• Create individual accounts • Issue recognition bonds • Perpetually roll over principal and enough interest to keep path of debt same as that of unfunded liability under current system
		Diversification **No:** Current system **Yes:** Borrow, invest proceeds in equities through trust fund	**Diversification** **No:** Require individual accounts to hold bonds **Yes:** Permit individual accounts to hold equities and bonds
	YES	• Raise taxes / cut benefits to decrease unfunded liability	• Create individual accounts • Issue recognition bonds • Raise taxes / cut benefits to make path of debt lower than path of unfunded liability under current system
		Diversification **No:** Invest trust fund in bonds **Yes:** Invest trust fund in equities	**Diversification** **No:** Require individual accounts to hold bonds **Yes:** Permit individual accounts to hold equities and bonds

stocks as well as bonds, thus diversifying without privatizing. Alternatively, workers could be given private accounts in which the money was always invested in government bonds, thus privatizing without diversifying. This is the case in Mexico's new individual account system: the Mexican government has required that all pension assets be invested only in inflation-indexed bonds (Mitchell and Barreto 1997). It is also possible to raise system funding without involving individual accounts; taxes could be raised or benefits cut, and the proceeds could be put into a central trust fund. Singapore's national Provident Fund, for example, is a nonprivatized, prefunded system in which the central government collects taxes sufficient to generate substantial assets, which it then invests on the system's behalf. Conversely, people could be given individual accounts without prefunding of benefit promises. A privatized but unfunded pension system has recently been established in Latvia, where payroll taxes are collected by the government, which then credits workers' so-called notional accounts with paper returns on contributions. Chile is the best-known example of a country whose program is both prefunded and privatized: here workers hold assets in individually managed accounts, and debt under the old system is being reduced over time.

Likewise in the United States, privatization without prefunding is quite possible; a Social Security reform that created a national 401(k)-type system of private accounts could be implemented with no change in Social Security debt. For example, the Social Security system could issue new explicit debt (recognition bonds), guaranteed by the federal government, with payouts set exactly equal to the benefit promises that have accrued to date under the current system. These bonds would be given to current participants in lieu of their accrued future benefit payments. All new contributions to Social Security would then go directly into private individual accounts.[4] If the recognition bonds were paid off in full with new government tax receipts, the debt would eventually disappear when the last of today's workers finally died. However, the Social Security system could instead borrow again in the future by issuing new bonds to meet the recognition bond coupon payments, and then do so again and again to meet the payments on these new bonds. Subject to some limits, the government could choose how much interest and principal to roll over and how much to pay off. If the government chose to keep the path of explicit debt equal to the path of unfunded liabilities under the current system (the implicit debt), the result would be a Social Security system that was privatized without being prefunded.

We examine here the claim that a privatized, diversified Social Security system could deliver higher returns without any additional prefunding. We do so in three steps. First, we analyze returns in a privatized system that confines investments to government bonds. Next, we examine returns in a privatized and diversified system in which investments in stocks are permitted. Finally, we analyze returns in a privatized and diversified system and allow for the possibility that there are some constrained households that do not currently have access on their own to diversified capital markets.

ARE PROJECTED RATES OF RETURN ON SOCIAL SECURITY LOWER THAN THOSE ON U.S. CAPITAL MARKETS?

A starting point for projecting future returns on U.S. capital markets is to examine historical returns. Table 12.2 reports the historical average of inflation-adjusted (that is, real) returns on stocks, bonds, and Treasury bills, as well as their variability. The average annual real return on stocks (as proxied by the S&P 500) was 9.4 percent; the corresponding return on intermediate-term government bonds was 2.3 percent.[5] Whether these provide reasonable forecasts for future years depends in part on one's judgment about whether the past will predict the future.

Cohort-specific rates of return under Social Security, from a study by Dean Leimer (1994), are presented in Figure 12.1. Historical data on current and past workers and retirees, as well as projections of future contributions and benefits, are used to compute rates of return, which we sometimes call by their more precise name, internal rates of return (IRRs). We note first that prospective (internal) rates of return depend on a host of predictions, including mortality, population growth, and real wage growth.[6] Second, the prospective IRR data are not those that would follow from forecasting taxes and benefits under *current*

Table 12.2. **Annual Inflation-Adjusted Returns on Stocks and**
          Government Bonds, 1926–1996

Asset	Arithmetic Average Real Return	Standard Deviation
S&P 500	9.4	20.4
Long-term government bond	2.4	10.5
Intermediate-term government bond	2.3	7.1
Short-term Treasury bill	0.7	4.2

Source: Data from Ibbotson and Associates 1998.

Social Security rules, since that system faces insolvency or actuarial imbalance. Instead, the IRR figures for the future assume that taxes will be increased enough to keep the system from running out of money.[7]

Figure 12.1 shows that early cohorts under the program received very high IRRs in real terms. Workers born in 1876 received a real return of over 35 percent a year. Workers born in 1900 received a 12 percent real return. The figure reveals that IRRs fell over time for subsequent cohorts. Leimer estimated the return to be 5.7 percent for those born in 1920 and about 2 percent for those born 1950–70. For workers born in 1975, he forecast that IRRs would be around 1.8 percent, dropping down to 1.5 percent for those born in 1998.

Young or middle-aged workers listening to the Social Security reform debate today could reasonably ask how their anticipated IRR from Social Security would compare with what could be earned by investing in U.S. capital markets. Leimer's data indicate IRRs of about 1.5 percent for future cohorts; theoretical models of a pure pay-as-you-go Social Security system in steady state suggest that the IRR would be expected to equal the growth of the wage base, which is currently forecast to be about 1.2 percent.[8] Either way, it is clear that projected IRRs are well below expected returns from investment in equities based on historical averages and that they fall short of average government bond returns in Table 12.2 as well. Thus, the popular rate-of-return argument in favor of privatization seems to apply whether or not the investments are diversified.

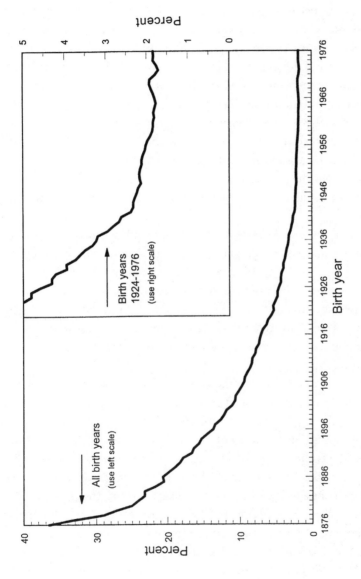

Fig. 12.1. Estimated real internal rates of return on Social Security contributions. *Source:* Leimer (1994) tax increase balanced budget scenario.

WHY ARE PROJECTED SOCIAL SECURITY RETURNS LOW?

Projected Social Security returns are low not because of waste or inefficiency but because the system developed as a primarily unfunded, pay-as-you-go system. In a pure pay-as-you-go system, all contributions received by the system are paid out in the same year as benefits to someone else, and no trust fund is accumulated. This means that there are some early beneficiaries who receive benefits even though they have not made any contributions. The U.S. Social Security system was not started as a pure pay-as-you-go system, because only those individuals who contributed some money to the system were eligible for benefits. Nevertheless, the accumulated trust fund was minimal, so that it was still the case that the present value of benefits received by those retiring soon after 1940 far exceeded the present value of contributions they had made.

The key to understanding why IRRs must fall in our nearly pay-as-you-go Social Security system is to exploit the connection between net present values (NPVs) and internal rates of return (IRRs). Whenever the NPV for a cohort is positive, the IRR for the cohort will be greater than the market rate, and vice versa. Therefore, stating that early generations received a positive net transfer from Social Security is equivalent to saying that they received above-market rates of return on their contributions.[9]

In Figure 12.1 we saw that the real rates of return for early cohorts (birth year 1876–1900) ranged from 12 to 37 percent.[10] Figure 12.2 presents estimates of cohort net present values, derived from Leimer's study, corresponding to these cohort rates of return.[11] The dotted line (the left scale) is the net present value, in 1997 dollars, of all contributions and benefits for individuals born in the indicated year. As expected for the beginning of a pay-as-you-go system, the present value of benefits exceeded taxes for the first wave of retirees. Each birth year cohort between 1880 and 1900 (those retiring approximately in 1945–1965) received a lifetime transfer (in 1997 present value dollars) of between $40 billion and $240 billion. The solid line in Figure 12.2 (the right scale) is the cumulative sum of all net transfers received by cohorts born before and including the indicated birth year. Cohorts born through 1900 received a cumulative net transfer of about $3 trillion.

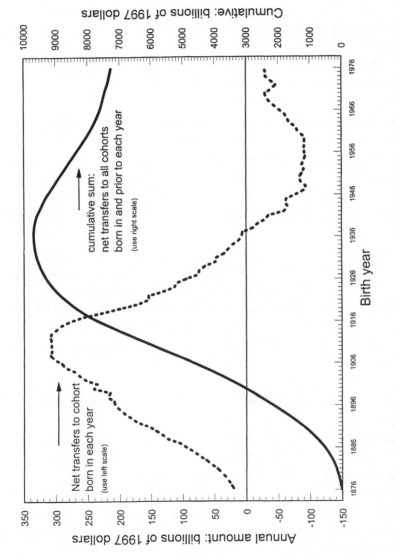

Fig. 12.2. Social Security net intercohort transfers. *Source:* Leimer (1994) tax increase balanced budget scenario and authors' calculations. All figures are present values as of 1997.

In part because the Social Security tax rates started out low in 1937 (the initial tax rate was 2 percent) and gradually rose over time, the positive transfers to retirees continued well past the first wave of beneficiaries. Those born between 1901 and 1917 received net transfers with present value of about $4.9 trillion. In addition, the twenty age cohorts born between 1918 and 1937 are scheduled to receive a further net transfer of $1.8 trillion, in present value. Adding up the $3 trillion, $4.9 trillion, and $1.8 trillion, we arrive at an estimate of the total net transfer to the first sixty age cohorts of $9.7 trillion, or roughly $10 trillion.

What do the positive net subsidies and high returns for early cohorts have to do with the low returns forecast for current and future cohorts? It can be shown that the present value across all cohorts (from the beginning of the system forward for the infinite future) of the net transfers received must sum to zero.[12] Inevitably, cohorts born after 1937 must give up in aggregate the whole $10 trillion, discounted back to 1997 dollars.[13]

In other words, since past cohorts received positive net transfers, some present and future cohorts must receive negative net transfers. The connection described above between net transfers and rates of return means that we can translate this statement about net transfers into a statement about rates of return. Because past cohorts received rates of return greater than market rates, current and future cohorts must receive rates of return lower than market rates.[14]

How big the negative transfer must be for any one cohort born after 1937 depends on how the total transfer is spread across all the cohorts. Observe that according to (our modifications of the numbers in) Leimer, the cohorts born between 1938 and 1977 are scheduled to receive negative transfers of about $2.5 trillion, reducing the total projected net transfer to cohorts born before 1978 to approximately $7.2 trillion. Of course much of this $2.5 trillion transfer has not yet occurred. The individuals born in 1975, for example, have just begun to work and so have not had time to make any significant transfers through the Social Security system. Roughly half of the working careers of cohorts born between 1938 and 1977 had passed by 1997. We might guess, therefore, that subtracting the present value of Social Security taxes already paid by cohorts born between 1938 and 1977 from the present value of Social Security benefits already accrued as a result of these taxes gives about half of $2.5 trillion. That would mean that the sum of the net tax burden on all contributions made after 1997 would equal $9.7 trillion minus $1.25 trillion, or about $8.5 trillion. In fact, the number must be equal to the unfunded liability, which was calculated independently by Stephen Goss (1999) at just under $9 trillion, thus providing a check on our numbers.

There is a simple way of estimating the transfers that might be made each year after 1997. Suppose the total negative transfer of $9 trillion is spread equitably among all the cohorts, in the sense that every cohort is (or will be) asked to give up the same percentage of its earnings each year of its working career. In a steadily growing economy, the required annual transfer in year t would then be approximately equal to $(r - g) \times$ (unfunded liabilities at end of year $t - 1$), where r is the riskless real rate of return and g is the growth rate of the economy (approximately equal to the sum of population growth and technological improvement).[15] Assuming that r is about 2.3 percent (as indicated in Table 12.2) and that g is about 1.2 percent, and using $9 trillion as the current unfunded liability, transfers in 1997 must be on the order of $100 billion. Measured as a percentage of Social Security taxes paid, which were about $400 billion in 1997, this transfer represents about 25 percent of annual payroll taxes.[16]

Spreading the remaining start-up cost of our pay-as-you-go Social Security system evenly over all cohorts requires each cohort to give up about 25 percent of every annual contribution, or 3 percentage points of the current 12.4 percent payroll tax. In other words, implicit interest payments explain why young workers may expect only 75 percent of their taxes back in (the present value of) benefits over their lifetimes.[17] As long as the Social Security debt is spread out over all subsequent cohorts, returns on Social Security will be lower for every cohort than returns paid by bonds.

ARE LOW SOCIAL SECURITY RETURNS
A VALID REASON TO SUPPORT PRIVATIZATION?

The second step in the causal argument supporting privatization seems the easiest and most straightforward—so much so that it is often taken for granted. If projected returns on Social Security are significantly lower than those offered in U.S. capital markets, doesn't it immediately follow that we would all be better off if we were allowed to invest Social Security contributions directly in private securities? Frequent arguments in the popular press and some studies by advocates of privatization suggest that this is the case.[18] Yet this conclusion is misleading for two reasons: it ignores transition costs (that is, how do we eliminate the implicit Social Security debt?); and it does not account for changes in risk borne by participants.

Transition Costs

Let us begin by ignoring issues related to risk, such as diversification. Since the rate of return on bonds is greater than the rate of return of Social Security, it would be easy to increase the return for future cohorts by simply ignoring past contributions and not paying any benefits accrued under the current system. The old Social Security system could be shut down, and all new Social Security tax receipts could be put into private accounts invested in bonds. Future cohorts would be able to earn market returns. But then the entire $10 trillion cost of subsidizing the first sixty cohorts would in effect be borne by the current middle-aged and old, who would then have paid into the system for years and received nothing in return.

Alternatively, one could shut down the old system and privatize but continue to pay all the Social Security benefits accrued to date, based on past contributions. As noted earlier, recognition bonds could be issued to workers and retirees for the full amount of the unfunded liability (that is, $9 trillion). If the government did not default on these bonds, new taxes would have to be raised to pay interest on the recognition bonds. Further, if the new taxes were set to keep the path over time of recognition bond debt the same as the path of implicit debt under the current system, then the new taxes would correspond exactly to the transfers we mentioned in the last section.[19] In other words, it can be shown that the new taxes raised would eliminate all of the higher returns on individual accounts.[20] Let us see why.

Consider a steady-state economy growing at the constant rate g with market interest rate r and with a pay-as-you-go Social Security system begun sometime in the distant past. As pointed out earlier, the implicit tax paid through Social Security in each year is $(r - g) \times$ (the unfunded liability at the end of the previous year). If suddenly at date t Social Security were privatized and transition costs were ignored (for example because accrued benefits were never paid), the IRR on the privatized system in which individual accounts were all held in marketed bonds would be equal to r. If, instead, recognition bonds were issued, their market value at date t would have to be equal to the unfunded liability in that year. To keep the debt growing at the same rate g as the economy, taxes in the next year would have to be raised in the amount $(r - g) \times$ (unfunded liability). The extra taxes needed to finance the payments on the recognition bonds would thus be identical to the transfers made each year in the old Social Security system. By choosing the tax rates appropriately, the tax burden could be made to fall on exactly the same people who were contributing more to Social Security than they were receiving in benefits.[21] Aside from the transfers, participants in the current pay-as-you-go Social Security system are in effect earning the bond rate of return on their money. In a privatized system in which households invested their forced saving in bonds, they would have to pay in new taxes exactly what they paid before in transfers.

In other words, the rate of return on a privatized system in which all private investment is in marketed bonds, net of new taxes needed to pay the appropriate interest on the recognition bond debt, would be identical to the low rate of return on the current system. This is true regardless of how large the difference is between r and g—this difference could be 1.1 percent, 3 percent, 10 percent, or even higher.[22] That is why it is fallacious to assume that all future participants in a privatized Social Security system could earn returns equal to those forecast for U.S. capital markets. Thus, we agree that returns to the current Social Security system are low, but we argue that there is no costless way of improving them for all current and future workers.

Suppose, alternatively, that taxes were raised disproportionately on current cohorts, and the receipts were used to buy out some of the recognition bond debt, so that the system reform increased the degree of funding.[23] Then later cohorts would face lower taxes to pay the interest on the remaining recognition bond debt. For these later cohorts, returns on Social Security contributions, net of recognition bond taxes, would be higher than under the current system. But for current workers, returns on a privatized system would be lower than under the current system. Thus, transition costs mean either that returns under a privatized system would be the same as the current system (privatization with no prefunding) or that returns in the privatized system would be lower than under the current system for some or all of the currently alive cohorts and then higher for later cohorts (privatization with prefunding). The debate should be focused on whether this is a trade-off worth making, not on whether there is a free lunch.[24]

Risk Adjustment

Advocates of Social Security reform might be tempted to say that people would invest their individual accounts in stocks—earning a higher rate of return—rather than in bonds. By now readers should be suspicious of arguments that promise something for nothing. After all, we just saw that although bonds earn a higher return than the Social Security system, privatizing and investing in bonds would give no higher return once the new taxes needed to redeem the outstanding liabilities of the current system were properly accounted for.

IRR computations usually overlook the fact that workers and retirees bear different risks in a privatized versus a publicly run Social Security system. It is important to keep in mind that when one asset is riskier than another, it should have a higher-equilibrium expected market return; this explains why stocks on average should earn a higher return than bonds. As a result, safer returns from a conventional Social Security system cannot be directly compared with riskier returns anticipated from an equities-based system, unless risk adjustment is done to make the programs comparable. By risk adjustment, we mean adjusting downward the expected value of risky returns (for example, stock returns) to recognize the increased risk associated with these securities.

Households that already hold both stocks and bonds in their portfolios and that have the expertise to buy and sell stocks and bonds should value an additional dollar of stocks the same as an additional dollar of bonds, even though stocks have a much higher expected rate of return. If they valued an additional dollar's worth of stocks more than an additional dollar's worth of bonds, they would have already sold some of their bonds and bought stocks with the money.[25] For this type of household, the risk-adjusted rate of return on an additional dollar of stocks is identical to that on bonds. Put differently, when considering a Social Security change that alters a small fraction of such a household's portfolio, it would be appropriate to compare the current Social Security system to a privatized system in which the individual accounts were required to invest only in government bonds.[26] And we have already seen in that case that privatization does not bring higher returns, correctly measured.

For a larger change in Social Security investment policy, such households could simply use their non–Social Security portfolio to completely offset the change in Social Security. For example, imagine a middle-aged household paying $5,000 a year in Social Security taxes (including employer contributions), which initially were being placed directly into a personal account (run by the government) in the U.S. Treasury bond market. Suppose the household was also saving outside of the Social Security account an additional $10,000 a year, $9,000 in stocks and $1,000 in treasury bonds. Overall, the household is putting 60 percent in stocks ($9,000 out of $15,000), and 40 percent in bonds ($6,000 out of $15,000). If the government suddenly switched the entire Social Security account into stocks, this household could restore the 60-40 split of its total saving by putting $4,000 into stocks and $6,000 into bonds out of its private saving. In fact, no matter how the Social Security account is invested, this household will be no better or worse off. The appropriate risk-adjusted return to such a household from a Social Security account, no matter how it is invested, is the bond return. For a household that is already diversified, the correctly measured return from a privatized and diversified Social Security system is no higher than the current system.[27]

The real economic benefit to privatization comes from the attendant diversification that would be made available to households that cannot participate on their own in diversified capital markets. According to economic theory, every household whose income is uncorrelated with stock returns should include some stock in its portfolio in order to take advantage of the higher returns stocks provide compared to bonds and other safe assets. The first dollars invested in stocks would definitely raise risk-corrected returns, because they would bring extra returns without adding much risk. Subsequent dollars invested in stock continue to raise returns, but at the cost of more and more risk, eventually lowering risk-adjusted returns. How much money should optimally be invested in stocks depends on the wealth and risk tolerance of the household.

Households that are constrained in their private portfolio from holding sufficient amounts of stock would be helped if a portion of their Social Security returns coincided with equity returns. What type of households would fit into this category, and how do we recognize them? First, there are households that will not accumulate any wealth outside of Social Security but that would like to borrow money to invest in the stock market if they could find a lender to loan them money at the bond rate.[28] Second, there are households that will invest 100 percent of their private wealth in the stock market and that would like to invest even more in the stock market if they could borrow at the bond rate. Finally, there are households that will accumulate wealth outside of Social Security but will choose not to invest in the stock market either because they are uninformed about the relative returns and risks or because it is not worth it to them to incur the fixed costs of becoming a stock market investor. Each of these groups would benefit from owning individual accounts invested in the stock market.[29] This provides us with an economic rationale for privatization and diversification.[30]

There remains the issue of how many "constrained" households there are that do not have sufficient access to the stock market. The second group is probably small. The first and third groups are a subset of the people who own no stocks. Fully 59 percent of the U.S. population (in 1995) did not hold stocks in any form.[31] Some of the nonstockholders, however, are young and have not yet accumulated much Social Security or private wealth. What we really want to know is what fraction of the population is unlikely to hold stock in the future, when they are accumulating Social Security wealth. Although we do not have direct estimates of this, about 50 percent of the population 44 to 54 years old and 60 percent of those 55 to 64 years old held no stock in 1995. But stock ownership has risen in the past and is likely to continue to rise in the future, so this is probably an upper bound on the fraction of the population that will not hold stock in the absence of Social Security privatization and diversification. Also, not all those without stock would benefit substantially by holding stocks. For some, their wage income or private business income might be sufficiently positively correlated with the stock market that they are better off not holding any equities. Others, who hold zero stock because they are very risk averse and face a small fixed cost, would see only a small benefit from increased holdings of stock in their Social Security account. Overall, we would guess that significantly fewer than half of households would benefit substantially, and therefore experience substantially higher risk-adjusted returns, from increased Social Security investment in stocks.

If there is a large number of constrained households, then Social Security diversification would have macroeconomic consequences as well. The most important general equilibrium effect of diversification would be an increase in the demand and thus in the price of stocks and a corresponding decline in their expected return. As the value of the stock market increased, current holders of stocks, which disproportionately include the wealthy and older workers who have had time to accumulate stock, would see their wealth increase. Young workers would find that they earned smaller returns on their future stock purchases than they would have in the absence of diversification.[32]

Although privatization and diversification may indeed bring benefits to some constrained households, and perhaps some indirect benefits to the economy as a whole, the presence of these households is not part of the currently popular rate-of-return argument for privatization. According to that argument, all households, and especially the youngest (25-year-old workers), are supposed to see higher returns from privatizing Social Security. Yet when properly measured, rates of return for unconstrained households will stay the same or actually decline for young unconstrained households.

Another risk consideration is that the government-run Social Security system provides insurance functions that an individual-account system probably would not provide, including insurance for shocks to earnings, length of life, disability, and inflation. For instance, the benefit formula is structured to provide a higher rate of return to low lifetime earner households than to high lifetime earner households. This is justified on the grounds that a social insurance plan can pool over the entire population certain risks that are difficult to insure privately, particularly disability, unemployment, and poverty. To the extent that private equivalents for these forms of social insurance would be more costly or nonexistent, privatizing the program would increase participants' risk exposure. Consequently, to the extent that social insurance affords benefits that private insurance could not, this raises the risk-adjusted return on a government-run Social Security system.

Another risk factor must be accounted for as well. A publicly run defined benefit program incurs political risk. This occurs because current workers cannot effectively contract with and bind as-yet-unborn cohorts of taxpayers to pay for them when they grow old. As a result, baby boomers feel unsure that they will wield the political clout to extract rising payroll taxes from their children and grandchildren, to support them when they are old. This is a risk that cannot be traded, so there is no way for those more willing to bear this risk to trade with those less willing to bear it. Although the simple models described above do not have a good way to price this type of risk, correcting for political risk would probably work in the direction of increasing the risk-adjusted returns and relative attractiveness of a privatized system.

CONCLUSION

In this chapter we argue that privatization, diversification, and prefunding are distinct and should be considered as such. We also argue that it is worthwhile separating a move toward system privatization into three steps. Suppose that individual accounts are created but that all benefits accrued to date from past Social Security contributions are honored and that the funding level of the system is held constant (because new explicit debt is issued to cover the unfunded liability of the present Social Security system). In the first step, consider a world with no uncertainty in which individuals are only allowed to invest the individual accounts in government bonds. Although the market return on bonds is greater than that projected on Social Security, once transition costs (to pay interest on the new debt) are accounted for, the rate of return on the two systems would be identical. We estimate that paying for the transition costs would require about a 25 percent tax on all payments into new accounts. This surtax would wipe out all of the extra returns attainable by holding bonds in people's individual accounts. Our 25 percent number depends on forecasts of future growth rates g of the economy and future real interest rates r. If those forecasts of r and g were to change, the tax would have to change. But the result that all of the gains to privatization would disappear in extra taxes to pay off the unfunded liability is true regardless of the specific values of r and g.

Next, consider adding idiosyncratic risk (for example, shocks to earnings and length of life). If the privatized system contains no special insurance provisions, and the private market is unable to provide these, then the risk-adjusted rate of return under privatization would be lower than under the current system.

Third, consider adding aggregate risk and allowing households to invest their individual accounts in equities. For households that already held both stocks and bonds elsewhere and were thus unconstrained in their portfolio choice, the risk-adjusted rate of return would be no higher than the risk-adjusted rate of return if the individual accounts were held entirely in bonds. For the others, namely, those who do not currently have as much invested in equities as they might like, the risk-adjusted rate of return on a portfolio with equities would be higher as a result of diversification into stocks, thus providing an important rationale for diversification. Nevertheless, this return would not be as much higher as a naive comparison of expected returns would suggest. If this group is large, there will also be general equilibrium effects that will likely lower the expected return on stocks, thus making worse off young households that would have invested in stocks anyway.

Finally, what if the system's funding were increased at the same time as individual accounts were created? Although the increase in funding would likely raise the rate of return on Social Security for future generations (and raise national saving in the process), it must be kept in mind that it would do so only at the cost of lower returns to current cohorts.

We argue that the Social Security reform debate should focus on the trade-off between returns for current cohorts versus future cohorts; the risk-bearing benefits to the economy of enlarging the population that holds a diversified portfolio to include constrained households; and whether diversification is better implemented via privatized personal accounts or through trust fund investments.

We recognize that privatization has several other important benefits, including increased portfolio choice, reduced political risk, possibly reduced labor supply distortions, and an intangible increased sense of ownership and responsibility. It is also possible that privatization may improve the political feasibility of implementing prefunding or diversification, thus increasing the chance of achieving the benefits to future generations and constrained households described earlier.

Indeed, some find these overwhelming reasons to favor privatization. These positives, however, must be balanced against the loss of social risk pooling mentioned above, somewhat higher administrative costs, and perhaps the social and personal costs of permitting workers to make "unwise" portfolio choices.[33] In any event, our main message is that the popular argument that Social Security privatization would provide higher returns for all current and future workers is misleading, because it ignores transition costs and differences across programs in the allocation of aggregate and household risk.

ACKNOWLEDGMENTS

This chapter was originally published as *Would a Privatized Social Security System Really Pay a Higher Rate of Return?* in *Framing the Social Security Debate: Values, Politics, and Economics,* edited by R. Douglas Arnold, Michael J. Graetz, and Alicia H. Munnell (National Academy of Social Insurance and Brookings Institution Press, 1998), 137–57. It is reprinted here with permission. It differs from the original only due to minor copyediting changes and updates to the references (to reflect revised dates and publication information for articles that were published subsequent to the original version of this chapter). This chapter draws on a longer paper by the authors (Geanakoplos, Mitchell, and Zeldes 1999). Useful comments were provided by Jeff Brown, Martin Feldstein, and Kent Smetters.

NOTES

1. Although we focus on the rate-of-return concept of money's worth in this chapter, additional measures are evaluated in more detail in our longer study (Geanakoplos, Mitchell, and Zeldes 1999).

2. There is debate over whether prefunding should refer to a change that reduces the total government debt rather than just the Social Security debt. Here we assume that any changes in Social Security do not change the non–Social Security debt or deficit.

3. The concept of unfunded liability is different from that of actuarial imbalance. Actuarial imbalance is defined as the present value of expected benefits over some period (often seventy-five years) minus the present value of expected tax receipts over the same period, minus the current value of the trust fund. The United States currently has a seventy-five-year actuarial imbalance of about 2.2 percent of payroll a year, or about $2.9 trillion in present value. See Goss 1999.

4. More gradual transitions to a system of individual accounts that leave (implicit plus explicit) debt unchanged are also possible.

5. These are arithmetic averages of annual returns from 1926 through 1996 taken from Ibbotson and Associates 1998. The 1994–96 Social Security Advisory Council projected that in the future stocks would earn a 7 percent real return, compared with 2 percent real return on bonds.

6. The internal rate of return (IRR) is defined as the interest rate that equates the present value of taxes paid to the system and the present value of benefits received, by cohort. Two other "money's worth" measures sometimes reported are the present value ratio (PVB/PVT), or the present value of benefits divided by the present value of taxes, and the net present value (NPV), or the present value of benefits received minus the present value of taxes paid. The IRR and its companion money's worth measures are appealing because they seek to summarize in a single measure how a household might evaluate the complex multiyear stream of Social Security payments and receipts. However, the measure's simplicity belies the extensive assumptions and calculations needed to arrive at a single summary number. For example, in order to conclude that workers born in 1930 anticipate a Social Security IRR of 4 percent, it is necessary to compute what that cohort paid in payroll taxes over all years of work (Leimer 1994). Not all those born in 1930 have retired as yet, so future earnings profiles, taxes, and retirement patterns must be forecast. Each group's tax payments must then be compared against the stream of Social Security benefits actually paid out to people of that birth year. Of course, many 1930-cohort members are still living, so future benefit payments and mortality patterns must again be estimated. For details see Geanakoplos, Mitchell, and Zeldes 1999.

7. Leimer also provides estimates under the assumption that benefits are reduced to maintain solvency.

8. For a discussion of the assumptions used to estimate future wage base growth rates as well as future Social Security benefit and tax paths, see Advisory Council on Social Security 1997.

9. Comparing the present value of a cohort's benefits and taxes is an application of the generational accounting approach to measuring fiscal policy. See, for example, Auerbach, Gokhale, and Kotlikoff 1994.

10. Recall that these are real or inflation-adjusted returns; nominal returns would obviously be even higher.

11. Leimer (1994) used the interest rates on trust fund assets (essentially intermediate-term U.S. Treasury bonds) to convert current dollars into 1989 dollars.

We convert the series into 1997 dollars using the corresponding interest rates between 1989 and 1997.

12. To see this, first consider a system that is pay-as-you-go, so that in each year aggregate taxes are equal to aggregate benefits, that is, benefits minus taxes equals zero. Hence, the present value of each year's benefits minus taxes must equal zero, and therefore the sum across all years of these present values must equal zero as well. So long as the present value of all benefits across all years and the present value of all taxes across all years are each finite, which must necessarily hold if the interest rate is on average higher than the rate of growth of the economy, we can rearrange and regroup benefits and taxes however we like. Grouping together benefits and taxes for each birth cohort, it must be, as claimed, that the present values of net transfers (benefits minus taxes), cohort by cohort, sum to zero.

This is also true with prefunding, and even with trust fund borrowing, provided that the trust fund assets are invested at the same interest rate used to compute present values. In this case, the present value of all benefits paid up to and including any year T is equal to the present value of all taxes up to and including year T plus the present value of the year T trust fund. Allowing T to go to infinity and assuming that the trust fund is not allowed to grow increasingly negative at rate r or faster and that the government would not want it to grow increasingly positive at rate r or faster, the present value of net transfers (benefits minus taxes) made to all birth cohorts must equal zero. See Geanakoplos, Mitchell, and Zeldes 1999 for more details.

The difference between a prefunded system and a pay-as-you-go system is that in the latter, the early cohorts must get positive transfers, leaving negative transfers for later cohorts, whereas in a prefunded system, the early cohorts may not get any positive transfers. Our current Social Security system has very little prefunding. The correspondingly small trust fund indeed earns a bond rate of return, so our analysis is relevant.

13. It is important to note that this discounting is at the real rate of interest. If, for example, the real rate of interest is 2.3 percent a year and inflation is 3 percent, and if the $10 trillion were paid back in one lump sum in thirty years, then it would cost $48 trillion in 2027 dollars. The relentless power of compounding interest is what makes the burden of the initial Social Security transfers many years ago loom so large today.

14. If the system had instead started as and remained a fully funded system, then early participants would have received market returns, that is, zero net transfers, as would all current and future workers.

15. The transfer in period $t + 1$ (TRANS_{t+1}) is the amount by which contributions in period $t + 1$ exceed the present value of the benefits accrued as a result of those contributions. Define $\text{UL}t$ as the unfunded liability at time t. It can be shown (Geanakoplos, Mitchell, and Zeldes 1999) that the change in the unfunded liability between t and $t + 1$ ($\Delta \text{UL}_{t,t+1}$) is equal to ($r \times \text{UL}_t$) − TRANS_{t+1}. In a steady-state

economy, the unfunded liability must grow at rate g, that is, $\Delta UL_{t,t+1} = g \times UL_t$. This implies that the transfer must be exactly $(r - g) \times UL_t$, as claimed in the text.

16. This number is, of course, only an approximation. To get it we assumed that the real interest rate would stay constant at 2.3 percent and that the wage base would grow steadily at 1.2 percent. Among other things, both assumptions ignore demographic changes. In the current baby boom era, both real interest rates and growth rates are higher than we assumed. If anything, however, it looks as if actual $r - g$ is higher than we presumed, which would imply that the necessary transfers might be even more than we suggest.

17. As a check, consider a hypothetical worker who pays level real Social Security taxes for forty years and receives level real benefits for the next twenty years at an internal rate of return of 1.2 percent (an estimate of g). If, instead, his contributions were reduced by 25 percent but his benefits remained the same, then his internal rate of return would be 2.12 percent, which is close to our estimate of r of 2.3 percent.

18. See, for example, Steve Forbes, "How to Replace Social Security," *Wall Street Journal*, December 18, 1996, and Beach and Davis 1998. There are sites on the World Wide Web that calculate for users the benefit stream they will likely receive from Social Security and compare it to the income stream attainable from investing their Social Security contributions in private capital markets. See, for example, the Cato Institute Web site at www.socialsecurity.org/calc/calculator.html.

19. In a steady state, the required path of debt would keep constant the ratio of outstanding recognition bond debt to GDP.

20. For a further discussion of this result, see Geanakoplos, Mitchell, and Zeldes 1999.

21. There are different ways of measuring accrued benefits, and each method would require a different tax scheme to make taxes in a privatized system just equal to transfers in the current Social Security system. We give one example. Suppose accrued benefits are defined on an equal present value basis, that is, suppose each dollar of contributions brings the same present value of accrued benefits (discounted back to the time when the dollar is contributed). Suppose this ratio is 0.75. Then a proportional tax of $(1 - 0.75) \times 12.4$ percent = 3.1 percent would leave everyone exactly as well off in a privatized system as he or she was in the current pay-as-you-go Social Security system.

22. Higher r makes privatized returns higher, but, as we have just seen, it also increases the interest burden of the unfunded liability.

23. A potential advantage of prefunding is that it would, according to most economists, increase national saving. There is no reason to believe that privatization without prefunding would necessarily increase national saving. See, for example, Mitchell and Zeldes 1996.

24. As argued, for example, by Feldstein (1998).

25. This is not to say that such a household would put its first dollar of savings into bonds instead of stocks but rather that after its (perhaps considerable) invest-

ment in stocks, the next dollar of stock would increase well-being no more than another dollar of bonds.

26. In practice, government bond returns are not equal to Social Security returns, and neither is riskless. We ignore these issues here.

27. This argument holds even if there is an inexplicably large equity premium, as some economists claim there is. Suppose the excess return on stocks above bonds is much more than can be justified by the risk differential, because many households are irrationally underinvesting in equities. In that case, we might be tempted on paternalistic grounds to force these irrational households to hold more stock. However, this is no simple matter. If Social Security were simply privatized, these households would likely choose not to hold any equities in their Social Security accounts for the same reasons they held too few stocks in the rest of their portfolio. If households were instead forced into equities in Social Security, they would likely undo this by reducing their holdings of equities in the rest of their portfolio.

28. Given the chance, these "liquidity constrained" households would prefer to use borrowing to increase current consumption. If borrowing could be used only to purchase other assets, however, these households would choose to borrow and purchase stocks.

29. This assumes that the fixed costs would be lower under an individual account system.

30. This raises the issue of whether diversification into stocks is better achieved through privatized individual accounts or through central trust fund investments. If constrained investors tend to be irrational or myopic in their investment decisions, then it would be more advantageous for them if the Social Security trust fund itself undertook stock investments on their behalf. Unconstrained investors could still keep control of all their asset holdings (inside and outside of their Social Security funds) by compensating in their private accounts for whatever the trust fund did that was not to their taste, as we saw above. However, households such as those that have chosen optimally to hold small amounts of stocks, perhaps because they are risk averse, might be forced to hold too much extra in stocks in their Social Security accounts. These households would be made worse off. The more heterogeneous constrained households are in their tolerance of risk, and the wiser we think constrained households would be in their investment choices, the more attractive is privatization as a means of achieving diversification. The more homogeneous constrained households are in their tolerance of risk, and the more myopic we think constrained households would be in their investment choices, the more attractive is trust fund investment as a means of achieving diversification.

31. This is based on calculations using the 1995 Survey of Consumer Finances. It includes stocks held directly, through mutual funds, and through defined contribution pensions. See Kennickell, Starr-McCluer, and Sunden 1997 and Ameriks and Zeldes 2000.

32. Social security diversification would bring some indirect benefits to the

economy if there were many constrained households. Unconstrained households would end up holding less stock, because some of it would be in the hands of Social Security accounts held by constrained households that could not buy stock previously. Thus, unconstrained households would bear less risk. They would be inclined to shift the mix of investment projects undertaken toward more risky ones. This might in turn raise future GDP.

33. See Mitchell 1998 for an analysis of administrative costs.

REFERENCES

Advisory Council on Social Security. 1997. *Report of the 1994–1996 Advisory Council on Social Security.* Vol. 1, *Findings and Recommendations.* Washington, D.C.: U.S. Government Printing Office.

Ameriks, J., and S. P. Zeldes. 2000. How Do Household Portfolio Shares Vary with Age? Working paper, Graduate School of Business, Columbia University.

Auerbach, A. J., J. Gokhale, and L. J. Kotlikoff. 1994. Generational Accounting: A Meaningful Way to Evaluate Fiscal Policy. *Journal of Economic Perspectives* 8, no. 1: 73–94.

Beach, W. W., and G. G. Davis. 1998. Social Security's Rate of Return. Heritage Foundation Study, Washington, D.C., January.

Feldstein, M. 1998. Transition to a Fully Funded Pension System: Five Economic Issues. In H. Siebert, ed., *Redesigning Social Security.* Institut für Weltwirtschaft an der Universität, Kiel. Tübingen, Germany: Mohr Siebeck.

Forbes, S. 1996. How to Replace Social Security. *Wall Street Journal,* December 18.

Geanakoplos, J., O. S. Mitchell, and S. P. Zeldes. 1999. Social Security Money's Worth. In O. S. Mitchell, R. J. Myers, and H. Young, eds., *Prospects for Social Security Reform.* Philadelphia: Pension Research Council and University of Pennsylvania Press.

Goss, S. C. 1999. Measuring Solvency in the Social Security System. In O. S. Mitchell, R. J. Myers, and H. Young, eds., *Prospects for Social Security Reform.* Philadelphia: Pension Research Council and University of Pennsylvania Press.

Ibbotson and Associates. 1998. *Stocks, Bonds, Bills, and Inflation Yearbook.* Chicago: Ibbotson and Associates.

Kennickell, A., M. Starr-McCluer, and A. E. Sundén. 1997. Family Finances in the U.S.: Recent Evidence from the Survey of Consumer Finances. *Federal Reserve Bulletin,* January.

Leimer, D. 1994. Cohort Specific Measures of Lifetime Net Social Security Transfers. ORS Working Paper no. 59, February, Office of Research and Statistics, Social Security Administration, Washington, D.C.

Mitchell, O. S. 1998. Administrative Costs in Public and Private Retirement Systems. In M. Feldstein, ed., *Privatizing Social Security.* Chicago: University of Chicago Press.

Mitchell, O. S., and F. Barreto. 1997. After Chile, What? Second-Round Social Security Reforms in Latin America. *Revista de Analisis Economico* 12 (November): 3–36.

Mitchell, O. S., and S. P. Zeldes. 1996. Social Security Privatization: A Structure for Analysis. *American Economic Review* 86 (May): 363–67.

Moore, S. 1997. *Prepared Testimony on the Future of Social Security for This Generation and the Next.* House Ways and Means Committee, Social Security Subcommittee, 105th Cong., 1st sess., June 24.

13

Changing Retirement Trends and Their Impact on Elderly Entitlement Programs

Joseph F. Quinn, Ph.D.

One of the most dramatic demographic trends in the post–World War II period has been the earlier and earlier withdrawal from the labor force of older American men. One simple definition of the average age of retirement is the age at which half of the population is in the labor force and half is out. According to this definition, the average retirement age for men was 70 in 1950 (see Table 13.1). By 1970 it had dropped to age 65, and by 1985 to age 62—a remarkable decline of eight years during a mere three and a half decades.

The same dramatic change can be seen by observing the labor force participation trends at any given age in Table 13.1. In 1950 more than 70 percent of all 65-year-old men in America were either employed or actively looking for work. Their participation rate fell by over twenty percentage points during the next two decades, and by nearly another twenty points during the subsequent fifteen years. By 1985 only 30 percent of 65-year-old men remained in the labor force—a decline of nearly 60 percent since 1950.

About 80 percent of men aged 62 were labor force participants in both 1950 and in 1960. In 1961 Congress lowered the age of eligibility for Social Security old age benefits from 65 to 62 (as it had for women in 1956), and a steady decline in participation rates ensued. By 1975

Table 13.1. Male Labor Force Participation Rates by Age, 1950–2000

Year	Age						
	55	60	62	65	68	70	72
1950	90.6	84.7	81.2	71.7	57.7	49.8	39.3
1960	92.8	85.9	79.8	56.8	42.0	37.2	28.0
1970	91.8	83.9	73.8	49.9	37.7	30.1	24.8
1975	87.6	76.9	64.4	39.4	23.7	23.7	22.6
1980	84.9	74.0	56.8	35.2	24.1	21.3	17.0
1985	83.7	71.0	50.9	30.5	20.5	15.9	14.9
1990	85.3	70.5	52.5	31.9	23.4	17.1	16.4
1995	81.1	68.9	51.3	33.5	22.4	20.6	16.0
2000	79.9	66.1	53.0	35.7	27.9	20.2	18.5

Source: Data from U.S. Bureau of Labor Statistics.

the age 62 rate was below two-thirds, and by 1985 it had dropped to one-half—a decline of nearly 40 percent in only twenty-five years.

Even larger percentage declines between 1950 and 1985 occurred for older men—drops of about two-thirds for those aged 68, 70, and 72. Declines are also observed below age 62, but they were much more modest—about 16 percent at age 60 and 8 percent at age 55.

Dora Costa (1998, chap. 2) has shown that this trend toward earlier and earlier retirement began long before 1950 and can be documented back to 1880 in the United States and several other industrialized nations.

One purpose of this chapter is to argue that a century-old trend is over and has been over since the mid-1980s. The era of earlier and earlier retirement among American men has come to an end. Significant changes in the retirement patterns of older American women occurred at about the same time. Although some reasons for the changes in trend are cyclical—the result of the robust American economy—there have also been fundamental societal changes that have altered the relative attractiveness of work and leisure late in life. Although the strength of the economy will undoubtedly continue to ebb and flow, with important implications for the demand for labor, including the labor of older Americans, the societal and institutional changes discussed below are not likely to be reversed. I argue, therefore, that an era has come to an end and that past trends may not be good indicators of what lies ahead.

The chapter also mentions the importance of "bridge jobs"—part-time or short-duration jobs that occur between full-time career employment and complete labor force withdrawal. Many Americans retire gradually, in stages. Although many older workers do leave the labor force as soon as they can afford to do so, many others continue working after they leave their career jobs—often part time, often self-employed, and often in a new line of work. Surveys suggest that this will continue in the future, as the baby boomers age and make their retirement decisions.

The timing and the nature of retirement in the future are vitally important to the nation. The ratio of workers (Social Security contributors) to retirees (Social Security recipients) has changed dramatically in recent decades—from about 5 to 1 in 1960 to about 3.3 to 1 today, with forecasts of only two workers per retiree by 2020. In a pay-as-you-go system, in which benefits are primarily paid from current contributions, one dollar of benefits costs each contributor twenty cents if there are five workers per recipient, but fifty cents if there are only two. These ratios have changed for two reasons: because the age distribution of the population is changing, with an increasing percentage of the population in the older cohorts, and also because the age of retirement has been falling, as outlined above. As we see in this chapter, however, future retirement trends are not set in stone. Rather, they will be influenced by important economic and demographic trends and by the incentives embedded in current and future public policy initiatives.[1] When and how people retire, in turn, will affect the strains on our public and private retirement systems and, even more important, the size, strength, and productivity of our economy.

EARLY RETIREMENT TRENDS: THEN AND NOW

Male retirement trends can be seen in annual Bureau of Labor Statistics data, published by gender and five-year age cohort. (See, e.g., U.S. Bureau of Labor Statistics 1965–2001, January issues.) Figure 13.1 shows labor force participation rates for two cohorts of older men for the time period 1964–85, along with simple time trends over that pe-

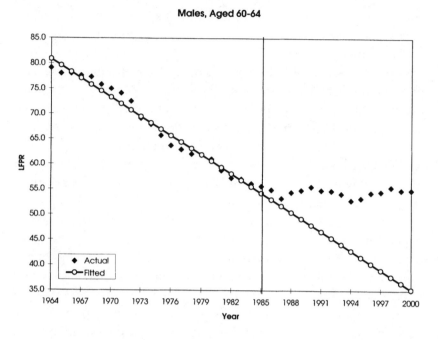

Fig. 13.1A. Labor force participation rates, actual and fitted values, males aged 60–64, 1964–2000.

riod extrapolated through 2000. For men aged 60 to 64, the participation rate fell from 79 to 56 percent between 1964 and 1985, an average decline of well over one percentage point per year and a total drop of about one-third during these two decades. For men aged 65 to 69, the rate declined by almost one percentage point per year, from 43 to 24 percent—a decline of more than 40 percent overall. Similar trends are observed for younger (aged 55 to 59) and older men (70 and above).

Since the mid-1980s, however, male retirement trends have been very different. Figure 13.1A and B compare the linear extrapolations based on the 1964–85 experience with actual data through 2000. Rates of labor force participation flattened out, then increased in recent years, and they are much higher today (by about twenty percentage points for men aged 60 to 64 and 65 to 69) than the pre-1986 trends would have predicted. The same phenomenon is observed among men at older and younger ages.

Males, Aged 65-69

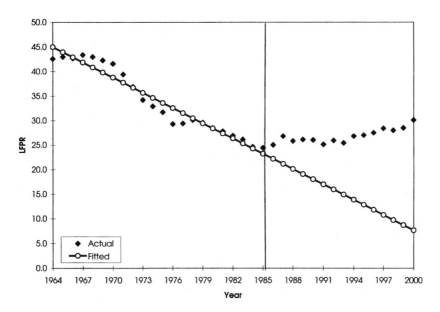

Fig. 13.1B. Labor force participation rates, actual and fitted values, males aged 65–69, 1964–2000.

The story for older American women is both different and the same. Older women's participation rates in the postwar period have reflected two offsetting phenomena—the early retirement trend of older Americans and the increasing labor force participation of married women. Before the mid-1980s, they appear to have canceled out. As seen in Figure 13.2A and B, we observe very modest changes in the labor force participation of women aged 55 to 59 and 60 to 64 between 1964 and 1985, and the same is true for women a bit older.

What is similar to the male phenomenon is the experience since then. As with the men, there are substantial breaks from trend for all older age cohorts in the mid-1980s, and in all cases actual participation rates since 1985 are significantly higher than the earlier trends would have predicted. The similarity of the break points in the male and female time series is striking.

A straight-line projection is an unsophisticated long-run extrapola-

Females, Aged 55-59

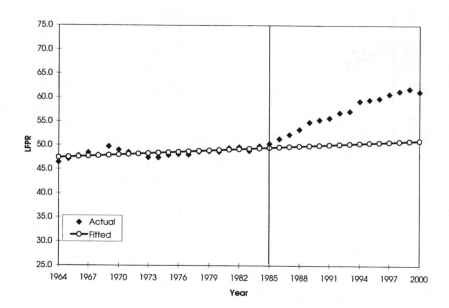

Fig. 13.2A. Labor force participation rates, actual and fitted values, females aged 55–59, 1964–2000.

tion tool. Nonetheless, these graphs do suggest that something is different now than it was about two decades ago.

WHY THE CHANGE IN RETIREMENT TRENDS?

There are two types of hypotheses about the reasons for these changes. One emphasizes permanent changes in the retirement environment and argues that we have entered a new era. The other says that the strength of the economy has been key, and it implies that the historical declines will resume if the economy falters. There is truth in both.

The Permanent View

There have been many important societal changes—changes unlikely to be reversed—that are consistent with increased work effort late in

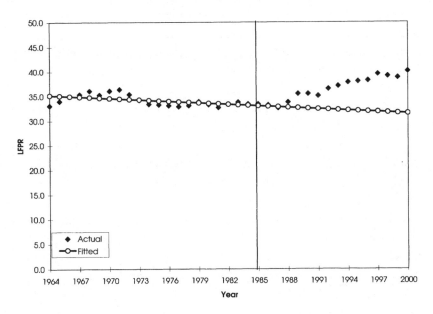

Fig. 13.2B. Labor force participation rates, actual and fitted values, females aged 60–64, 1964–2000.

life. For example, mandatory retirement was first delayed from age 65 to age 70 in 1978 and then eliminated in 1986 for the vast majority of American workers. This increased the options facing those individuals who had been constrained by the prior policy and who wanted to keep working; it also sent an important message to society as a whole that there was no one age appropriate for retirement.

In addition, Social Security rules have been changed to make work late in life more attractive (Quadagno and Quinn 1997). The income that a recipient could earn before losing any Social Security benefits was indexed to wage growth in 1975, and in 1978 higher exempt amounts were introduced for beneficiaries aged 65 through 71. In 1983 the earnings test was eliminated for those aged 70 and 71, and in 1990 the benefit loss for each dollar earned over the exempt amount was reduced from 50 to 33 cents for recipients aged 65 to 69. In 2000 Congress eliminated the earnings test altogether for those above the normal retirement age, which is currently moving from 65 to 66 over a six- year period. For those over 62 but younger than the normal retirement age, the exempt amounts are increasing dramatically, and by 2002 these younger recipients will be able to earn up to thirty thousand dollars per year without any loss of benefits (Social Security Administration 2000, tables 2.A20, 2.A29).

Important changes are also under way in the private sector, including a shift in the relative importance of defined contribution (DC) and defined benefit (DB) pension plans. The proportion of employer pension participants whose primary coverage is DC increased from 13 to 42 percent between 1975 and the mid-1990s. Including secondary plans, which are nearly all DC, the proportion of participants with a DC plan more than doubled from 26 to 53 percent over this same time period (EBRI 1997, table 10.2; Olsen and VanDerhei 1997, table 2). Most DC plans are age-neutral by design and do not contain the age-specific work disincentives that DB plans often have.

The nature of jobs in America is also in transition, with manufacturing on the decline and service employment on the rise. Although there is considerable variation in the nature of jobs within these broad occupational categories, it is probably easier, on average, for older employees to remain working in service occupations. Steuerle, Spiro, and Johnson (1999, fig. 1) estimate that the percentage of American workers in physically demanding jobs declined from 20 percent in 1950 to 11 percent in 1970 and 7.5 percent in 1996.

Finally, older Americans are living longer and are healthier. The life expectancy of American men at age 65 increased by three years (to 15.8 years) between 1950 and the present; and for women at age 65, life expectancy increased by over four years (to 19.3 years). Further increases are projected throughout the twenty-first century (U.S. House 1998, table A-2). Manton, Stallard, and Coder (1995) find significant declines in morbidity among the elderly population between 1982 and 1989. Crimmins, Reynolds, and Saito report significant improvements between 1982 and 1993 in the ability of men and women in their 60s to work—changes large enough that "the percentage unable to work at age 67 in 1993 is lower than the percentage unable to work at age 65 in 1982" (1999, S31). Many workers at traditional retirement ages anticipate a decade or two of healthy lifespan ahead, and many are deciding that some combination of work and leisure is preferable to all of one or all of the other.

These societal changes suggest that the future may not look like the past. The relative attractiveness of work and retirement late in life has been changed in favor of work, and older Americans seem to be responding accordingly.

The Cyclical View

An alternative hypothesis is that a strong American economy temporarily delayed the inevitable further decline in elderly labor force participation rates. The unemployment rate declined from nearly 10 percent in 1983 to about 5 percent in 1989, and by 2000 it had fallen to 4 percent—the lowest unemployment rate since the late 1960s (Council of Economic Advisers 2001, table B-42). Strong labor demand creates employment options for workers of all ages.

To test this hypothesis, I ran some simple regressions on the labor force participation rates of each of the age-gender cohorts mentioned above, using the same time period (1964–85). I included a time trend, as before, and added the overall civilian unemployment rate as a proxy for the business cycle.

The regression results suggest that the cyclical explanation does have merit. In seven of the eight age-gender equations, the coefficient of the unemployment rate has the expected negative sign. Tighter labor markets (that is, lower unemployment rates) are associated with higher labor force participation among older workers. The coefficients are significantly different from zero for three of the groups likely to be contemplating retirement—men aged 60 to 64 and 65 to 69, and women aged 55 to 59.

In Figure 13.3A and B we illustrate actual and predicted participation rates, using the expanded equation, for one age cohort each of men and women. As expected, the differences between actual and predicted rates are moderated by the business cycle effects, but large differentials still remain. For men aged 60 to 64, for example, the differential between predicted and actual participation rates in 2000 is now 15 percentage points compared to 20 points in Figure 13.1; for women aged 55 to 59, the 2000 differential declines from 9 to 6 points. The

Males, Aged 60-64

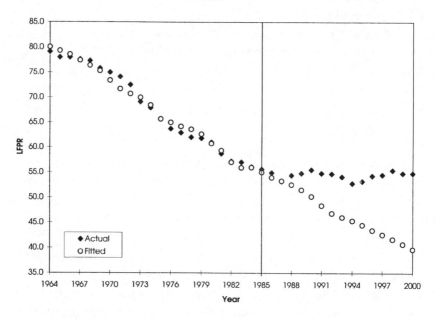

Fig. 13.3A. Labor force participation rates, actual and fitted values, including the business cycle, males aged 60–64, 1964–2000.

same was true for the other gender-age groups as well—smaller differentials but the same qualitative results. The conclusion remains unaltered: although the business cycle is important, other changes have had an important influence on retirement patterns as well.

This conclusion is reinforced by one last regression specification, which includes the data from 1964 through 2000 but permits the trend line to alter slope after 1985. As seen in Table 13.2 (p. 306), even after including the impact of the business cycle, *the change in trend* after 1985 is positive and significantly different from zero for all eight cohorts. For men aged 60 to 64, for example, the trend increases by over one percentage point per year after 1985, from −1.19 (which represents a decline of well over a percentage point per year from 1964 to 1985) to −0.09 (almost zero). For men aged 65 to 69, the slope also increases by over a point after 1985 and reverses sign, going from −0.86 points to

Females, Aged 55-59

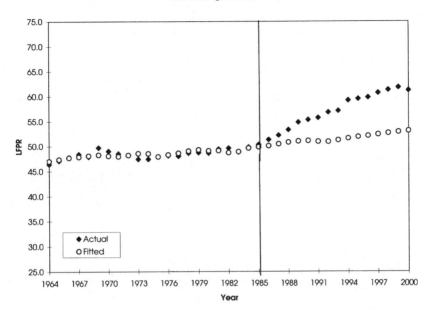

Fig. 13.3B. Labor force participation rates, actual and fitted values, females aged 55–59, including the business cycle, 1964–2000.

+0.18 per year. For the three youngest cohorts of women, the *increases* in trend after 1985 are in the range of 0.4 to 0.6 point per year, and the net results (the old trend plus the change in trend) show net increases in participation since 1986 for all four groups of older women.

Figure 13.4A and B compares actual and predicted participation rates for the same cohorts of men and women who appear in Figure 13.3, but here we include the change in trend after 1985, along with the unemployment rate. The difference from the earlier figures is striking. With the addition of the change in trend, the predicted rates track the actual almost perfectly, and the differences between the two only rarely exceed one percentage point.

A change in trend is a description, not an explanation, but it is consistent with the societal and public policy changes discussed above— the elimination of mandatory retirement, new Social Security incen-

Males, Aged 60-64

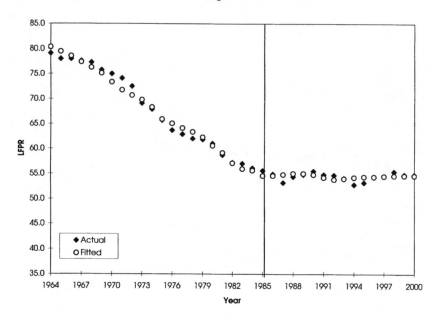

Fig. 13.4A. Labor force participation rates, actual and fitted values, males aged 60–64, including the business cycle and change in slope, 1964–2000.

tives, the trends in the type of employer pension plans, and changes in the occupational mix, health, and longevity. It makes sense that some older Americans would choose to work longer, and they do.

DO OLDER AMERICANS WANT TO WORK?

Survey evidence suggests that many older Americans would like to work more than they do. McNaught, Barth, and Henderson (1989) examined the responses of 3,500 men (aged 55 to 64) and women (aged 50 to 59) in a 1989 Harris survey. Between 14 and 25 percent of those who were no longer employed said that they preferred to be working if a suitable job were available. Quinn and Burkhauser (1994) analyzed those in that same sample who were still working and found that about 10 percent said they expected to stop working before they really wanted to. One interpretation of this response is that they expected to stop

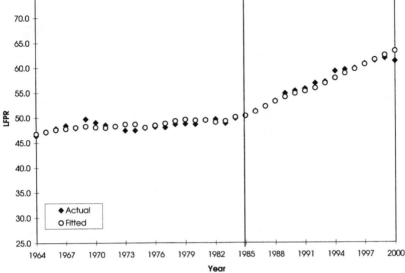

Fig. 13.4B. Labor force participation rates, actual and fitted values, females aged 55–59, including the business cycle and change in slope, 1964–2000.

working given the inflexibility of working hours and the financial incentives that they faced (e.g., from the old Social Security rules and from defined benefit pension plans) but that they would continue working under other circumstances.

In a more recent AARP survey of 2,000 baby boomers aged 34 to 52, 80 percent said they expected to keep working at least part time after age 65—one-quarter because they would need the income and one-third for the enjoyment it would bring (Roper Starch Worldwide 1998). In a 1998 Employee Benefit Research Institute survey, 61 percent of workers said they would work for pay after retirement, many for financial reasons and many others (more than half) to improve their quality of life (Yakoboski, Ostuw, and Hicks 1998). The stark contrast between these estimates (80% and 61%) and the current labor force participation rate of Americans aged 65 to 69 (about 30% for men and 20% for women) gives one pause about using these survey results as a

Table 13.2. Labor Force Participation Rate Regressions by Gender and Age

	Trend (1964–1985)	Δ Trend after 1985	(Trend + Δ Trend)
Men			
55–59	−0.552	0.395	−0.157
	(0.029)	(0.065)	
60–64	−1.188	1.100	−0.088
	(0.043)	(0.099)	
65–69	−0.865	1.040	0.175
	(0.052)	(0.119)	
70+	−0.422	0.476	0.054
	(0.018)	(0.041)	
Women			
55–59	0.198	0.599	0.797
	(0.032)	(0.073)	
60–64	−0.089*	0.542	0.453
	(0.036)	(0.081)	
65–69	−0.140	0.438	0.298
	(0.027)	(0.062)	
70+	−0.085	0.174	0.089
	(0.008)	(0.019)	

Note: All coefficients are significantly different from zero at the 0.01 level, except *, which is significant at the 0.05 level. Standard errors in parentheses.

predictor of the future, but they do suggest that new attitudes toward work late in life are developing.

As we will see below, changes in the nature of retirement are already under way. Many workers do not leave the labor force in the old stereotypical fashion, directly from a full-time career job. Many retire more gradually, using transitional bridge jobs on the way out.

HOW DO OLDER AMERICANS LEAVE THE LABOR FORCE?

This research is based on the Health and Retirement Study (HRS), an ongoing longitudinal study of the retirement process in the United States.[2] In 1992 more than 12,000 men and women in about 8,000 households were surveyed, and they are being reinterviewed at two-year intervals. We used the first three waves of the HRS—data from the 1992, 1994, and 1996 surveys. By 1996 the age-eligible respondents were aged 55 to 65. Many had crossed the important age 62 threshold, and a few had reached age 65.

With a goal of understanding how older American workers withdraw from the labor force, we analyzed these data in two ways. The first was retrospective. We asked what these respondents were doing in 1996 and how they got there. How many were still working on full-time long-tenure career jobs? How many were working on or had worked on bridge jobs? The second approach was forward looking. We identified a sample (about 5,800) with a long-tenure career job somewhere in their work history and then moved forward from this job to ask how they had left these jobs, if they had done so. Did those who moved leave the labor force or move to a bridge job? In both cases—looking back from 1996 and forward from their last career job—we find that a substantial minority of older Americans use bridge jobs as part of the labor market exit process.[3]

We define a career job as a full-time job (1,600 or more hours per year) that the respondent has held or is expected to hold for at least ten years. A bridge job, therefore, can either be a job of shorter duration or a part-time job of any duration.

At the time of the 1996 survey, 62 percent of the sample were working, compared to 70 percent in 1994 and nearly 80 percent in 1992, when they were four years younger. By using the longitudinal nature of the data set and retrospective questions in the 1992 survey, we could analyze the last job of those no longer working and determine whether it was a bridge or a career job. We also investigated the current jobs of those still employed and judged whether these looked like bridge or career jobs.[4]

Of the nearly 4,300 men in this sample, 40 percent were still working full-time on their career jobs in 1996. We will have to follow them through subsequent waves of the HRS to see exactly how and when they retire. Nearly a quarter (23%) were working on what we define as a bridge job (and about two-thirds of them had had full-time career jobs just before this bridge job), and 36 percent of the men were not working at all. Of the latter, about one-third (10 percentage points) had last worked on a bridge job; the remainder had left the labor market directly from a full-time career job—stereotypical retirement. If we combine these two figures—the 23 percent working on a bridge job in 1996 and the 10 percent who were no longer working but who had last worked on a bridge job—we get a lower bound estimate of about one-third for the proportion of men using a bridge job between career employment and complete labor force withdrawal.[5]

The experiences of the women in the sample suggest even more bridge job activity late in life. A slightly higher percentage of the women had already stopped working by 1996 (40%), and most of these (21 percentage points) last worked on a bridge job. Of those women still at work, a higher proportion (25% of the female sample) were working on bridge jobs. For the women, the lower bound estimate of bridge job activity is 45 percent, assuming that none of the full-time career workers still employed will move to a bridge job in the future.

This snapshot reveals considerable bridge job activity among older Americans in 1996. At a minimum, about one-third of these men and nearly one-half of these women used bridge jobs before complete labor force withdrawal.[6]

Thus far, we have implicitly assumed that part-time or short-duration jobs indicate gradual or partial retirement. For some this is true, but for others it may not be. Some workers may have had a history of short-duration or part-time jobs. What is there to suggest that a part-time job that we observed in 1996 indicates any more about retirement than the previous ones did?

To focus on those for whom a part-time or short-duration job would represent a change, we concentrate here on just the subsample of persons with a full-time career job (ten years' duration) somewhere in their work history.[7] We then proceed forward in time to see how, if at all, the individual leaves that career job.

Almost half of these men and women were still working on their full-time career jobs in 1996, and we will have to utilize subsequent waves of the HRS to learn when and how they leave. Of the remainder—those who had left their career jobs by 1996—nearly half moved to a bridge job rather than directly out of employment. It is interesting to note that the exit patterns of career men and career women look more similar than do those of men and women in general.

We also compared the exit patterns of the majority (87%) who were wage-and-salary workers with the 13 percent who were self-employed on their career jobs. Prior research suggests that self-employed and wage-and-salary workers retire in different ways and that crossovers between classes of worker are common late in life (Quinn 1980; Quinn, Burkhauser, and Myers 1990). The HRS data confirm both of these conclusions.

More than a quarter of the wage-and-salary workers had stopped work directly from their career jobs by 1996, compared to only 16 percent of the self-employed. Of the wage-and-salary workers who moved to a bridge job, nearly a quarter became self-employed. Of the self-employed who took a bridge job, about a third switched to wage-and-salary work. Although the proportion of career self-employed people who switched to a wage-and-salary job is higher than the reverse, there is still a substantial net increase in the number of self-employed because of the much larger proportion of career wage-and-salary workers to begin with. This is one reason why self-employment is more prevalent among older workers than it is in the labor force in general. For some older Americans, self-employment provides the means for gradual retirement, with additional flexibility of hours and type of work.

Additional research reported in Quinn 1999 analyzed the correlates of three types of job change activity among those on a career job in 1992: remaining on that career job through 1996, moving to a bridge job, and moving directly out of the labor force. Both tabular and multi-variate techniques were used.

As expected, the percentage remaining on their career jobs until 1996 declines with age, and the percentage who stopped working rises, with large jumps at key Social Security ages (i.e., the age 62 or the age 65 threshold). The importance of bridge job activity among those who left their career jobs declines with age. Among those men and women still less than 60 in 1996, over half of those who left their career jobs moved to bridge jobs; among those aged 62 or older, it was less than one-third.

Health status, measured in three different ways, also has the expected effects on both men and women.[8] In all cases, the worse the health status, the less likely people were to continue working on career jobs through 1996, the more likely they were to stop working, and the less likely they were to move to a bridge job if they did leave a career job.[9]

We also investigated the influence of two important components of the employee benefit package—health insurance coverage and pension status. We hypothesize that those who have health insurance on their career jobs but would lose it if they left will be less likely to depart, as will those participating in a pension plan but not yet eligible to claim benefits. The data provide support for both of these hypotheses. As expected, men and women with health insurance coverage at risk were the most likely to remain on their career jobs through 1996, and two-thirds of them did. Those who would maintain health coverage from some source after departure were the most likely to leave employment altogether. Those with no coverage at all were the most likely to move to another job. This may be related to the lack of health insurance coverage on the first job, or the latter may be correlated with a generally unattractive compensation package.

When we concentrated on only those who left their career jobs between 1992 and 1996, we found that those who did maintain health insurance coverage from some source were less likely to move to a bridge job than others, suggesting that health insurance may be one reason that some seek new work after leaving career employment.

With respect to pensions, we differentiated between defined benefit and defined contribution participation in the individual's primary plan and determined whether each person would be eligible to receive pension benefits by 1996, the end of the transition period. Several reasonable generalizations emerged. First, those participating in a pension plan (DB or DC) but not eligible to receive benefits by 1996 were much more likely than others to remain on the career job through 1996. This could be a straightforward pension effect, or it might also reflect the impact of age, since those not yet eligible for benefits tend to be younger than those who are eligible. Second, those eligible to receive benefits (DB or DC) by 1996 were the most likely to move directly from a career job to no job. Furthermore, the effects of DB eligibility appear to be stronger than the effects of DC eligibility. This may reflect the fact that DB plans often have strong age-specific incentives to leave the career job, whereas DC plans, by their nature, do not.

Finally, we compared the career job exit behavior of individuals in different wage rate categories and found a result noted before, at least among men: those at both ends of the socioeconomic spectrum are more likely to use transitional jobs on the way out (Quinn, Burkhauser, and Myers 1990). These findings are consistent with the hypothesis that there are two very different types of bridge job holders—those who continue working because they have to, and those who do so because they want to, even though they could afford to retire. It is interesting to note again that in the AARP survey of baby boomers mentioned above, about a quarter said they expected to keep working at least part time after age 65 because they would need the income, and about a third said they would continue working because of the enjoyment it would bring.

SUMMARY

Evidence suggests that the postwar era of earlier and earlier retirement has come to an end in the United States. After decades of decline, participation rates for older American men have been flat since the mid-1980s and have increased in recent years. For older women, the trends before 1986 were flat, but since then participation rates have risen substantially. Many more older men and women are currently working than the earlier trends would have predicted.

One important factor has been the strong economy, which increased the demand for labor, including older workers. But evidence suggests that there is more happening here. Changes in retirement trends are consistent with changes in the retirement environment that have altered the relative attractiveness of work and leisure and encouraged continued employment late in life. Mandatory retirement has been eliminated, and Social Security no longer penalizes the average person who continues to work after the normal retirement age. On the employer side, defined contribution pensions, which do not contain the strong age-specific work disincentives that many defined benefit plans do, are growing in popularity.

In addition, older Americans are living longer and are generally healthier than were earlier cohorts. Many can anticipate a decade or two of productive activity after age 62 or 65, and many have decided that some combination of work and leisure, for a while at least, is preferable to either continued full-time career employment or complete labor force withdrawal.

Research suggests that bridge jobs are an important part of the retirement process. Many older Americans retire gradually, using part-time or short-duration jobs on the way out. Many turn to self-employment. Surveys indicate that many of today's workers expect to keep working after they retire or turn 65. There is evidence that this can be good for workers. Kim and Moen find that "for men, post-retirement employment appears to be beneficial for their psychological well-being. Those who are retired and re-employed report the highest morale and lowest depression" (1999, 22). (They found no such relationship, however, for women.) Continued employment can also benefit the economy, since it will increase the productive capacity of the nation in the future, when the baby boom cohorts begin to retire. Toder and Solanki (1999, 26) estimate that if future cohorts were to adjust their retirement behavior to maintain a constant number of years in retirement as longevity increases, the ratio of labor supply to (needs-weighted) population would be about the same in 2040 as it is today, rather than declining about 8 percent without the retirement change.

A central tenet of economics is that people respond to incentives and that some of those near the margin will change their behavior if the incentives they face are altered. Public policy has changed in ways that make continued work at older ages more attractive and therefore more likely. Workers have responded as expected. Future initiatives, outlined in Burtless and Quinn 2001, can make work late in life even more attractive. If employers are willing to structure compensation and job characteristics to meet the needs of these potential employees, society can tap a growing pool of older, experienced, and willing workers for years to come. This would be beneficial for the nation as a whole, for employers, and for many of these older Americans as well.

ACKNOWLEDGMENTS

This chapter is drawn from two prior papers, "Has the Early Retirement Trend Reversed?" Boston College Department of Economics Working Paper no. 424, May 1999; and "New Paths to Retirement," which is Quinn 2000 in the References. I would like to thank Kevin Cahill of Abt Associates for excellent research assistance.

NOTES

1. For more detail and discussion on policies that would encourage more work late in life, see Burtless and Quinn 2001.

2. See Juster and Suzman 1995 for more detail on this outstanding data set. The age-eligible respondents were all aged 51 to 61 in 1992, during the first wave of data, but spouses could be older or younger. The HRS contains detailed information on each individual's demographic background; health and disability status; family structure; current, past, and prior employment; retirement plans (for those still working); health and life insurance coverage; housing status; income; and wealth.

Since we are focusing on the transition from work, we analyzed only those respondents with work experience after age 49, resulting in a sample of nearly 8,000 individuals—about 4,300 men and 3,700 women.

3. This research is described in more detail in Quinn 2000.

4. For an individual still working, job tenure is increasing with time, and we will not know the eventual tenure of that job until the respondent leaves it. Since part-time jobs are considered bridge jobs regardless of tenure, their eventual length does not matter, but for full-time jobs, it does. Some full-time workers on jobs with less than ten years duration in 1996 will have more than ten years tenure when they eventually leave. Rather than classify all current jobs with less than ten years duration in 1996 as bridge jobs and thereby exaggerate the phenomenon, we assumed that full-time workers younger than 62 would remain on their current jobs until age 62 and those still employed after age 62 would remain until age 65. We then classified the 1996 jobs as either career or bridge depending on their (estimated) eventual tenure.

We made these assumptions because over half of all covered workers claim Social Security benefits at age 62, and nearly all of the rest claim at age 65 (Social Security Administration 2000, table 6.B5.). Most could not receive benefits while maintaining full-time status on a career job.

5. This estimate of one-third may overcount a few full-time workers who will continue beyond our age 62 and age 65 assumptions, and thereby turn what we have labeled bridge jobs into career jobs. But it also counts none of those men still working on full-time career jobs, even though many of them will move to a bridge job in the future. Since this second bias is likely to be larger than the first, we are confident that this estimate of one-third is a lower bound.

6. The definition of a full-time career job adopted here, requiring full-time employment for at least ten years, is arbitrary, as is any definition. This definition may treat as a bridge job some experiences that really should be viewed as new careers. To test the sensitivity of our results, we also experimented with definitions requiring only eight or five years duration.

The definitions do make a difference, but the qualitative conclusions remain unchanged—bridge job activity is an important part of the labor force withdrawal process in America. When we decrease the tenure definition for a career job from ten to eight years, the extent of bridge job activity declines about 5 percent. When we drop the definition all the way to five years, the extent of bridge activity declines about 20 percent. But even under this severe definition, our lower bound estimates suggest that more than a quarter of the men and more than a third of the women pass through bridge jobs late in life. These estimates will undoubtedly rise as we observe in subsequent waves of the HRS the actual behavior of those still on their career jobs.

7. By searching the HRS data on the current, last (for those not working), and prior jobs, we can identify a full-time career job for 84 percent of the men and for 60 percent of the women we analyzed above.

8. We measured health in three different ways, all based on 1992 HRS responses: (1) a dichotomous variable based on whether the respondent claimed "any impairment or health problem that limits the kind or amount of paid work you can do," (2) a three-way variable based on a self-description of current health status (excellent or very good, good, fair or poor), and (3) a variable based on the individual's ability to perform a series of activities of daily living.

9. In fact, the influence of health on labor market transitions is undoubtedly stronger than it appears in this research, since this subsample includes only those on a career job in 1992. Those with more serious health limitations are more likely to have been out of the labor force by 1992 and therefore do not even appear in this analysis.

REFERENCES

Burtless, G., and J. F. Quinn. 2001. Retirement Trends and Policies to Encourage Work among Older Americans. In P. Budetti, R. Burkhauser, J. Gregory, and A. Hunt, eds., *Ensuring Health and Income Security for an Aging Workforce*. Kalamazoo, Mich.: W. E. Upjohn Institute for Employment Research, 375–415.

Costa, D. L. 1998. *The Evolution of Retirement: An American Economic History, 1880–1990*. Chicago: University of Chicago Press.

Council of Economic Advisers. 2001. *Economic Report of the President*. Washington, D.C.: U.S. Government Printing Office.

Crimmins, E. M., S. L. Reynolds, and Y. Saito. 1999. Trends in Health and Ability to Work among the Older Working-Age Population. *Journal of Gerontology* 54B, no. 1: S31–40.

Employee Benefit Research Institute. 1997. *EBRI Databook on Employee Benefits*. 4th ed. Washington, D.C.: Employee Benefit Research Institute.

Juster, F. T., and R. Suzman. 1995. An Overview of the Health and Retirement Survey. *Journal of Human Resources* 30 (suppl.): S7–56.

Kim, J. E., and P. Moen. 1999. Work/Retirement Transitions and Psychological Well-Being in Late Midlife. Working paper no. 99-10, Cornell Employment and Family Careers Institute, Ithaca, N.Y.

Manton, K. G., E. Stallard, and L. Corder. 1995. Changes in Morbidity and Chronic

Disability in the U.S. Elderly Population: Evidence from the 1982, 1984, and 1989 National Long Term Care Surveys. *Journal of Gerontology* 50B, no. 4: S194–204.

McNaught, W., M. Barth, and P. Henderson. 1989. The Human Resource Potential of Americans over 50. *Human Resource Management* 50:455–73.

Olsen, K., and J. VanDerhei. 1997. Defined Contribution Plan Dominance Grows across Sectors and Employer Sizes, While Mega Defined Benefit Plans Remain Strong. EBRI Special Report no. 190, October, Employee Benefit Research Institute, Washington, D.C.

Quadagno, J., and J. F. Quinn. 1997. Does Social Security Discourage Work? In E. Kingson and J. Schulz, eds., *Social Security in the Twenty-first Century,* 127–46. New York: Oxford University Press.

Quinn, J. F. 1980. Labor Force Participation Patterns of Older Self-Employed Workers. *Social Security Bulletin,* April, 17–28.

Quinn, J. F. 1999. Retirement Patterns and Bridge Jobs in the 1990s. EBRI Issue Brief no. 206, February, Employee Benefit Research Institute, Washington, D.C.

———. 2000. New Paths to Retirement. In O. S. Mitchell, P. B. Hammond, and A. M. Rappaport, eds., *Forecasting Retirement Needs and Retirement Wealth,* 13–32. Philadelphia: University of Pennsylvania Press.

Quinn, J. F., and R. V. Burkhauser. 1994. Public Policy and the Plans and Preferences of Older Americans. *Journal of Aging and Social Policy* 6, no. 3:5–20.

Quinn, J. F., R. V. Burkhauser, and D. A. Myers. 1990. *Passing the Torch: The Influence of Economic Incentives on Work and Retirement.* Kalamazoo, Mich.: W. E. Upjohn Institute for Employment Research.

Roper Starch Worldwide, Inc. 1998. Boomers Look toward Retirement. Presentation for the American Association of Retired Persons, Washington, D.C., June 2.

Social Security Administration. 2000. *Social Security Bulletin,* Annual Statistical Supplement.

Steuerle, E., C. Spiro, and R. W. Johnson. 1999. Can Americans Work Longer? Straight Talk on Social Security and Retirement Policy, August, Urban Institute, Washington, D.C.

Toder, E., and S. Solanki. 1999. Effects of Demographic Trends on Labor Supply and Living Standards. Occasional Paper no. 2, Urban Institute Retirement Project, Washington, D.C.

U.S. Bureau of Labor Statistics. (1965–2001, January issues). *Employment and Earnings.* Washington, D.C.: U.S. Government Printing Office.

U.S. House Committee on Ways and Means. 1998. *1998 Green Book.* Washington, D.C.: U.S. Government Printing Office.

Yakoboski, P., P. Ostuw, and J. Hicks. 1998. What Is Your Savings Personality? The 1998 Retirement Confidence Survey. EBRI Issue Brief no. 200, August, Employee Benefit Research Institute, Washington, D.C.

14

Aligning Incentives for a National Retirement Policy

Lynn Etheredge

Over the past sixty years, national retirement policy has relied on three major tools: Social Security, Medicare, and pensions. In 2001 more than $500 billion of federal revenues will go to the Social Security trust funds and more than $225 billion to the Medicare trust funds—the two fundamental retirement programs that cover almost every American. About $400 billion of net contributions and earnings will go into employer-based retirement plans, which supplement Social Security and Medicare for about half of the workforce, and the federal government will encourage these plans through $90 billion of tax subsidies (U.S. House Committee on Ways and Means 2000; U.S. Congress, Joint Committee on Taxation 2001). When the baby boom generation is fully retired, more than 70 million individuals will depend on Social Security, Medicare, and pensions for their standard of living, health benefits, and economic security, for an average of about twenty years (more than forty years for some). Although these elements of national retirement policy are all primarily financed by employer and employee payroll contributions, each has evolved independently.

The federal government has started to redesign national policies and programs to prepare for the baby boom generation's retirement. Major reforms of Medicare were enacted in 1997, and further changes, based on recommendations of a National Bipartisan Commission on the Future of Medicare, are now being considered. The debate started by the Advisory Council on Social Security's 1997 report may lead to that program's greatest changes since its 1935 enactment. Recent developments show an openness to new ideas about expanded consumer choice and flexibility in benefit options, such as allowing retirees to choose between traditional Medicare and private health plan benefits or to receive higher cash incomes and reduced benefits (Medicare+Choice, Medicare Medical Savings Accounts); investing some part of Social Security taxes in private pension accounts (two proposals by the Advisory Council on Social Security); allowing individuals to choose to pay taxes on IRA contributions when they are made so that benefits will be tax free during retirement (the Roth IRA); permitting more retirement needs to qualify for tax favored savings (exclusion of employer-paid premiums for qualifying long-term care insurance); and eliminating some of the benefit reductions applied to retirees who continue to work (Social Security earnings test).

These new measures signal the beginning of the long overdue process of revamping Medicare, Social Security, and pension policy so they can be a viable national retirement system for the baby boomers. However, four major problem areas remain:

1. *Work versus Retirement.* Government policies have encouraged a trend toward earlier retirement and discouraged older workers from continuing substantial work. Although trends toward earlier retirement have recently turned around, in 1999 59 percent of workers elected to receive Social Security retirement benefits at age 62 and 93 percent of workers by age 66 (U.S. House Committee on Ways and Means 2000). Life expectancy has been steadily increasing; individuals now turning 65 can anticipate a retirement period, on average, of at least another fifteen to twenty years. But analysts are beginning to question the sense of encouraging more than 70 million (mostly healthy) baby boomers to leave the workforce early—lowering the gross domestic product and government revenues, as well as their own earnings and financial resources. Retirement ages are rising for full Social Security benefits (so far, with little effect). However, amid these changes, a comprehensive review of early retirement and work incentives in Social Security, Medi-

care, and pension policies is overdue. Social Security and Medicare benefits could offer options to encourage work efforts on the part of older Americans.

2. *Pension coverage and savings.* The national personal savings rate has continued to decline and is now at its lowest rate in more than forty years (Yakoboski 2000). One of the key contributing factors has been that growth of employer-based pensions has stalled out, leaving half of the private sector workforce—more than 50 million workers—without current pension coverage[1] (U.S. House Committee on Ways and Means 2000). These persons lack the automatic payroll withholding and tax advantages (and the employer matching contributions) that encourage savings among workers with employer-sponsored pension benefits. Many will receive little or nothing in pension benefits and will be mostly dependent on what the federal government decides to spend for Social Security and Medicare benefits, supplemented by other savings or part-time earnings. As Victor Fuchs points out in chapter 17 in this volume, rising health costs not covered by Medicare will likely erode the living standards of many older persons. With large fiscal problems looming over both Medicare and Social Security, private savings (particularly tax boosted savings, such as pensions) are important for financing health care needs, higher living standards, and financial security.

3. *Benefits.* Overall, Medicare covers less than one-half of the elderly's health expenses, and most individuals patch together Medicare with supplementary (Medigap) plans. An improved health insurance benefit menu, including rollover financing options from pension plans for supplemental benefits (such as outpatient prescription drugs), could offer additional coverage, savings, portability, better financing, and more choices. Insurance underwriting practices and tax policies now limit market functioning and some types of benefit exchanges. It is important to foster growth of long-term care coverage, the largest gap in insurance protection for most retirees.

4. *Financing.* Social Security and Medicare's Hospital Insurance trust fund are both inadequately funded to provide benefits through the baby boomers' retirement. Increased revenues will be needed for the Medicare program; a constant 1.45 percent (employer/employee) tax rate can hardly be expected to finance more than 70 million additional enrollees. The financial difficulties of Social Security and Medicare—in-

tended to be a near-universal floor for all citizens—raise questions about the $90 billion per year of taxpayer-paid subsidies for private pensions, particularly about financing private pension benefits that are far more than Social Security's average benefit of about ten thousand dollars per retired worker in 2001. If there will be inadequate taxpayer financing for basic Medicare and Social Security benefits, perhaps economies should come from pension subsidies.

In this chapter I present several ideas for how a new policy framework that features better coordination of Medicare, Social Security, and pension policies could produce needed progress on the intractable retirement policy issues described above.

WORK VERSUS RETIREMENT

The rules government makes about the eligibility age(s) for Medicare, Social Security, and pension benefits, and how these benefits are affected by work, are critical issues for present and future retirees. Today, these rules are inconsistent and can penalize individuals who work longer and more than statutorily designated retirement ages and earnings limits. Given the increasing span of retirement, rising medical care costs, and uncertain financing for Social Security and Medicare benefits, many individuals would be better off if these incentives were changed and they had options to encourage work, at least part-time work, for several more years before full retirement. Government tax revenues would rise with the greater earnings that would result.

Eligibility

Medicare eligibility begins at age 65. Retirees cannot start Medicare at an earlier age, even with reduced benefits or higher premiums, and affordable private insurance is often not available for early retirees with health problems. Persons who defer starting Medicare until after age 65 do not receive higher benefits (or lower premiums) later. For Social Security, individuals can receive full earned benefits starting at age 65 (as of 2022, age 67). They can also elect to receive actuarially reduced benefits starting as early as age 62. Persons who delay Social Security until after "normal" retirement age (65 to 67) qualify for "deferred retirement credits" that will similarly enhance their monthly benefit checks. For a person who would receive an annual benefit of $10,000 beginning at normal retirement age, a one-year delay in starting the benefit would result in an increase of about $50 per month. There are now no options for lump sum payment of the $10,000 benefit.

Pension plans—including tax advantaged retirement plans such as 401(k)'s, Keoghs, Simplified Employee Pensions (SEPs), and IRAs— offer more flexibility than Medicare or Social Security do. For example, 401(k) plans, the rapidly growing employee directed plans, allow persons to take lump sum withdrawals as early as age 59.5 (or annuities at an earlier age) without penalty and to defer starting withdrawals until age 70.5. For defined contribution plans, such as 401(k)s, an individual is entitled to the full value of the account, whenever it is withdrawn.[2]

Work Incentives

Medicare, Social Security, and pensions also differ in the incentives to work that they offer recipients. Although the Senior Citizens' Freedom to Work Act of 2000 (P.L. 106-182) eliminated the earnings test after age 65, Social Security benefits, for a primary recipient and family members, are still reduced for individuals under age 65 by one dollar for every two dollars of earnings over $10,000. These are punitive tax rates, and they apply to the older persons most likely to be interested in continuing full-time work or, in "bridge" jobs, engaging in part-time work. They are in addition to the income and Social Security taxes owed on earnings. In contrast, taxable pension incomes are subject to the same tax rates as earned incomes, except that there is a 10 percent penalty for early withdrawal (before age 59.5). A 10 percent surtax on pension incomes of more than $160,000 per year from tax advantaged pensions was repealed in 1997.

Persons lose most Medicare financing for health benefits when they work after age 65 for an employer of twenty or more workers that offers health insurance benefits. In these instances, Medicare becomes a "secondary payer" and pays only for covered benefits that are not paid by the employer's plan. This shifts most of Medicare's costs to employers and these older workers and raises employers' costs for employing workers after age 65. There are no offsetting benefits for older workers. Workers for smaller employers and for firms that do not offer health insurance do not have reduced benefits.

Crafting a More Coherent Policy

A more coherent national retirement policy should allow for early retirement of those who cannot work. Given the financial problems of financing the baby boom generation's retirement, however, better work incentives should be a top priority.

A set of early retirement options, with actuarially reduced benefits, for those who are unable to find suitable work or choose to retire early could be coordinated for Medicare, Social Security, and pensions. Adopting a common standard for all three would allow more flexibility in personal decision making.[3]

On the opposite side of the coin, delayed retirement options up to age 70.5, coordinated for Medicare and Social Security, could provide actuarially fair and enhanced benefits for later retirees. If a worker delayed receiving Social Security and Medicare for one year, for example, he or she might be allowed to elect either a lump sum "retirement bonus" check of $10,000 or more, payable on the day of retirement, or enhanced monthly benefits. The government would be able to afford these financial incentives because it would save approximately $13,000 for each year that a person's retirement was delayed ($10,000 Social Security benefits, plus $3,000 Medicare benefits, plus interest) and would also collect additional taxes from the worker's earnings.

These lump sum options for later retirement could add substantially to the "nest egg" of many retirees. They thus might be a more effective inducement for continued work than small increases in monthly retirement checks. In 1996 the lowest-income quintile of households headed by individuals age 65 to 69 had only $3,750 of net worth in nonhousing assets, the second-lowest-income quintile of households had $20,750, and even the third-lowest-income quintile of households had only $48,150 (U.S. Bureau of the Census 2001). The enhanced benefit options would apply for each year of delayed retirement up to 70.5—for example, a $30,000 bonus for three years' delay in retirement (and twice that amount for a household with two workers delaying retirement). Such bonus options offer a readily available means for older workers to build up financial reserves.

Older individuals should incur no penalties for earning income as economically productive members of society. The remaining Social Security benefit reductions for work-related earnings (50% tax rates for age 62 to 65) ought to be eliminated. For post-65 workers with employer health insurance as their primary coverage, Medicare could make a premium contribution (via an employer tax deduction) for the added costs of covering these workers, so that they would not be disadvantaged in the labor market.

Measures such as these would provide senior citizens with better (and fairer) incentives for substantial work efforts. The longer-term payoff, for retirees and government budgets, would depend on how much additional earnings, savings, and revenues resulted.

EXPANDED PENSIONS

A second key challenge for an integrated national retirement policy is to create new retirement savings options for individuals who do not have employer-provided pensions. The availability of good supplementary pension income is the critical difference between a retirement that is just "getting by" on Social Security and Medicare and one with a much better standard of living, ability to afford health care, and financial security. The majority of retirees, lacking significant private pension incomes, are almost totally dependent on these two programs. Some 60 percent of retirees, for example, receive 75 percent (or more) of their income from Social Security, and nearly all of the elderly depend on Medicare as their primary health insurance coverage (Employee Benefits Research Institute 1997). As Fuchs illustrates (see chapter 17), so long as health care costs not covered by Medicare (Medigap, prescription drugs, and long-term care) are rising much faster than Social Security increases (3.5 percent in 2001), these individuals will likely have declining standards of living during their retirement years unless they have additional savings as well as work options.

The major federal government policy to build pension coverage has been to encourage employers to offer pension plans to workers.[4] The tax code subsidies of about $90 billion a year are intended to give higher pension benefits to executives so that their companies will offer pension benefits for workers and encourage participation.[5] Experts report uncertainty as to how well justified these subsidies' higher-income tilt is, but most pension benefits are paid to middle- and upper-middle income persons (Salisbury and Jones 1994; Friedland, Etheredge, and Vladeck 1994). Since there has not been a thorough congressional review of national pension policy since the enactment of the Employee Retirement and Income Security Act (ERISA) of 1974, many elements of pension policy merit reexamination. As of 1998, employer-based retirement plans had assets of $7.4 trillion (Salisbury 2001).[6] As of January 2001, the combined assets of the Social Security and Medicare trust funds were $1.3 trillion.

An improved national retirement policy should make available voluntary pension coverage for the majority of workers—more than 50 million persons—without employer sponsored pensions. These workers are most often without coverage simply because their employer does not offer a pension plan. In broad terms, national retirement policy thus faces the same issues that national health policy faces. Our social welfare policies have primarily emphasized employer-based coverage and have left tens of millions of persons, whose employers do not want to offer health insurance and pension benefits, without comparable benefits and tax assistance. Many of these workers are now multiply disadvantaged, second-class citizens; they lack both health insurance and pension coverage and also do not share in the more than $150 billion annually of federal tax subsidies offered for workers who do have such benefits.

An integrated approach to Social Security and pensions would offer a practical method for making good pension plans available for all workers. The Social Security payroll contribution collection system can be used to direct investments to both government social insurance and individual pension plans.[7] Persons who do not have an employer sponsored pension plan (and their employers) could make payroll contributions via this collection system to (1) qualified private pension plans (a Teachers Insurance and Annuity Association, or TIAA, model); (2) stock, bond, and money market index funds (a federal employees' pension model); (3) Social Security, for supplemental benefits; or some combination of these choices.[8] Such contributions would benefit from the same contribution limits, tax benefits, and legal protections that employer pensions enjoy. Thus there would be two parallel retirement savings systems: persons with employer sponsored pensions would make payroll contributions to those plans; persons without such pensions would make payroll contributions to individual pension accounts.[9]

Using this approach, the average worker, who is now limited to a $2,000 annual contribution to an IRA, could benefit from the much higher contributions now allowed for workers with employer sponsored plans ($10,500 of employee contributions for a 401[k] plan in 2000). Other advantages for workers would include payroll withholding (which is usually not available for IRAs) and tax benefits (pension contributions would be excluded from taxable income on the taxpayer's 1040 tax form, as is done with IRAs), as well as ERISA-type regulation. Such funds would also be immediately vested and universally portable.

Although younger workers with children may not be large savers, the baby boom generation will be more able to save, once children are grown and mortgages are paid, and might take advantage of such new opportunities as they become better educated about retirement needs. There is certainly time for baby boomers to build up substantial savings, if they have tax advantaged means similar to those of workers with employer pension plans. A two-worker couple starting to invest $5,000 per year in a tax advantaged pension plan at age 50 would have approximately $135,000 by age 65 (assuming 8% annual interest). To the extent that these new savings arrangements were successful, they would offer a highly leveraged return on federal investment. If $10 billion annually of new savings for future retirees was generated, the tax costs (at 15% income tax rate) would be $1.5 billion, which entails much less expense for building up resources for the baby boom generation than would the alternative of increasing taxes by $10 billion for government trust funds.

CAFETERIA BENEFITS

An integrated retirement policy also could offer a broader range of choices to fill the gaps in health and long-term care insurance coverage. The gaps in Medicare acute care coverage, such as the lack of outpatient prescription drug coverage and inadequate catastrophic insurance protection, are well known. Most elderly persons now fill in such benefits with private Medigap policies or employer provided supplemental coverage. It would be desirable to include many of these standardized Medigap options in basic Medicare or to offer Medigap options as part of the new national "open season" during which individuals can choose between Medicare and competing health plans. Such arrangements would reduce administrative expenses, improve portability, and allow better comparison shopping between Medicare (with Medigap) and Medicare+Choice plans.

Prescription Drugs

It would be particularly desirable to have an expanded, government structured "cafeteria menu" of options that included guaranteed choice for prescription drug coverage. Two of the criticisms against prescription drug coverage in the past no long apply. First, nearly all pharmacies now use electronic claim submission, so the high administrative costs of paper claims for small benefits is no longer a factor. Second, most pharmacy benefits (such as those for federal employees) are now offered through pharmacy benefit management (PBM) companies that negotiate price discounts, so a national system of Medicare price controls for prescription drugs would not be needed.

Long-Term Care

The most serious insurance market failure for the elderly is the lack of a good system of long-term care benefits. Few retirees can have full economic security until these gaps can be closed. Private long-term care insurance covered only 8 percent of the national nursing home expenses of $90 billion in 1999, and Medicare paid for only 11 percent of nursing home costs. Individuals can qualify for Medicaid—which paid 47 percent of nursing home expenses—only by spending down nearly all of their assets. Nearly 27 percent of nursing home expenses were paid out of pocket (Heffler et al. 2001). Because Medicaid nursing home expenses remain one of the largest long-term government budget costs of both federal and state governments, both government and retirees would benefit from a better-developed market for private long-term care coverage.

Congress recently attempted to accelerate the growth of private long-term care insurance by excluding employer paid premiums for qualified plans (as well as such plans' benefits) from recipients' income tax. Although some employers offer long-term care benefits, most are still fully employee paid, and it is questionable whether this product will grow quickly as a new, employer financed retirement benefit. Indeed, employers are tending to cut back on many retiree commitments, including health benefits. Similarly, it is questionable whether a large Medicare benefit improvement to cover most nursing home care should be anticipated; the Congressional Budget Office forecast for Medicare expenses to rise by about 3 percent of GDP by 2030 would require revenue increases comparable to about a $270 billion annual tax increase in the year 2000 (when GDP was about $9 trillion) just to cover current benefits (CBO 1998). Thus, for long-term care benefits, it is particularly useful to consider whether more flexible use of pension fund assets could be part of the answer.

Two measures that might rapidly increase private long-term care coverage are as follows. First, federally qualified pension plans could be required to offer a menu of payout options that includes a "rollover" for a portion of pension accounts to pay premiums for qualifying long-term care policies. If persons were allowed to make such election into their early 60s, at the time most will be considering their retirement needs and resources, they would not need to use their long-term care coverage for about fifteen years. This change would, by itself, create a very large potential market for private long-term care insurance. These reforms should integrate long-term care insurance into the same public market as other Medicare benefits, with qualification standards, consumer rights, quality assurance, and performance "report cards" for beneficiaries. Adding long-term care insurance as a cafeteria option for pension arrangements would instantly make available a very large potential purchasing pool for these benefits, if the products were deemed to be of value, and would be less expensive than building up still another funding stream of taxpayer subsidized savings available only for long-term care insurance.[10]

Second, private long-term care insurance would be more affordable (and much less risky) if Medicaid spending down and Medicare were redesigned to mesh with private long-term care insurance, for example, to cover benefits after a two-year period for individual self-pay or private insurance. One possible source for whatever additional financing would be needed, in an integrated system, would be a 0.25 percent tap on tax qualified retirement fund balances. Because pension plans have been developed to provide retirement security and because the tap would eliminate a major gap in financial security that few individuals can now close by themselves, this approach could gain widespread acceptance. With about a $9.5 trillion balance in employer and individual tax favored retirement accounts, such a tax rate would raise about $24 billion annually, which could be combined with state matching funds. Persons who purchase qualifying private long-term care insurance could also be exempt from state Medicaid spend-down requirements.

Government would lose tax revenues to the extent that (taxable) pension incomes became (nontaxed) long-term care premium payments. Government's major long-term gain would result if a large market in private long-term care insurance could be "jump-started" in this way, sharply reducing future Medicaid expenses and tax deductions for catastrophic long-term care expenses. Additional government financing from a tap on pension fund assets would improve budget resources.

FUNDING PRIORITIES

A comprehensive national retirement perspective also raises important questions about priorities for taxpayers' support of Social Security, Medicare, and pensions. Social Security and Medicare were designed to be nearly universal benefits, guaranteeing basic standards of living and economic security. Pension benefits were a supplement. Nevertheless, both Social Security and Medicare benefits are now in financial jeopardy, and there are proposals for benefit cuts. If cutbacks are on the table for basic benefits, however, taxpayer support for supplemental pension benefits should be subjected to new scrutiny. Major overhaul of the pension system could jeopardize what has proved to be a useful private savings vehicle for retirement. However, economies could be considered in taxpayer financing for pensions if savings are needed to ensure financial integrity of the Social Security and Medicare programs.

Lynn Etheredge

A new national retirement policy for the baby boom generation needs to make major progress on the four critical problems of better work incentives, expanded pension coverage, more health and long-term care benefits, and sound financing of Medicare and Social Security. A strategy based on coordinated reforms of Medicare, Social Security, and pension policies offers a number of promising options for consideration.

ACKNOWLEDGMENTS

The author thanks Alicia Munnell, John Rother, Dallas Salisbury, and Larry Thompson for thoughtful critiques of an earlier version of this chapter. The chapter was supported by a grant from the Robert Wood Johnson Foundation to the Health Insurance Reform Project at George Washington University. This is an updated version of a paper that was originally published in *Health Affairs* 18, no. 1: 80–91, and is reprinted here with permission.

NOTES

1. Some of these workers will earn retirement benefits at other points in their career. Some workers will withdraw and spend funds before retirement.

2. For defined benefit plans, earlier retirement is often available with reduced benefits; later retirement may not result in similarly higher benefits.

3. Actuarially reduced (or enhanced) benefits would be budget neutral for trust fund expenditures over time. Medicare benefit reductions could be through higher premiums.

4. Pension policy has been supplemented in recent years by IRAs, Roth IRAs, and a Medical Savings Account (MSA) demonstration.

5. The intentional inequities include "integration" rules that allow employers to reduce pensions for lower-wage workers to offset their Social Security benefits; employer contributions based on percentage of earnings, which makes for higher contributions for higher-income workers; and the greater tax advantages of tax excludable income for higher-income executives. Disparities are limited by various "top heavy" rules and other provisions. Social Security and Medicare intentionally favor low- and moderate-income workers.

6. Of this amount, $5 trillion was in private sector plans and $2.4 trillion in government plans. All retirement plan assets, including IRAs, were $9.5 trillion.

7. One of the options proposed by the Advisory Council on Social Security was to direct part of OASDI contributions to individual pension accounts. Improvements in Social Security Administration procedures would be needed to implement individual account proposals.

8. Collection and redirection of contributions would occur via the banking system, so the pension contributions would not need to become government rev-

enues and outlays. Funds could also be remitted directly by employers to pension plans, if more convenient. Pension experts believe that payroll withholding methods are essential for broad participation in retirement plans; most employees do not now have payroll withholding for their IRA contributions, which is one reason why participation is low.

9. Employers that now offer pension plans would not be likely to drop them, since an employer sponsored plan offers higher contribution limits (up to $30,000 for executives); greater employer design flexibility; and tax exclusions of employer contributions from Old Age, Survivors, Disability and Health Insurance (OASDHI) taxes, a 15.3 percent advantage.

10. A rollover option excludes the pension funds from income taxes that would need to be paid on the original pretax contributions if the pension funds were withdrawn and then used to pay the premiums.

REFERENCES

Congressional Budget Office (CBO). 1998. *Long-Term Budgetary Pressures and Policy Options*. Washington, D.C.: U.S. Government Printing Office, May.

Employee Benefit Research Institute. 1997. *EBRI Databook on Employee Benefits*. 4th ed. Washington, D.C.: Employee Benefit Research Institute.

Friedland, R., L. Etheredge, and B. Vladeck, eds. 1994. *Social Welfare Policy at the Crossroads*. Washington, D.C.: National Academy of Social Insurance.

Heffler, S., K. Levit, S. Smith, C. Smith, C. Cowan, H. Lazenby, and M. Freeland. 2001. Health Spending Growth Up in 1999: Faster Growth Expected in the Future. *Health Affairs* 20, no. 2: 193–203.

Salisbury, D. 2001. *EBRI Research Highlights: Retirement and Health Data (Special Report)*. SR 36 Issue Brief no. 229, January, Employee Benefit Research Institute, Washington, D.C.

Salisbury, D., and N. Jones, eds. 1994. *Pension Funding and Taxation*. Washington, D.C.: Employee Benefit Research Institute.

U.S. Bureau of the Census. 2001. *Household Net Worth and Asset Ownership, 1995*. Current Population Reports, P70-71, February. Washington, D.C.: U.S. Government Printing Office.

U.S. Congress, Joint Committee on Taxation. 2001. *Estimates of Federal Tax Expenditures for Fiscal Years 2001–2005*. JCS-1-01, April 5. Washington, D.C.: U.S. Government Printing Office.

U.S. House Committee on Ways and Means. 2000. *2000 Green Book*. WMCP 106-14, October 6. Washington, D.C.: U.S. Government Printing Office.

Yakoboski, P. 2000. Retirement Plans, Personal Saving, and Savings Adequacy. EBRI Issue Brief no. 219, March, Employee Benefit Research Institute, Washington, D.C.

IV

POLITICAL

REALITIES

15

Enacting Reform

What Can We Expect in the Current Political Context?

Norman J. Ornstein, Ph.D.

The 2000 U.S. elections were the most consequential in the modern era. For the first time since 1952, every power center in Washington—the White House, the Senate, the House of Representatives—was simultaneously up for grabs. The presidential contest was an open one, with no incumbent running; from the start, it was both fluid and unpredictable. The Senate's Republican margin changed from five seats to four soon before the election with the tragic death of Georgia Republican senator Paul Coverdell: there were enough Republican seats up for grabs and genuinely contestable to leave its majority unsettled. The House of Representatives had its smallest partisan margin in forty-six years, making a shift of a mere 7 seats to the Democrats out of 435 enough to change the majority. At the same time, in the state legislatures, where postelection redistricting would shape the U.S. House for the next decade, more than twenty chambers were close enough that a shift of five or fewer seats would change party control.

The stakes were thus remarkably high—and made higher because of the dynamics of the previous decade. Bill Clinton's election in 1992 fundamentally altered patterns of power in American politics. His election represented a break from twelve consecutive years of Republican control of the White House and from an era of Republican dominance spanning twenty of the previous twenty-four years. More significant, his reelection represented the first time a Democrat had been reelected to a second term since Franklin Roosevelt. Furthermore, the Republican victory in 1994 created the first GOP congressional majority in forty years, and the continued Republican majority with the 1996 election represented the first time since 1928 that the Republicans had won two consecutive terms in control, a pattern they continued with the 1998 elections. From 1952 to 1992, basically, each political party in America had its own sphere of influence. The 1994 and 1996 elections in effect turned both of those spheres upside down, adding to the determination of Republicans to win back the White House in 2000 and the Democrats to win back Congress. Each party looked to November 7, 2000, to create a new pattern of superiority, one that could be parlayed into a longer-term dominance well into the new century.

It took thirty-six days beyond November 7 for the dust to settle from this high-stakes election—and nothing fundamental was resolved. Although Republicans did win the White House, it was under extraordinary circumstances, after a nearly unprecedented period of tension and wrangling; and even then, after five of nine Supreme Court justices effectively declared George W. Bush the winner, it was with the barest majority of 271 electoral votes. The Republicans retained their majority in the House of Representatives but saw their margin shrink yet again, to 5 votes out of 435. And the Senate ended up in a tie for the second time in American electoral history, the first since 1880.

After the election, seventeen states had Republican majorities in their legislative chambers, sixteen had Democratic majorities, and the rest were split. In major surveys, the public party identification showed a virtual dead heat between Republicans and Democrats. In the presidential popular vote, Democrat Al Gore edged out Republican Bush by roughly 0.5 percent of the votes cast. By most standards, the nation is divided as evenly as possible in partisan political terms. The overall votes cast nationwide for the House of Representatives were close to dead even. Though Republicans, for the first time since 1952, took control of the White House and both houses of Congress, the control of the Senate was nominal and effective control of the House quite limited. Even as George W. Bush was being inaugurated as the forty-third president of the United States, politicians and consultants were turning their attention to 2002, when both houses of Congress were slated to be up for grabs again, with Democrats eager to take back majorities, bullish on their chances, and looking for any political advantage or leverage.

Contrast George Bush's arrival as president with that of Ronald Reagan. Reagan won the White House in a landslide and brought with him the first Republican Senate in a quarter century along with a robust gain of thirty-three GOP seats in the House of Representatives. Bush won by the slimmest of margins and had "negative coattails," with his party losing seats in both houses of Congress. Bush also lost the bulk of his presidential transition to the postelection maneuvering.

But despite a dauntingly unfavorable environment, George W. Bush moved swiftly to assume control of the White House, organizing a White House staff and selecting a cabinet with alacrity and settling quickly on two initial top priorities—education and tax cuts. Other issues, including health policy and Social Security, despite their prominence in the campaign (more on this later), were relegated largely to second- or third-stage status. Indeed, in keeping with his strategic focus, Bush subordinated other priorities to the achievement of his most important, especially the tax cuts. To provide maximum flexibility for the latter, his budget refused, for example, to include Medicare in the fully protected "lockbox" category that Democrats and moderate Republicans demanded.

Bush's initial approach, his strategy for his first hundred days, was reminiscent of Reagan's, and in the first two months he had at least as much promise of success. Reagan in fact had started swiftly, then stumbled and faced heavy odds against his top priorities of budget and tax cuts until the assassination attempt against him in late March of his first year altered dramatically the political dynamic. Bush's chances for a smoother beginning and a reasonably successful first hundred and eighty days seemed quite respectable from an April 2001 vantage point.

But in the broader sense, the political dynamic of 2001–2, combined with larger structural issues, created a more intractable political environment for those second- and third-stage issues.

Consider first the dynamics of this time period. In most post–World War II elections, there was no serious question about the partisan control of Congress. Democrats kept the majority in the House for forty consecutive years from 1954 until 1994 and held the majority in the

Senate for a quarter century, from 1954 until 1980. That meant that those Congresses were sensitive to upcoming elections but saw the stakes more in individual than institutional terms—what would happen in their own contests for reelection, not would they be committee or sub-committee chairs or relegated to dreaded minority status. The 2000 election, and the 2002 and (almost certainly) the 2004 contests as well, will have a starkly different dynamic, one with the razor-thin majorities of both houses of Congress clearly at stake and in play. That means high stakes under any circumstances. But the stakes are made higher yet by another factor, the result not of the short-term politics of the next election but of a longer trend inside Congress.

The typical post–World War II Congress was characterized by a classic "normal distribution" in ideological terms. Most members could be characterized as in the broad center of the political spectrum. To use a football field analogy, most lawmakers would have been clustered near the midfield stripe, between the thirty-five- and forty-yard lines. The centrist tendencies in both parties fit well most of the senior members, meaning that on many committees, a shift in majority would have led to a shift in chairmanships that would result in little if any ideological change. For example, a move in the 1960s from Wilbur Mills (D-Ark.) as chairman of the House Ways and Means Committee to John Byrnes (R-Wis.) would have had no discernible policy consequences.

The 107th Congress, by contrast, has a classic bimodal distribution. Perhaps 15 percent or so of the members are near the midfield line. In the House of Representatives, especially, there are substantial numbers of lawmakers around each ten- and twenty-yard line—and lots of members behind each goalpost! Why is the 107th Congress so ideologically polarized—like its predecessor, and almost certainly like its successor? There are many reasons. Forty years of one-party rule tends to generate more partisan and ideological polarization, especially on the part of the perpetual minority. Contemporary political culture, which has a take-no-prisoners quality, including a trend to criminalize political differences, tends to drive out moderates. The permanent campaign reinforces a culture in which colleagues on the other side of the aisle become permanent enemies instead of frequent adversaries and occasional allies. Polarization makes compromise more difficult, which also tends to discourage moderates and accelerate their departure rates.

Consider one other important factor. Despite the incredibly high stakes, the election that brought this Congress in had a strikingly small number of truly contested seats—probably no more than thirty-five or forty in the House. The year 2000 reinforced a paradoxical pattern that has been in the making for more than two decades: as the elections have become more and more consequential, House seats have become increasingly safe.

Safe seats generate lawmakers more sensitive to their party primaries than to any real competition in general elections. Primaries are usually dominated by each party's ideological base. Thus, we have more House members representing their bases and more members very sensitive to avoiding any alienation from the base. Safe seats also mean more homogeneity in districts, which in turn means less dissonant feedback from constituents and more ideological and partisan reinforcement for lawmakers.

The ideological differences are most distinct among senior members and leaders; contrast current Ways and Means chair Bill Thomas (R-Calif.) with current ranking member Charles Rangel (D-N.Y.), for example, or investigations panel chair Dan Burton with ranking Democrat Henry Waxman. The same is true of party leaders; think of the gulf between Dick Armey and Tom DeLay, on the one hand, and Dick Gephardt and David Bonior on the other. Thus, the election stakes, in terms of outlook, agenda-setting, staff, and power, are enormous, and the obstacles to genuine bipartisanship, especially in the House, are great.

The change in Congress is not simply ideological and partisan. Congress has also been characterized by substantial change in membership generally, resulting in a striking generational shift. The change did not come with one huge election shift or through the ouster of large numbers of incumbents in elections. Rather, it came incrementally through a regular pattern of change, fueled as much by voluntary departures as election defeats. In the 107th Congress, three-fourths of the members are new since the 1990s began. Forty-five of the 100 senators are in their first term. This is both a post–Cold War Congress and a Generation X Congress. The number of military veterans is sharply down, and the number of members more self-absorbed and less institution-minded is sharply up. A prime quality for the exercise of strong leadership is the existence of followership. Republicans found impressive discipline in the House in the first months of the 107th Congress, because of their uniform desire, fresh after eight years of their nemesis Bill Clinton, to keep their new president strong. But signs of individualization were evident from the get-go in the Senate and seemed to be emerging in the House after sixty days or so.

No House leader could easily find majorities with a 5-vote margin; no Senate leader could easily pass legislation in a tied setting, especially when 60 votes, not 50, are required to overcome a filibuster. There would be ample headaches for strong leaders, but the majority leaderships in both houses have struggled mightily to achieve any characterization in the same zip code as "strong."

Add in two further complications. All these politics are occurring during a time of slowdown, after an unprecedentedly strong and sustained economic performance. We continue to have projections of huge budget surpluses, but it is clear that the demands on government will increase if the slowdown turns into full-fledged recession, and especially if it lasts for any length of time. We will see an expanded set of budget cross-pressures, including public demands for more social services, such as prescription drug benefits and steps to take care of a larger number of uninsured Americans; demands on the federal government from states that see their own surpluses melting away and their public demands rising; the top priority of very large tax cuts and the political pressures to cut taxes even more; and the possibility that the projections of surpluses intended to fund all these things will decline sharply as economic figures are adjusted.

The politics of surpluses meshes directly with the politics of the budget. It turns out that the politics of surpluses, even when projections show them expanding in the face of economic slowdown, is every bit as frustrating and divisive as the politics of deficits. Discretionary spending caps, in an era with strong leaders, normal levels of contentiousness, and lower-stakes elections, would be a minor obstacle to a bipartisan desire to satisfy each party's policy goals and most members' political needs. It would be relatively easy to move back to a form of budget incrementalism from the era of decrementalism.

But today's very different broad politics make for different budget politics. Caps and budget rules combine with the need to satisfy party ideological bases and to find traction against the other side for the next election. This creates a witch's brew of contentiousness, with tax cuts, Social Security, Medicare, defense, and the gamut of domestic priorities all thrown into the mix. After several years when discretionary spending grew by near-double-digit amounts, President Bush, in response to unrealistically low caps set in the balanced budget agreement of 1997, proposed a 4 percent increase for fiscal 2002. But even his Senate Budget Committee chairman, Pete Domenici (R-N.Mex.), said soon after the president's announcement that that amount was too low.

No matter the outcome for fiscal 2002, the result is going to be continuing severe pressure on discretionary spending, domestic and defense, relieved largely via budget chicanery and legerdemain, and continuing upward pressure on the twin tower entitlements of Social Security and Medicare. The problems, of course, could grow worse with a potential bidding war on tax cuts—and much worse if future adjustments in projections of budget surpluses are downward rather than upward.

Barring truly extraordinary developments, closely divided Congresses are likely to be the norm, not the exception, for some time to come. Weak leadership in Congress, even larger proportions of junior members, and continued sharp ideological and partisan divisions are a given; lengthy periods of divided government are a likely concomitant. Absent a cataclysm, neither party is at all likely to gain enough standing to emerge as a clear majority force; each side will be scrambling to find voter blocs and issues by which to gain predominance. Budget politics may shift some if Democrats recapture the majority in the House, but the fundamental difficulties—entitlements growing as a share of the budget and everything else squeezed down—will remain.

If outside players, a few lawmakers, or even the lame duck president occasionally raise the issue of developing long-term approaches to Social Security and Medicare—including slowing their rates of growth— the pressure within each party will be to add inoculation against a Social Security or Medicare political flu and to use any evidence available to label the other side as insufficiently concerned about either program. The impetus to a bidding war—adding more benefits or reducing direct costs, rather than reining in growth—will be great.

That is particularly true with Medicare. Talk of Medicare reform, especially reform that would expand the use of managed care in the

Medicare program, is not off the table, but it is far removed from the top priority items on either the presidential or congressional agendas. The primary Medicare agenda is a substantive one, but the focus is expansive, with the prescription drug issue leading. President Bush's first bid in this area, an immediate infusion of cash to those states with programs to help the poorest elderly, was summarily rejected by key players in both parties in Congress. The sharp partisan differences in approach to prescription drug benefits for the elderly, with Democrats insisting on running any program through Medicare and Republicans demanding a central role for private insurers, either through tax credits or direct subsidies for recipients, make compromise difficult. The most likely compromise discussed on Capitol Hill is to adopt some version of Ways and Means chairman Bill Thomas's idea for direct subsidies to the elderly to pay for private prescription drug insurance—with substantial additional money added in to satisfy enough recalcitrant Democrats. Whichever way a compromise goes, it will be far more likely to expand the scope of the Medicare program than to be included as part of a package that restrains future growth.

The year 1999 began with a vigorous debate ongoing about major reform of the Social Security system, including a variety of financing options and even talk of partial privatization. Some broad compromise, including perhaps a version of President Clinton's USA accounts and some investment of funds in market index funds, seemed feasible. But impeachment politics took any serious prospect of bipartisan negotiation off the table.

Social Security did become a campaign issue of sorts in 2000, with candidate Bush endorsing the idea of partial private accounts, funded by diverting 2 percent of employee FICA taxes, and candidate Gore opposing the notion (as he opposed any possible increase in retirement age or any significant structural change in the program). Not surprisingly, President Bush has not made this idea an early priority. In any event, the sharp stock market drop has dulled any public appetite for private accounts, and even more extended projections of solvency in the trust funds have dulled any appetite for serious Social Security reform.

Of course, there could be a crisis in the program, but, as various chapters in this volume make clear, that is not likely in the near future. Rather, the most interesting long-term dynamic here is the broader one facing budget politics. Social Security, Medicare, and the long-term care component of Medicaid together make up over 40 percent of the federal budget. If no significant changes are made in these programs and in other budget areas, these three programs would constitute more than 50 percent of the budget in a decade and would make up about 70 percent of the budget by 2030! Few lawmakers currently see Social Security and Medicare as components of a zero-sum game; the domestic and defense discretionary budget caps are viewed separately from the budget growth freedom given to the entitlements. That will change as the budget squeeze becomes more palpable.

My late beloved colleague Herb Stein said many insightful things; one of the best is "If something can't go on forever, it will stop." The likelihood of a federal budget in which Social Security, Medicare, and Medicaid make up 70 percent of the whole budget is slim. But if, when, and how this inexorable trend becomes exorable is a key element of our politics in the next decade.

There are, of course, ample reasons to examine Social Security, Medicare, and Medicaid on their own merits. If President Bush succeeds in his first year in accomplishing his two central initial goals, education reform and tax cuts, he may decide to make such an examination his top priority, creating an atmosphere for a broad, bipartisan negotiation over one or more of these programs. If that does not occur, the issues of Social Security, Medicare, and Medicaid will emerge only as politicians in both parties feel the squeeze their growth puts on other programs in government. The squeeze will not be on *every* other program; programs funded separately, via trust funds, like the highway program, will be insulated. Unabated growth in highway spending means even more pressure on programs like Head Start, student loans, environmental cleanup, the FBI, strategic defense, embassy security, agricultural aid, the national parks, and so on.

One alternative would be to let all programs grow, allowing the federal budget to take an increasing share of GNP. If anything, our politics and ethos are moving in the opposite direction. Another would be to let the disputes be confined to discretionary programs—pit Headstart against education, not Headstart and education against Medicare. As the discretionary programs find their growth stilted, and as they also have to compete with new ideas and priorities as well as surprises and emergencies, the bloodshed required to narrow the trade-offs would become too great to sustain.

So we have the following dynamics. We have two major parties, neither of which has a clear standing as a majority, each facing the likelihood of close contests on a fairly regular basis for control of each house of Congress and for the White House, each struggling to build a base in the electorate and in Washington to relegate the other side to a more permanent minority status. Each party's congressional base is becoming more ideologically cohesive, as the two sides become more polarized, a polarization that does not reflect broader public attitudes or issue positions. Ideological polarization has been accompanied by increased partisan tension, animosity, and distrust, which have abated somewhat thanks to the personal style of President George W. Bush but still rest just beneath the surface.

Each side desperately seeks traction—issues to mobilize its own base, demoralize the other side, and turn voters in the middle against its opponents. A direct corollary is that each side seeks inoculation against issues that will damage it among swing voters. These sentiments exist for a wide range of issues, including abortion, gun control, nuclear proliferation, and global warming. But few issues have anywhere near the potential for gain or damage as Social Security and Medicare.

Each side will therefore continue to be greatly tempted to nail the other party as insufficiently concerned about Social Security and Medicare or as predatory—trying in an underhanded way to damage or reduce the programs to accomplish other goals, such as higher government spending for the poor or more tax breaks for the rich. If a higher level of trust existed between the parties, the willingness of prominent Democrats and Republicans to risk compromise would be greater. Without any trust, the pressure is more one-sided, to appear more generous than the other side and to trap the opposition into appearing insensitive or predatory.

Things might be different if the parties had strong leaders who could transcend these petty politics, cut deals across party lines, and bring the votes to the table to enact them. No such leaders are evident. There does exist the possibility that President Bush will change the dynamic permanently, joined by eager lawmakers tired of rancor and bickering. Speaker J. Dennis Hastert, unlike his Whip, would prefer civility to partisan division and conflict. But even a president inclined to forge bipartisan majorities cannot easily overcome larger forces. When Gerald Ford became president after the trauma of Nixon's impeachment, he began by stating his credo to Congress: "cooperation, conciliation, compromise." Within a year, he was vetoing bills at a faster rate than any other modern president. No one will bring miracles.

The political dynamics I describe above do not exist in a vacuum. The GOP move in 1999 to protect every dollar in the Social Security reserve mostly has served to accelerate the time when lawmakers are forced to recognize the cruel zero-sum politics pitting entitlements against discretionary programs. When they do, they will feel compelled to find ways to reexamine Social Security and Medicare, not as budget issues but in terms of reform needs. If there is no real crisis looming in Medicare, the broader trends in health care, including more uninsured, the backlash against managed care, the reluctance of many managed care companies to participate in Medicare, the resumption of medical inflation, and the squeeze on medical providers generated by the 1997 budget agreement, will push senior citizens to demand changes in Medicare, which in turn will push lawmakers to act. The changes they push will fit the usual public definition of health reform—more benefits for less money.

If the focus among politicians in Washington is largely on Medicare and Social Security, the long-term care issue is looming in the background and will likely emerge independently in the next five years or so. Most lawmakers continue to think of Medicaid as a program of health care for the able-bodied poor; the reality is that it has evolved into a program more for the elderly, blind, and disabled, with its single largest expenditure going for long-term care for the elderly. The over-85 age group is the fastest growing in America; the over-100 age group is the fastest growing subgroup within that category. As more Americans reach elderly status, and more elderly persons live longer, the demands for long-term care, both in institutions and at home, will grow. Medicaid has become the backdoor way by which the society finances the majority of long-term care expenses.

Without the surface appeal of Medicare or Social Security, Medicaid has no protective armor; it will face the same budget pressures as the discretionary budget. But before long, the demands of both seniors and their children to ease their burden in the long-term care area will push lawmakers to add funding to Medicaid, even as countervailing pressures build to cut it back. So it too will have the push-pull dynamic that will hit Social Security and Medicare, with just a slight delay and with one large caveat. Members of Congress will face great temptation to push more of Medicaid's costs off onto the states. They will call it "the New Federalism." Even if they remove federal mandates as a sop, the underlying entitlement to long-term care subsidy will remain, putting states in a very difficult position. The states, of course, will vigorously fight this initiative, adding an additional ring to the legislative circus ahead.

Up to this point, I have not mentioned the elderly as a voting bloc, or the role and importance of various interest groups. Each of these forces is highly significant, but it is most important to realize that the politics I describe above exist regardless of the voting intentions of any demographic group or the actions of any lobbying organization.

As for elderly voters, Robert Binstock is right—there is no "elderly" vote, if we mean a group of people largely predisposed to vote in the same way, motivated by the same set of issues. What we know about elderly voters is that their orientations are shaped less by the fact that they are elderly and more by the era in which they came of age politically. Thus, those voters who came of age during the Depression—the Roosevelt seniors—are different from those who came of age a decade or more later—those whom pollster Celinda Lake calls the Reagan seniors. Gender and marital status matter as well: the female elderly have different emphases and different views than the male elderly, and the married elderly have different views than the single elderly, just like their nonsenior counterparts.

To be sure, self-interest does matter here, and elderly voters are more sensitive to events or disruptions in programs in which they have a direct stake. But their political behavior is variegated, not uniform. Lake notes that Reagan seniors, those in their 60s, are the most Republican of any age cohort, whereas the Roosevelt seniors, over 70, are the most Democratic of any age cohort. Within each category, however, senior women favor Democrats more than senior men do. But both the Reagan and the Roosevelt seniors favor the Democratic Party to protect Social Security and Medicare, and men in both senior categories are more concerned about Medicare than Social Security and more confident that the Democratic Party will protect it. That does not mean, however, that they will shift their voting patterns; other issues, including moral values, are of equal or greater importance.

Groups representing "the elderly" or groups of seniors, from AARP to the National Committee to Preserve Social Security and Medicare to United Seniors, also have some significance. AARP, through the breadth of its membership and the expertise of its staff, has real influence in the policy process, but it cannot determine the agenda or dictate outcomes. The National Committee has less ongoing or sustained influence, but after its aggressive role in fighting the Medicare Catastrophic Act, it serves as a counterforce to bold action, including any means testing.

Other groups will certainly be active on these issues. No doubt the securities industry will actively lobby for its own interests when issues of Social Security privatization or any form of investing assets in stocks arise. But the industry will play little if any role in raising these issues to the point of active negotiations by the president and Congress.

Rather, the challenge to developing any comprehensive approach to the problems of an aging society is to find a way to turn political actors away from their intense focus on party positioning and the shrinking options they face in budget politics to adopt a larger framework. It requires coming up with a reasonable, even compelling substantive proposal, making it both understandable and attractive to the larger electorate, finding ways to get it on the agenda of the attentive public and then on the agenda of political actors. Then it will take either a strategy to restore some level of mutual trust and respect across bitter political adversaries or a major crisis to force them together. In short, there are no easy answers or routes here.

16

The Politics of Enacting Reform

Robert H. Binstock, Ph.D.

At the turn of the century, our nation is in a substantial quandary with respect to public policies on aging. Our federal, state, and local governments spend a great deal of money to provide older Americans with income, access to health care and long-term care, and assistance in many other aspects of their lives. But we face substantial economic and political challenges in maintaining existing government benefits to older people in the decades ahead because of the impending aging of the baby boom cohort. Moreover, there are and will be many elderly persons who—unable to do much to help themselves—need even more assistance than current government programs provide if they are to have an adequate level of well-being.

A possible way out of this quandary, suggested in various chapters of this volume, is to enact comprehensive policy reforms that will be more flexible and efficient than our current patchwork of programs and more responsive to the needs of our aging society. Yet the nature of our political system, and its underlying ideology and culture, generally militate against consideration of comprehensive policies, let alone their adoption and effective implementation. There are some rare circumstances, however, that facilitate attention to sweeping policy initiatives. Such circumstances can occasionally be fashioned by politicians and other advocates for causes; can arise from broad social, economic, and political developments; or can come about through a confluence of political leadership and societal developments.

This chapter considers political factors that bear on whether major policy reforms for an aging society can be seriously considered, and perhaps adopted, in the years immediately ahead. It begins with a discussion of the changing political contexts of policies on aging during the twentieth century and how those changes are relevant to the politics of old-age policies today. Next it looks at forces in the American political system, perennial and contemporary, that make it difficult for comprehensive policies focused on the aging of the baby boom to be addressed in the near term. It then proposes some approaches that might improve the feasibility of some potential near-term responses to the challenges posed by our aging society.

THE CHANGING POLITICAL CONTEXTS OF OLD-AGE POLICIES

American political ideology has its roots in laissez-faire liberalism, a tradition in which the individual and the market are reified (Hartz 1955). Consequently, our use of government to provide a social safety net for our populace, in comparison with that of other developed countries, is limited (see chapter 2, by Gruber and Wise, in this volume). For example, a recent study of 29 industrialized nations found that 24 of them provide government-assured health insurance to at least 99 percent of their citizens (Anderson and Poullier 1999). But the U.S. rate is only 33 percent, by far the lowest; Mexico and Turkey are the only other nations among the 29 that have no form of universal health insurance.

Our use of the power of government to provide a safety net has largely been confined to only a few select groups that have been politically legitimized as "deserving" for one reason or another (see Binstock 2001). Veterans receive government provided health care from the Department of Veterans Affairs. Blind and disabled persons, as well as selected groups of very poor persons, have health insurance coverage through Medicaid, Medicare, and other programs, as well as benefits from additional in-kind and cash income transfer policies. But the politically legitimized group of Americans that benefits the most from social programs is older people.

The United States was comparatively late in beginning the construction of a social safety net for aged persons. The Social Security Act of 1935 was enacted some quarter of a century after similar public pension programs had been established in most of the industrial world (Hudson and Binstock 1976). Since then, however, we have created something that could be termed an *Old-Age Welfare State,* comprising a number of different programs that use old ages as sweeping, convenient markers for designating categories of Americans as in need of governmental assistance. The result is that today nearly two-fifths of the annual federal budget is spent on benefits to older persons.[1]

If the present political context of policies on aging were the same as it generally was when the Old-Age Welfare State was constructed, from the 1930s through the mid-1970s, perhaps the adoption of a comprehensive policy to provide for the aging of the baby boom would not be as politically difficult as it will be today. But the politics of old-age policies has gone through several changes in the last quarter century. And policy options for our aging society confront different political circumstances.

Compassionate Ageism: Piecemeal Construction of an Old-Age Welfare State

From the New Deal until about twenty years ago, public policy issues concerning older Americans were framed by an underlying *ageism* (see Palmore 1990), the attribution of the same characteristics, status, and just deserts to a heterogeneous group that has been artificially homogenized, packaged, labeled, and marketed as "the aged." The stereotypes of ageism—unlike those of racism and sexism—have not been wholly prejudicial to the well-being of their objects, the aged. Indeed, ageism has been expressed through a number of policies, such as Medicare health insurance, that treat all older persons the same by providing them with benefits and protection primarily on the basis of old age (see Kutza 1981).

Prior to the late 1970s, the predominant stereotypes of older Americans were compassionate. Elderly persons tended to be seen as poor, frail, socially dependent, objects of discrimination, and above all "deserving" (see Kalish 1979). For more than forty years—dating from the Social Security Act of 1935—American society accepted the oversimplified notion that all older persons are essentially the same, and all worthy of governmental assistance. The lowest levels of economic status, health, and functional capacities that could be found among aged individuals became familiar as common denominators (Neugarten 1970).

The American polity implemented this compassionate construct by adopting and financing major age-categorical benefit programs and tax and price subsidies for which eligibility is not determined by need. Through the New Deal's Social Security, the Great Society's Medicare and Older Americans Act (an omnibus social service program), special tax exemptions and credits for being aged 65 or older, and a variety of other measures enacted during President Nixon's New Federalism, the elderly were exempted from the screenings that are applied to welfare applicants to determine whether they are worthy of public help.

During the 1960s and 1970s, just about every issue or problem affecting some number of older persons, that could be identified by advocates for the elderly, became a governmental responsibility: nutrition, legal, supportive, and leisure services; housing; home repair; energy assistance; transportation; employment assistance; job protection; public insurance for private pensions; special mental health programs; a separate National Institute on Aging; and on, and on, and on. By the late 1970s, if not earlier, American society had learned the catechism of compassionate ageism very well and had expressed it through a great many policies; a committee of the U.S. House of Representatives, using loose criteria, was able to identify 134 programs benefiting the aging, overseen by 49 committees and subcommittees of Congress (U.S. House of Representatives 1977).

"Greedy Geezers" and the Construct of "Intergenerational Equity"

Starting in 1978, however, the long-standing compassionate stereotypes of older persons began to undergo an extraordinary reversal. Older people came to be portrayed as one of the more flourishing and powerful groups in American society and, at the same time, attacked as a burdensome responsibility. Throughout the 1980s and into the 1990s the new stereotypes, readily observed in popular culture, depicted aged persons as prosperous, hedonistic, politically powerful, and selfish. For example, "Grays on the Go," a 1980 cover story in *Time,* was filled with pictures of senior surfers, senior swingers, and senior softball players. Older persons were portrayed as America's new elite—healthy, wealthy, powerful, and "staging history's biggest retirement party" (Gibbs 1980).

A dominant theme in such accounts of older Americans was that their selfishness was ruining the nation. The *New Republic* highlighted this motif with a drawing on the cover caricaturing aged persons, accompanied by the caption "greedy geezers." The table of contents "teaser" for the story that followed announced, "The real me generation isn't the yuppies, it's America's growing ranks of prosperous elderly" (Fairlie 1988). This theme was echoed widely, and the epithet "greedy geezers" became common in journalistic accounts of federal budget politics (e.g., Salholz 1990). In the early 1990s *Fortune* magazine declaimed that "the Tyranny of America's Old" was "one of the most crucial issues facing U.S. society" (Smith 1992).

Why the Reversal of Stereotypes?

The immediate precipitating factor for this reversal of stereotypes may have been the serious cash flow problem in the Social Security system that emerged within the larger context of a depressed economy during President Carter's administration (see Estes 1983; Light 1985). A high rate of unemployment substantially reduced the payroll tax base for Social Security revenue, and a very high rate of inflation produced corresponding sharp increases in benefits through the program's cost-of-living adjustments.

Two additional elements contributed importantly. One was the tremendous growth in the amount and proportion of federal dollars expended on benefits to aging citizens, which at that time had come to be more than one-quarter of our annual budget and comparable in size to expenditures on national defense. Journalists (e.g., Samuelson [1978]) and academicians (e.g., Hudson [1978]) began to notice and publicize this phenomenon in the late 1970s. By 1982 an economist in the Office of Management and Budget had pointed up the comparison with the defense budget by reframing the classical trade-off metaphor of political economy from "guns vs. butter" to "guns vs. canes" (Torrey 1982). Another element in the reversal of the stereotypes of old age was dramatic improvements in the aggregate status of older Americans, in large measure due to the impact of federal benefit programs. Social Security and Medicare, for example, have helped to reduce the proportion of elderly persons in poverty from about 35 percent four decades ago (Clark 1990) to 9.7 percent today (U.S. Bureau of the Census 2000). The success of such programs had improved the economic status of aged persons to the point where journalists and social commentators could—with only superficial accuracy (see Quinn 1987)—describe older people, on average, as more prosperous than the general population.

Intergenerational Equity: The Contemporary Dimension

In this unsympathetic climate of opinion, "the aged" emerged as a scapegoat for an impressive list of American problems, and the concept of so-called intergenerational equity—really, intergenerational *inequity*—became prominent in public dialogue. At first, these issues of equity were propounded in a contemporary dimension.

Demographers and advocates for children blamed the political power of elderly Americans for the plight of youngsters who had inadequate nutrition, health care, education, and insufficiently supportive family environments (e.g., Preston 1984). One children's advocate even proposed that parents receive an "extra vote" for each of their children, to combat older voters in an intergenerational conflict (Carballo 1981). Former secretary of commerce Peter Peterson (1987) suggested that a prerequisite for the United States to regain its stature as a first-class power in the world economy was a sharp reduction in programs benefiting older Americans. Widespread concerns about spiraling U.S. health care costs were redirected, in part, from health care providers, suppliers, administrators, and insurers—the parties that were responsible for setting the prices of care—to elderly persons for whom health care was provided. A number of academicians and public figures, including politicians, expressed concern that health care expenditures on older persons would soon absorb an unlimited amount of our national resources and crowd out health care for others as well as various worthy social causes (see Binstock and Post 1991). Some of them even proposed that old-age-based health care rationing would be necessary, desirable, and just (e.g., Callahan 1987).

By the end of the 1980s, the themes of intergenerational equity and conflict had been adopted by the media and academics as routine perspectives for describing many social policy issues (see Cook et al. 1994) and had also gained currency in elite sectors of American society and on Capitol Hill. For instance, the president of the prestigious American Association of Universities asserted, "The shape of the domestic federal budget inescapably pits programs for the retired against every other social purpose dependent on federal funds" (Rosenzweig 1990).

Indeed, the construct of intergenerational inequity had gained such a strong foothold in the thinking of policy elites that they took it for granted as they analyzed American domestic policy issues. For example, in 1989 a distinguished "executive panel" of American leaders convened by the Ford Foundation designated older persons as the only group of citizens that should be responsible for financing a broad range of social programs for persons of all ages. In a report entitled *The Common Good: Social Welfare and the American Future*, the panel recommended a series of policies, costing a total of $29 billion (Ford Foundation 1989). And how did the panel propose that this $29 billion be financed? Solely by taxation of Social Security benefits. In fact, every financing alternative considered in the report assumed that elderly people should be the exclusive financiers of the panel's package of recommendations for improving social welfare in our nation. Apparently the Ford panel felt that the reasons for this assumption were self-evident; it did not even bother to justify its selections of these financing options, as opposed to others (also see, e.g., Beatty 1990).

In this political climate, some of the long-standing features for structuring old-age programs began undergoing significant revisions. A number of policy changes were made to reflect the diverse economic situations of elderly individuals (although the redistributive aspect of Social Security's benefit formulas had been recognizing such diversity for many years). Some of them took benefits away from "greedy geezers." Others directed benefits toward poor older persons.

The Social Security Reform Act of 1983 began this trend by making Social Security benefits subject to taxation for the first time, at higher income levels. The Tax Reform Act of 1986, even as it eliminated the extra personal exemption that had been available to all persons 65 years and older when filing their federal income tax returns, provided new tax credits to very-low- income older persons on a sliding scale. The Older Americans Act programs of supportive and social services, for which all persons aged 60 and older are eligible, became gradually targeted by Congress to low-income older persons. The Qualified Medicare Beneficiary and the Specified Low-Income Medicare Beneficiary programs, established by the Medicare Catastrophic Coverage Act of 1988, required Medicaid to pay Part B premiums, deductibles, and copayments for low-income older persons. And the Omnibus Budget Reconciliation Act of 1993 continued this trend by adding to taxation of Social Security benefits.

These policy changes clearly established the principle that the diverse economic circumstances of older people can be addressed through politically feasible legislative reforms. Consequently, they set the stage for the legitimacy of complicated provisions of this kind that might be embodied in policy options to address the aging of the baby boom.

The Aging of the Baby Boom: Older People versus Society

The construct of intergenerational equity also had a future dimension, focusing on impending changes in the age structure of American society that would be brought about by the aging of the baby boom cohort, 76 million persons born between 1946 and 1964 (Hobbs 1996). One aspect of this issue was highlighted by the "generational accounting" analyses of economist Laurence Kotlikoff (1992), which, though controversial (see Haveman 1994), received considerable attention. Kotlikoff suggested that future generations of older people would do less well than contemporary older people in terms of the taxes they pay for income security purposes and the subsequent lifetime payments they would receive through public programs.

But the more prominent aspect was concern about the consequences for society of sustaining the Old-Age Welfare State in the twenty-first century when the baby boom will become eligible for old-age benefit programs. This dimension was initially highlighted by the efforts of Americans for Generational Equity (AGE). Formed as an interest group in 1985, with backing from the corporate sector as well as from a handful of congressmen who led it, AGE recruited some of the prominent "scapegoaters" of older people to its board and as its spokespersons.

According to its annual reports, most of AGE's funding came from insurance companies, health care corporations, banks, and other private sector businesses and organizations that are in financial competition with Medicare and Social Security (Quadagno 1989).

Central to AGE's credo were the propositions that tomorrow's elderly will be locked in an intergenerational conflict with younger age cohorts regarding the distribution of public resources and that substantial changes would be needed in the policies that make up the Old-Age Welfare State. The organization disseminated this viewpoint from its Washington office through press releases, media interviews, a quarterly publication, a book (Longman 1987), and periodic conferences with such titles as "Children at Risk: Who Will Support an Aging Society?" and "Medicare and the Baby Boom Generation." Although AGE faded from the scene at the end of the decade, its message concerning the economic and social consequences of an aging society was taken up shortly thereafter by the Concord Coalition (1993), an organization founded by former senators Paul Tsongas and Warren Rudman.

Since the mid-1980s, concerns about the societal consequences of an aged baby boom have been expressed in an apocalyptic fashion. For instance, biomedical ethicist Daniel Callahan, concerned about future health care expenditures for older people, characterized the elderly population as "a new social threat" and a "demographic, economic, and medical avalanche . . . one that could ultimately (and perhaps already) do [sic] great harm" (1987, 20). Accordingly, he proposed old-age-based health care rationing—specifically, that Medicare reimbursement for life-saving care be categorically denied to anyone aged 80 and older. The Bipartisan Commission on Entitlement and Tax Reform (1994) depicted health care costs for older people as an unsustainable economic burden for our nation. And economist Lester Thurow saw baby boomers and their self-interested pursuit of government benefits as a fundamental threat to our political system:

No one knows how the growth of entitlements can be held in check in democratic societies. . . . Will democratic governments be able to cut benefits when the elderly are approaching a voting majority? Universal suffrage . . . is going to meet the ultimate test in the elderly. If democratic governments cannot cut benefits that go to a majority of their voters, then they have no long-term future. . . . In the years ahead, class warfare is apt to be redefined as the young against the old, rather than the poor against the rich. (1996, 47)

Fortunately, Thurow's assumption that older persons function as a cohesive bloc of self-interested voters is seriously uninformed, as is indicated below, and his assertion that older voters will be a majority is highly problematic (Binstock 2000).

The Era of the Market and Personal Responsibility

Apocalyptic visions of our aging society are generated, of course, by extrapolation—simply plugging in 76 million aged baby boomers into our existing framework of policies on aging. But as we know, extrapolation is perhaps the poorest mode of prediction (see Bell 1964). Especially with respect to public policies, which change continually. Demography is not destiny. Studies have shown, for example, that there is no association between population aging and the proportion of national wealth that industrialized nations spend on health care (see Binstock 1993; Reinhardt 1999; Gruber and Wise, chapter 2 in this volume). The structural features of health care systems—and behavioral responses to them by citizens and health care providers—are far more important determinants of a nation's health care expenditures than population aging and other demographic trends.

Yet responsible extrapolative projections, such as those undertaken by the Social Security trustees, the Centers for Medicare and Medicaid Services, the Congressional Budget Office, and other respected sources, are extremely valuable in getting politicians to address important policy issues such as those generated by the aging of the baby boom. And this is now the case with respect to the future of Social Security and Medicare and, to a lesser extent, the difficult challenges that individuals, their families, and society will face in providing long-term care in the decades ahead.

As in the past, the issues of income security, health care, and long-term care for older people are being addressed in piecemeal fashion, but this is occurring in a very different political context from those that we have briefly reviewed. Since the early 1990s, fiscal responsibility has been embraced in national politics; policy proposals are scrutinized with respect to the budgetary and fiscal implications of financing them. The aging of the baby boom is not viewed as a threat to society so much as a supportive challenge that has to be met in one way or another. To paraphrase Pogo (Walt Kelly's comic strip protagonist), many politicians are beginning to recognize that the baby boom—"the enemy"—"is us." Although today's elderly population may still be viewed by some as self-interested "greedy geezers," the aged baby boomers of the future are viewed as a social responsibility. Issues of contemporary intergenerational equity—trading off current expenditures on older people with other social causes—are not articulated as frequently today as they were in the 1980s. And the era of compassionate ageism in which expansive government policies created the Old-Age Welfare State has given way as the Era of the Market and Personal Responsibility has ascended.

The present emphasis on the market and personal responsibility has been reflected, of course, in recent policy changes and reform proposals affecting Social Security, Medicare, and long-term care financing. Proposals for partially privatizing Social Security abound, with many of them involving some measure of personal responsibility by workers in making market investment decisions. Medicare's strategy of promoting enrollment in managed care organizations shifts financial risk from government to the private sector. Current proposals to reform Medicare by financing enrollees' medical care with vouchers would substantially increase personal responsibility as well as expand the role of the market. And in the arena of long-term care, congressional bills of the late 1980s and early 1990s—designed to expand government's role in financing long-term care—have been replaced by policies that provide partial tax credits and deductibility for premiums paid for private long-term care insurance. These policy changes and ideas have laid the groundwork for new approaches in policies on aging that would combine a complex mixture of public programs and private mechanisms, incentives, and disincentives.

POLITICAL FORCES AND
COMPREHENSIVE POLICY OPTIONS

In many ways the stage is set for comprehensive policy options for dealing with the aging of the baby boom. But there are a number of political forces that would make serious consideration and adoption of such policies very difficult. Some of these forces are fundamental to the structure of our political system. Others have to do with timing, the propensities of politicians, and the various interests that have a stake in the status quo of the Old-Age Welfare State.

Fundamental Barriers to Comprehensive Policy Reform

To begin with, it is important to be mindful of some fundamental characteristics of American politics that make it very difficult for complex, sweeping policies to be adopted and implemented. First, we are ideologically predisposed against governmental action that is more or less comprehensive in its approach. To be sure, there have been some historical exceptions, some of which are discussed below. But generally speaking, when we do address social issues through government intervention, our approach has been piecemeal and incremental.

Second, as a reflection of our ideology, fragmentation of public power is endemic to our political system. Not only do we have some eighty thousand governments in this country with overlapping responsibilities, but also, as our introductory textbooks in American government make clear (see Woll and Binstock 1991), the framers of our governments took pains to make sure that the power of each was internally fragmented. Even if we confine ourselves to thinking about the possibilities of getting a national comprehensive policy on aging adopted by the federal government, we are contemplating the political challenge of assembling a majority from 435 fragments of power in one legislative chamber and 100 in the other, and then achieving agreement among them. If the desired policy is not the president's initiative, of course, there is still the step of gaining presidential acquiescence or, at least, avoiding a veto. If our nation had centralized, disciplined political parties, the challenges of concerting these fragments for comprehensive policies would be much easier. But, for a variety of reasons, we do not have such parties.

Assuming the adoption of a comprehensive policy for our aging society, there also remain the substantial challenges of effective implementation. Depending on the details of such a policy, these challenges can be formidable—even when implementation simply depends on public sector actions alone. Consider, for example, the Qualified Medicare Beneficiary and the Specified Low-Income Medicare Beneficiary programs, enacted in 1988. As noted above, they require state Medicaid programs to pay cost sharing and premium obligations for low-income Medicare enrollees. Ten years later, 2.2 billion of an estimated 5.1 million potentially eligible persons were not enrolled, due to less than ambitious outreach efforts in some states (U.S. General Accounting Office 1999). When effective implementation depends on private sector actions also—as might well be the case if a comprehensive old-age policy were to be adopted in the contemporary political context— fulfillment of policy expectations can be even worse. Perhaps the worst case of this kind might be the problems of implementation experienced with Lyndon Johnson's Great Society programs (see, e.g., Elmore 1982; Pressman and Wildavsky 1979). Contemporarily, one needs to simply think of issues in the implementation of Medicare HMOs (see, e.g., U.S. General Accounting Office 2000b) or the problems of fraud in the operations of Medicare and Medicaid (see, e.g., U.S. General Accounting Office 2000a). It is because of such problems of implementation that a relatively self-implementing program like Social Security has been characterized by many commentators as our most successful social program.

The Aging of the Baby Boom Is Not an Immediate Crisis

Although the challenges of sustaining the Old-Age Welfare State for aged baby boomers are now on the policy agenda, they are not immediate crises. Moreover, the terrorist attacks on New York and Washington, D.C., on September 11, 2001, have pushed old age policies, as well as many other issues, into the background. Consequently, unless the overall U.S. political context changes substantially, a comprehensive policy initiative for dealing with the challenges of our aging society is unlikely to receive much serious attention for the foreseeable future.

Even if the various old-age policy issues are considered on a piecemeal basis, no crisis seems immediately near. In 2001 the problem of funding Social Security retirement benefits at 100 percent of their current levels was not projected to occur until 2038, almost forty years in the future (Board of Trustees 2001). The same set of projections indicated that Medicare Part A would be sufficiently funded through 2029. (In any event, the "Wolf!" cry that "Medicare will go broke" has been heard too often for even senior citizens to be concerned.) Middle-class problems of paying for increasingly expensive long-term care have been with us for many years, largely absorbed by family burdens of providing unpaid care and the depletion of life-long asset accumulations. Individuals and their families have been experiencing the crisis of long-term care, but it has not been perceived as a policy crisis in Washington (except in the programmatic areas of growing Medicaid and Medicare home health expenditures, dealt with to some extent by the Balanced Budget Act of 1997). Political perceptions of long-term care as a societal crisis will not be likely to increase sharply until members of the baby boom reach advanced old ages.

Meanwhile, elections are always imminent as crises for most politicians. So their immediate attention to old-age policies is in terms of symbolic gestures and incremental proposals that they believe are important for positioning themselves favorably with the electorate. We have witnessed the meaningless "lockbox" politics of Social Security, in which members of Congress and the presidential administrations have been acting as if spending a very small amount of the funds that the OASI trust fund invests in government bonds (rather than using them to pay down the national debt) would have a significant effect on the economy or on the long-term viability of Social Security (Mitchell 1999). Attention to Medicare has been most prominently focused on the incremental (but politically appealing) step of providing coverage for prescription drugs (Toner 2000). And President Bill Clinton proposed a very minor long-term care initiative to provide a negligible amount of financial assistance to a small number of people, coupled with some meagerly funded information and counseling programs (see Binstock and Cluff 2000).

Who Gains and Who Loses If Action Is Postponed?

Except for the rare individual who aspires to be a statesman—either in contemporary or historical perspectives—today's politicians would lose little, if anything, by failing to deal with the policy challenges posed by an aged baby boom several decades hence. Most of them will be long gone from public life when the chickens come home to roost. In contrast, if they support policies radical enough to deal adequately with the aging of the baby boom, involving rather immediate changes in policies on aging, they could very well incur substantial opposition and retribution from older voters and other vested interests that have a substantial stake in the status quo.

The list of parties with vested interests in the status quo of the patchwork Old-Age Welfare State is substantial. In addition to older people themselves, it includes the insurance industry, health care providers, long-term care providers, the "retirement living" industry, "elderly law" attorneys, financial counselors, pension funds, organized labor, and the aging services network, to name some—and even AARP (formerly the American Association of Retired Persons), which markets supplemental health insurance and other goods and services to its more than 30 million members, with an aggregate revenue of several hundred million dollars (see Morris 1996). If a comprehensive policy option included a substantial immediate payroll tax increase, employers, too, would undoubtedly generate formidable opposition.

Some powerful vested interests would be supportive of policy approaches that involve substantial privatization of the Old-Age Welfare State. Among them, of course, would be the financial securities industry and various kinds of financial counselors, as well as publicly held corporations that could anticipate aggregate new investments of hundreds of billions of dollars through a measure that partially privatized Social Security. Similarly, the insurance industry has a lot to gain in the policy proposal offered by Lynn Etheredge (see chapter 14 in this volume) that would allow pension plans to be "rolled over" into an account that pays for long-term care insurance premiums.

What about the vested interest of today's older voters in the Old-Age Welfare State? They cast 20.3 percent of the votes in the 1996 presidential election (Binstock 2000). But in reality, older people do not vote in a cohesive fashion, even though politicians and their advisers tend to think that they do and are often afraid that they might.

A ubiquitous journalistic cliché for warning politicians is that "Social Security is the third rail of American politics—touch it and you're dead!" (e.g., Third Rail 1982). This view is also applied to Medicare and other old-age benefit programs. Empirically, however, this cliché has not held up. One reason is that older voters (and younger voters) cannot vote on Social Security, Medicare, or any other policy issues (except in referenda on state and local issues). They vote for candidates, responding to a variety of factors—including the personal characteristics of candidates and their positions on a number of issues and a variety of other campaign stimuli—as mediated through ideological predispositions and party attachments. Even when old-age policy issues are prominent in presidential election campaigns (the arena most salient to old-age policies), the positions of candidates generally appear to be the same. In 2000, for instance, both George W. Bush and Al Gore made government insurance coverage of prescription drugs a major feature of their campaigns; though their proposals differed somewhat with respect to technical details, the differences were difficult for journalists to sort out, let alone most older or younger voters (see Toner 2000). Similarly, in 1996, Medicare was a prominent campaign topic. On the one hand, both President Clinton and Senator Bob Dole labored hard to convey the impression that they (and their congressional party members) had been trying to "save" Medicare and would do so in the future. On the other hand, they tried to label their opponents as potential destroyers of Medicare or indifferent to the fate of the program and those whom it serves (Transcript 1996; Excerpts 1996). In 2000 and 1996, older voters distributed their votes among the candidates in roughly the same proportions as did other age groups; and this has been a typical distribution in presidential elections for many decades (Connelly 2000).

Even in the rare instances when it has been possible to differentiate substantially between candidates with respect to their old-age policy stances, no impact on older voters has been discernible. A classic case in point was Ronald Reagan's reelection in 1984. During the election campaign, Democrats portrayed him (with good reason) as having been an "enemy" of Social Security during his first term. Yet, in the balloting, older persons gave him 63 percent of their votes (as compared with 54% in 1980), about the same as the overall average and the proportions in other age groups (Binstock 1992).

The fundamental reason why older voters do not vote much differently from younger age groups is that their political attitudes and behavior are not predominantly shaped by common self-interests that derive from the attribute of being elderly. A heterogeneous birth cohort—comprising every economic, social, and political characteristic in American society—does not suddenly become homogenized when it reaches the old-age category. Old age is only one of many personal characteristics of aged people, and many older persons may not identify themselves in terms of it when voting, or even more generally.

Even if one assumes that rational self-interest is the major determinant of voting behavior (a problematic assumption—see Simon 1985), the self-interests of older people in relation to old-age policy issues, and the intensity of their interests, may vary substantially. Consider, for example, the relative importance of Social Security as a source of income for aged persons who are in the lowest and highest income quintiles. Social Security provides 81.8 percent of income for those in the lowest quintile but only 17.7 percent for those in the highest (Radner 1995). Some older persons have much more at stake than others do in policy proposals that would reduce, maintain, or enhance Social Security benefit payments.

For these and other reasons, older persons have not been a cohesive political force. As political scientist Hugh Heclo observed, "'The elderly' is really a category created by policy analysts, pension officials, and mechanical models of interest group politics" (1988, 393).

Nonetheless, politicians behave as if older voters are a powerful political force. And this has important implications for the feasibility of any policy option that would involve a rather immediate change in the distribution of current benefits to the aged. Although older voters have not behaved cohesively, and old-age advocacy groups have not demonstrated a capacity to swing a decisive bloc of older voters, the perception of being powerful is, in itself, a source of political influence (see Banfield 1961). Incumbent members of Congress are hardly inclined to risk upsetting the existing distribution of votes that puts them in office and keeps them there. Few politicians, of course, want to call the "electoral bluff" of the elderly or any other latent mass constituency if it is possible to avoid doing so. Hence, members of Congress and their staffs take heed when their offices are flooded with letters, faxes, phone calls, and e-mail messages expressing the (not necessarily representative) views of older persons. And they provide AARP and other old-age organizations with ready access to policy discussions.

To be sure, the old-age interest groups have had little to do with the enactment and amendment of major old-age policies such as Social Security and Medicare. Rather, such actions have been largely attributable to the initiatives of public officials in the White House, Congress, and the bureaucracy who have been focused on their own agendas for social and economic policy (e.g., on Social Security [see Derthick 1979; Light 1985]; on Medicare [see Ball 1995; Cohen 1985; Iglehart 1989; Marmor 1970]; cf. Pratt 1976; Pratt 1993). Nor have the old-age organizations been able to prevent significant policy reforms that have been perceived to be adverse to the interests of an artificially homogenized constituency of "senior citizens" (see Binstock 1994a; Day, 1998). Indeed, the political legitimacy of old-age interest groups has been eroding over the past ten years (see Binstock 1997; Day 1998; Street 1999). To some extent this erosion can be traced to the ineffective roles they played in specific political episodes such as the enactment of the Medicare Catastrophic Coverage Act in 1988 and its partial repeal in 1989 (Himmelfarb 1995) and the saga of health care reform efforts in 1993 and 1994 (Binstock 1994b).

Yet politicians remain wary of old-age organizations and "share [the] widespread perception of a huge, monolithic, senior citizen army of voters" (Peterson and Somit 1994, 178). So they continue to court the votes of older persons, eager to capitalize on (and wary of) the possibility that their voting behavior may become more cohesive, and ready to listen to the views of old-age interest groups despite their recent decline in political legitimacy. In electoral campaigns they strive to position themselves on old-age policy issues in a fashion that they think will appeal to the self-interests of older voters, and they usually take care that their opponents do not gain an advantage in this arena. And incumbents, of course, are especially concerned about how their actions in the governing process can be portrayed during the next election.

As a consequence, an old-age policy option that would involve rather immediate and relatively radical changes in the benefits that today's older persons receive through the Old-Age Welfare State would probably have little chance of adoption. With the aging of the baby boom still a distant and abstract crisis, members of Congress are unlikely to endorse cuts in current old-age income benefits, a risky privatization of current trust fund reserves or other privatizing approaches, a drastic reorganization in the financing or delivery of Medicare (or both), or an earmarked tax on older people to finance long-term care.

WHAT MIGHT ENHANCE CONSIDERATION OF COMPREHENSIVE REFORMS?

Many of the proposals for substantial reform of Social Security, Medicare, and long-term care that have been put forth in recent years—by various commissions, committees, politicians, and policy analysts—have received serious attention on the public policy agenda. But because of the political factors delineated above, as well as for other reasons, all but the most incremental of them may be very difficult to adopt.

For policy options that deal more comprehensively with the aging of our society, the difficulties of getting serious attention and securing adoption are even greater. The broader and more comprehensive a proposal may be, the more likely it is to be opposed by vested interests entrenched in the status quo, many of which are reinforced in their opposition by their "iron triangle" relationships cultivated over the years with members of the bureaucracy and Congress (see Berry 1997). What factors and circumstances could make possible serious near-term consideration, and perhaps adoption, of a comprehensive policy reform?

Advance Planning, Distant Startup, and Gradualism

Today's politicians might espouse and support a policy option that, though enacted now, calls for changes that would begin to take place in the medium-term future—and perhaps be implemented gradually from that point on. Such a policy would be unlikely to offend older or younger voters, and many of the various business and professional interests that have a stake in the policy status quo would have sufficient time to adapt.

The Social Security Reform Act of 1983 provides an excellent illustration of this approach. Among other things, it enacted a change in the normal retirement age for full Social Security benefits, from age 65 to age 67. Yet the change was not scheduled to begin until twenty years later, in 2003, and to take an additional twenty-four years to be fully implemented in 2027. This policy change elicited little outrage, unrest, or opposition, either from voters or from vested interests (such as employers, whose successors would have to pay more months and years of payroll taxes for whatever employees they might have in the future). In contrast, the portion of the Medicare Catastrophic Coverage Act of 1998 that required older persons to begin paying immediately out of their own pockets for insurance for extended hospital stays, at a rather steep rate, was repealed almost immediately following vociferous outcries from a minority of older persons (see Himmelfarb 1995).

The change in Social Security's normal retirement age is a felicitous political model. It combined advanced planning with a far distant and gradually implemented policy change to deal with the aging of the baby boom. Consequently, it engendered little opposition from old-age advocacy groups or any other parties. Unfortunately, from a policymaking point of view, the years when the baby boom will reach old age are not now far distant. Yet there is still some time left for the use of advance planning and gradualism to moderate political opposition.

Whatever comprehensive policy option one has in mind, whether a social insurance approach or a more complicated package of public and private sector features, it will probably involve measures for increasing dedicated revenue. Following the 1983 model, a sales tax, a value-added tax, or even an increase in the payroll tax (or more than one of such levies) could be scheduled to begin at minuscule rates some ten or so years from the date of authorizing legislation. Then the tax (or taxes) could be scheduled to increase very gradually over a number of years. Similarly, on the expenditure reduction side, upward changes in the age of eligibility for benefits could also be phased in very gradually after a startup some years hence.

An approach of this kind might not be sufficient, in itself, to enable a policy option to receive serious attention and possibly be adopted.

My assessment is that such changes would be unlikely to incur much of an outcry from voters because such changes would seem distant and relatively negligible. But conservative politicians would be unhappy with the principle of "raising taxes." Employers would certainly oppose an increase in their share of a payroll tax (although there is no inherent reason why the increase could not be confined to the employee share). And business and consumer groups could be expected to raise an outcry, although the distance and gradualism of implementation for such policies would be moderating factors.

Brokering the Ideal Option

Even if a comprehensive reform incorporated features of advance planning, distant startup, and gradualism, more would be needed. Its proponents would be well advised to engage in modifying their ideal proposal. For such a proposal to remain intact throughout the legislative process, its proponent(s) must have sufficient political influence to overcome the fragmentation of power as embodied in members of Congress and the interests to which they are responsive. This requires the effective mobilization of appointment powers, veto threats, promises, favors, charisma, authority, previously accumulated obligations, and other sources of influence to obtain majorities without sacrificing the substance of a proposal. It is very rare, especially in national politics, that political leaders are able to amass such influence in the strength and depth required to successfully achieve "proposal costless" social legislation. It could be argued that President Franklin Roosevelt had such influence during the mid-1930s. At the local level, some political machine bosses of the past seem to have had such influence (Banfield 1961).

In most circumstances, success in securing social legislation is "proposal costly." The details of what was initially an ideal proposal must be modified to obtain the support and mute the opposition of vested interests and their legislative representatives. Proposal-costly brokering is typically a long, arduous, frustrating task, and often—in the end—it is unsuccessful. Even when the legislation is ultimately adopted, it may effectively undermine its proponents' original intent. A classic example of such an outcome was Lyndon Johnson's Model Cities program. The original idea was to see what could be done to revitalize decaying inner cities through a massive infusion of federal funds to rebuild just two cities, as a demonstration that would show whether spending sufficient dollars on urban problems would be a solution. By the time this proposal was brokered to gain adequate congressional support for passage, the policy provided just $212 million for 150 cities (Banfield 1973). Brokering certainly secured passage of the legislation, but at the cost of the program's goal.

A good model for how to broker legislative support in an effective fashion can be found, once again, in the history of the 1983 Social Security amendments. The cash flow problem in Social Security required that some new policy had to be enacted in 1983 in order to increase revenues or curtail benefits, or both. All of the proposals that were being put forward to solve this problem were unpopular with at least one significant political faction. Within this context President Reagan appointed a National Commission on Social Security Reform comprising leaders from a variety of different public and private power bases—Democrats and Republicans from both houses of Congress, business, organized labor, and professional elites—and charged them with putting forth a proposal to solve the problem. The recommendations that the commission reported—the bargained outcome of conflicts and accommodations among the interests represented by its members—were adopted without much difficulty and only minor modifications (see Light 1985). As witnessed by the failure of the National Bipartisan Commission on the Future of Medicare to make any recommendations in 1999, however, this prebrokered approach is hardly a guaranteed recipe for success (see Commonwealth Fund 1999).

The Clinton administration's handling of its efforts to secure health care reform in 1993–94 provides an excellent example of unsuccessful brokering of a legislative proposal and, perhaps, a lesson to guide successful brokering in the future. Before the proposal entered the legislative process, the administration included in it substantive features designed to elicit support from various interest groups. For example, in the hope of gaining support from organized advocates for older people, it included substantial funding for a new federal long-term care program and Medicare coverage of outpatient prescription drugs. But AARP never endorsed the president's proposal. The administration's plan also offered to reduce the corporate burden of providing retiree health insurance by including $12 billion of (first-year) federal funds dedicated to this purpose. But the community of large corporations never supported the Clinton proposal.

What if the administration had held back these "plums" until a more effective time to use them, during the legislative process? At a critical time, would AARP have strongly endorsed the Clinton plan if the president had then offered a long-term care initiative and prescription drug coverage in return? Would large employers have been willing to offer support in return for $12 billion of corporate relief? One cannot say for sure. But holding back goodies to trade at the appropriate time in the process of brokering for support is certainly a better strategy than giving them away up front.

"Crisis" as a Context for Getting Attention

What about the prospects of securing a policy proposal that is relatively unbrokered—pristine enough to not be undermined with respect to its goal of adequate support for aged baby boomers? At various times in U.S. history, relatively radical social legislation has been politically feasible because the economic and social contexts of the time generated a sufficient sense of public crisis to overcome the fragmentation of power endemic to the American political system and the many vested interests in the status quo. Certainly the New Deal was the product of such a sense of crisis. One might also argue that the Great Society programs were the product of a sense of crisis, whether that sense had its roots in the national reaction to the assassination of President Kennedy or in President Johnson's capacity to generate a sense of crisis concerning the plight of the poor and the social unrest in our inner cities—or both.

Perhaps near-term attention to a comprehensive old-age policy approach would be feasible if the aging of the baby boom were more successfully marketed as a crisis. Many policy analysts and elite commentators have written and spoken about the aging of the baby boom as a looming crisis in American society (e.g., see Peterson 1999). As suggested earlier, some of them have been rather apocalyptic in their approach.

But there is little indication, if any, that the general public or even the media have engaged with issues generated by the aging of the baby boom in a crisislike frame of mind. This is understandable in the nature of the case: a far distant period portrayed by a lot of boring demographic and program expenditure projections. In comparison, for example, contemporary old-age-related issues are receiving substantial attention—such as the possibility that Social Security might be invested in the market, the shutdowns of Medicare HMOs and their "bait and switch" reductions and withdrawals of prescription drug coverage, and the financing and caregiving burdens of long-term care.

Anthony Downs has argued that there is an "issue-attention cycle" in American politics, rooted both in the nature of certain domestic problems and in the way major communications media interact with the public. With respect to the aging of the baby boom, we are in what he terms the "preproblem" stage of the cycle: the problem exists "but has not yet captured much public attention, even though some experts or interest groups may already be alarmed by it" (1972, 39).

What does it take to move from the "preproblem" stage to a "critical problem" stage? Downs suggests the following:

A problem must be dramatic and exciting to maintain public interest because news is "consumed" by much of the American public (and by publics everywhere) largely as a form of entertainment. As such, it competes with other types of entertainment for a share of each person's time. Every day, there is a fierce struggle for space in the highly limited universe of newsprint and television viewing time. Each issue vies not only with all other social problems and public events, but also with a multitude of "non-news" items that are often far more pleasant to contemplate. (1972, 42)

How could the aging of the baby boom be made more dramatic and more successful in the competition for news coverage? I am far from being an expert in communications and marketing, but I will sketch out one approach at the risk of seeming unsophisticated in this realm of affairs.

The fundamental strategy would be to undertake a media campaign that portrays the aging of the baby boom as *a crisis for baby boomers, their families, and society—rather than a Social Security crisis and a*

Medicare crisis. The central focus would be on *people* rather than *programs.* The key would be to convey the costs of policy inaction in terms of what it would mean tomorrow for older people, the nature of family obligations and lifestyles, and the fabric of familiar social institutions that are integral to daily life.

Such a campaign—perhaps undertaken by a president or some other political figure who can readily command media attention, or by some very well-funded organizational entity—should be strategically targeted to the 76 million baby boomers and should be strong enough to compete with advertising campaigns that tell this audience how to avoid growing old.

The goal of its initial phase would be to convey to baby boomers (perhaps in a congratulatory fashion) that they will live for many, many years as older Americans. (If old-age-related marketing to baby boomers seems far-fetched, we should be mindful that AARP has already been engaged in doing this for several years. Witness the special issue of *Modern Maturity* that pictured Susan Sarandon on the cover and featured a survey of the sex habits of Americans aged 45 and older [Jacoby 1999], and the subsequent launching of a new AARP magazine, *My Generation,* targeted to baby boomers [Carlson 2001].) Next, or perhaps as a complementary aspect of this first "congratulatory" phase, the aim would be to effectively inform baby boomers about the Old-Age Welfare State, or as the title of a book by Elizabeth Kutza (1981) expresses it, *The Benefits of Old Age.*

The next element would be to develop and convey scenarios that depict what life will be like for aged baby boomers if nothing is done to reconfigure the Old-Age Welfare State and thereby sustain supports for baby boomers in old age at levels reasonably comparable to what older Americans experienced in the last three decades of the twentieth century. Perhaps scenarios depicting what life will be like if nothing is done to improve upon such supports could even be included. What will the budgets of elderly couples and aged widows be like in terms of how much they have to spend on food, shelter, clothing, utilities, transportation, medical care, and long-term care? Will far more older persons have to be financially supported by their children than is the case today? Will American society witness the return of three- and perhaps four-generation households? For those who are less than wealthy, what limits might exist on their access to medical care and high-cost, high-tech medical interventions, particularly at advanced old ages? In our increasingly long-lived society, how many baby boomers will be caring for or paying for the care of their functionally disabled parents who are of advanced old age? What will happen to the life-long savings of baby boomers who become functionally disabled and have no families to provide essential supportive personal care? For those who do not have adequate savings to pay for long-term care—or those who deplete their savings—and have no caring family, what can they expect in the way of help from government and the private and voluntary sectors of our society? And those who have families as caregivers? What will life be like for their caregiving (and often employed) spouses, siblings, adult children and children-in-law, and perhaps their grandchildren? When "soccer moms" are transformed into unpaid nurses' aides engaged in endless caregiving? And on and on.

The generation and promulgation of scenarios that answer these questions might fairly be termed "scare tactics." But they would not be a great deal scarier than today's reality for many older persons and their families. Responsible visions of the future might be sufficient to help baby boomers and their families feel that a sufficient "crisis" looms in societal support for the basic needs of older people and their families to warrant policy action in the near-term future. If an issue as abstract, unfamiliar, and seemingly distant in consequences as Global Warming can reach the policy agenda, then a comprehensive policy to deal with the challenges of population aging surely could if the not-too-distant consequences are conveyed in terms of daily lives rather than projected program deficits.

If the scenery for the play of daily life in our aging society can be effectively painted for the American public, what else is needed to mobilize popular support for dealing with the aging of the baby boom? As implied above, the daily issues confronting older people are not now, and will not then be, hermetically sealed from the rest of society. Perhaps the way to gain widespread political support is to paint a comprehensive policy reform for an aging society as a "family policy" (see Harrington 1999). If it proves to be effective, in many ways that is what—in effect—it will be. At the same time it would be wise to (1) soft-pedal the theme of "providing for deserving old people," the theme that nurtured the growth of the Old-Age Welfare State; (2) avoid the resurgence of the "greedy geezer" (read "greedy boomers") label; and (3) refrain from debates concerning intergenerational equity.

CONCLUSION

Our capacity to respond adequately to the challenges of an aging society through governmental action is not dependent on sustaining the particular programs that were established through some four decades in which we constructed an Old-Age Welfare State. Nor is it dependent on such matters as the ratio of workers to dependents in our society. Ultimately, of course, the fundamental issues are whether we will have sufficient economic resources to transfer to baby boomers in their old age and whether we will have the political will to do so.

In the 2030s, when all baby boomers will have reached the ranks of old age, our economy may not be prosperous. If we postpone until then the challenge of dealing with the aging of the baby boom, confronting it may be economically and politically overwhelming. We might have a substantial crisis. The circumstances of daily life for older people might well resemble what earlier cohorts of older persons experienced prior to the construction of the Old-Age Welfare state. Perhaps even Thurow's vision of class warfare between the young and the old might actually develop.

Although the adoption of a forward-looking policy may seem politically difficult at the moment, my view is that it can be done in the near future. We can take advantage of the fact that we still (but not for long) have time to employ the strategy of a distant or semidistant startup for new measures, with gradual implementation. We need to convey a sense of crisis, in a futuristic dimension, by focusing on the crises that will be entailed for people, not programs. And we require political leadership that can frame the issues of the baby boom's old age in terms that enable us to understand that all of us—not just those of us who will be old at the time—will be affected. In short, if we can be brought to understand that "the beneficiaries 'R' us," we may have the political will to take action.

NOTE
1. Author's calculations, based on data in CBO 2000; Health Care Financing Administration 2000; Social Security Administration 2000. The total of benefits to older persons includes those paid to persons under age 65, on the basis of old-age eligibility, such as Old Age Insurance benefits to early retirees under Social Security.

REFERENCES
Anderson, G. F., and J.-P. Poullier. 1999. Health Spending, Access, and Outcomes: Trends in Industrialized Countries. *Health Affairs* 18, no. 3: 178–92.
Ball, R. M. 1995. What Medicare's Architects Had in Mind. *Health Affairs* 14, no. 4: 62–72.
Banfield, E. C. 1961. *Political Influence: A New Theory of Urban Politics.* New York: Free Press.
———. 1973. Making a New Federal Program: Model Cities, 1964–68. In A. Sindler, ed., *Policy and Politics in America,* 125–58. Boston: Little, Brown.
Beatty, J. 1990. A Post–Cold War Budget. *Atlantic Monthly* 256, no. 2: 74–82.
Bell, D. 1964. Twelve Modes of Prediction: A Preliminary Sorting of Approaches in the Social Sciences. *Daedalus* 93:845–80.
Berry, J. 1997. *The Interest Group Society.* 3rd ed. New York: Longman.
Binstock, R. H. 1992. Older Voters and the 1992 Presidential Election. *Gerontologist* 32:601–6.
———. 1993. Healthcare Costs around the World: Is Aging a Fiscal "Black Hole"? *Generations* 17, no. 4: 37–42.
———. 1994a. Changing Criteria in Old-Age Programs: The Introduction of Economic Status and Need for Services. *Gerontologist* 34:726–30.
———. 1994b. Older Americans and Health Care Reform in the 1990s. In P. V. Rosenau, ed., *Health Care Reform in the Nineties,* 213–35. Thousand Oaks, Calif.: Sage Publications.
———. 1997. The Old-Age Lobby in a New Political Era. In R. B. Hudson, ed., *The Future of Age-Based Public Policy,* 56–74. Baltimore: Johns Hopkins University Press.
———. 2000. Older People and Voting Participation: Past and Future. *Gerontologist* 40:18–31.
———. 2001. The Politics of Caring. In L. E. Cluff and R. H. Binstock, eds., *The Lost Art of Caring: A Challenge to Health Professionals, Families, Communities, and Society,* 219–42. Baltimore: Johns Hopkins University Press.
Binstock, R. H., and Cluff, L. E. 2000. Issues and Challenges in Home Care. In R. H. Binstock and L. E. Cluff, eds., *Home Care Advances: Essential Research and Policy Issues,* 3–34. New York: Springer.
Binstock, R. H., and Post, S. G., eds., 1991. *Too Old for Health Care? Controversies in Medicine, Law, Economics, and Ethics.* Baltimore: Johns Hopkins University Press.

Bipartisan Commission on Entitlement and Tax Reform. 1994. *Commission Findings*. Washington, D.C.: U.S. Government Printing Office.

Board of Trustees, Federal Old-Age and Survivors Insurance and Disability Insurance Trust Funds. 2001. *2001 Annual Report of the Board of Trustees of the Federal Old-Age and Survivors Insurance and Disability Insurance Trust Funds*. Washington, D.C.: U.S. Government Printing Office.

Callahan, D. 1987. *Setting Limits: Medical Goals in an Aging Society*. New York: Simon and Schuster.

Carballo, M. 1981. Extra Votes for Parents? *Boston Globe*, December 17, 35.

Carlson, E. 2001. AARP Unveils New Magazine: *My Generation* Will Target Baby Boomers. *AARP Bulletin*, January, 18.

Clark, R. L. 1990. Income Maintenance Policies in the United States. In R. H. Binstock and L. K. George, eds., *Handbook of Aging and the Social Sciences*, 382–97. 3rd ed. San Diego: Academic Press.

Cohen, W. J. 1985. Reflections on the Enactment of Medicare and Medicaid. *Health Care Financing Review*, annual suppl.: 3–11.

Commonwealth Fund. 1999. *After the Bipartisan Commission: What Next for Medicare?* Pub. no. 353, October. New York: Commonwealth Fund.

Concord Coalition. 1993. *The Zero Deficit Plan: A Plan for Eliminating the Federal Budget Deficit by the Year 2000*. Washington, D.C.: Concord Coalition.

Congressional Budget Office (CBO). 2000. *The Budget and Economic Outlook: An Update*. Washington, D.C.: U.S. Government Printing Office.

Connelly, M. 2000. Who Voted: A Portrait of American Politics, 1976–2000. *New York Times*, November 12, wk4.

Cook, F. L., V. M. Marshall, J. E. Marshall, and J. E. Kaufman. 1994. The Salience of Intergenerational Equity in Canada and the United States. In T. R. Marmor, T. M. Smeeding, and V. L. Greene, eds., *Economic Security and Intergenerational Justice: A Look at North America*, 91–129. Washington, D.C.: Urban Institute Press.

Day, C. L. 1998. Old-Age Interest Groups in the 1990s: Coalitions, Competition, and Strategy. In J. Steckenrider and T. Parrott, eds., *New Perspectives on Old-Age Policies*, 131–50. Albany: State University of New York Press.

Derthick, M. 1979. *Policymaking for Social Security*. Washington, D.C.: Brookings Institution.

Downs, A. 1972. Up and Down with Ecology: The "Issue-Attention Cycle." *Public Interest* 28 (summer): 38–50.

Elmore, R. 1982. Implementation of Federal Education Policy: Research and Analysis. In R. Corwin, ed., *Research in the Sociology of Education and Socialization*, vol. 3, 97–119. Greenwich, Conn.: JAI Press.

Estes, C. L. 1983. Social Security: The Social Construction of a Crisis. *Milbank Memorial Fund Quarterly / Health and Society* 61:445–61.

Excerpts from the Second Televised Debate between Clinton and Dole. 1996. *New York Times*, October 18, C22–23.

Fairlie, H. 1988. Talkin' 'bout My Generation. *New Republic* 198:19–22.

Ford Foundation, Project on Social Welfare and the American Future, Executive Panel. 1989. *The Common Good: Social Welfare and the American Future.* New York: Ford Foundation.

Gibbs, N. R. 1980. Grays on the Go. *Time* 131, no. 8: 66–75.

Harrington, M. 1999. *Care and Equality: Inventing a New Family Politics.* New York: Alfred A. Knopf.

Hartz, L. 1955. *The Liberal Tradition in America.* New York: Harcourt, Brace.

Haveman, R. 1994. Should Generational Accounts Replace Public Budgets and Deficits? *Journal of Economic Perspectives* 8 (winter): 95–111.

Health Care Financing Administration. 2000. Medicare and Medicaid Statistical Supplement, 2000. *Health Care Financing Review, Statistical Supplement.*

Heclo, H. 1988. Generational Politics. In J. L. Palmer, T. Smeeding, and B. B. Torrey, eds., *The Vulnerable,* 381–411. Washington, D.C.: Urban Institute Press.

Himmelfarb, R. 1995. *Catastrophic Politics: The Rise and Fall of the Medicare Catastrophic Coverage Act of 1988.* University Park: Pennsylvania State University Press.

Hobbs, F. B. 1996. *65+ in the United States.* U.S. Bureau of the Census, Current Population Reports, Special Studies, P23-190. Washington, D.C.: U.S. Government Printing Office.

Hudson, R. B. 1978. The "Graying" of the Federal Budget and Its Consequences for Old Age Policy. *Gerontologist* 18:428–40.

Hudson, R. B., and R. H. Binstock. 1976. Political Systems and Aging. In R. H. Binstock and E. Shanas, eds., *Handbook of Aging and the Social Sciences,* 369–400. New York: Van Nostrand Reinhold.

Iglehart, J. K. 1989. Medicare's New Benefits: "Catastrophic" Health Insurance. *New England Journal of Medicine* 320:329–36.

Jacoby, S. 1999. Great Sex: What's Age Got to Do with It? *Modern Maturity* 42, no. 5: 40–45, 91.

Kalish, R. A. 1979. The New Ageism and the Failure Models: A Polemic. *Gerontologist* 19:398–407.

Kotlikoff, L. J. 1992. *Generational Accounting: Knowing Who Pays, and When, for What We Spend.* New York: Free Press.

Kutza, E. 1981. *The Benefits of Old Age.* Chicago: University of Chicago Press.

Light, P. C. 1985. *Artful Work: The Politics of Social Security Reform.* New York: Random House.

Longman, P. 1987. *Born to Pay: The New Politics of Aging in America.* Boston: Houghton Mifflin.

Marmor, T. R. 1970. *The Politics of Medicare.* London: Routledge and Kegan Paul.

Mitchell, A. 1999. Democrats Put on Defensive by G.O.P. Ads: Social Security Pressed in Push to Win Seats. *New York Times,* October 28, 1.

Morris, C. R. 1996. *The AARP: America's Most Powerful Lobby and the Clash of Generations*. New York: Times Books.

Neugarten, B. L. 1970. The Old and the Young in Modern Societies. *American Behavioral Scientist* 14:13–24.

Palmore, E. B. 1990. *Ageism: Negative and Positive*. New York: Springer.

Peterson, P. G. 1987. The Morning After. *Atlantic Monthly* 260, no. 4: 43–49.

———. 1999. *Gray Dawn: How the Coming Age Wave Will Transform America— and the World*. New York: Times Books.

Peterson, S. A., and Somit, A. 1994. *Political Behavior of Older Americans*. New York: Garland.

Pratt, H. J. 1976. *The Gray Lobby*. Chicago: University of Chicago Press.

———. 1993. *Gray Agendas: Interest Groups and Public Pensions in Canada, Britain, and the United States*. Ann Arbor: University of Michigan Press.

Pressman, J. L., and A. B. Wildavsky. 1979. *Implementation: How Great Expectations in Washington Are Dashed in Oakland*. Berkeley: University of California Press.

Preston, S. H. 1984. Children and the Elderly in the U.S. *Scientific American* 251, no. 6: 44–49.

Quadagno, J. 1989. Generational Equity and the Politics of the Welfare State. *Politics and Society* 17:353–76.

Quinn, J. 1987. The Economic Status of the Elderly: Beware the Mean. *Review of Income and Wealth* 33, no. 1: 63–82.

Radner, D. R. 1995. Income of the Elderly and Nonelderly, 1967–1992. *Social Security Bulletin* 58, no. 4: 82–97.

Reinhardt, U. 1999. The Political Economy of Health Care for the Elderly Population. In K. Dychtwald, ed., *Healthy Aging: Challenges and Solutions*, 203–29. Gaithersburg, Md.: Aspen.

Rosenzweig, R. M. 1990. Address to the President's Opening Session, 43rd Annual Meeting of the Gerontological Society of America, Boston, November 16, p. 16.

Salholz, E. 1990. Blaming the Voters: Hapless Budgeteers Single out "Greedy Geezers." *Newsweek,* October 29, 36.

Samuelson, R. J. 1978. Aging America: Who Will Shoulder the Growing Burden? *National Journal* 10:1712–17.

Simon, H. A. 1985. Human Nature in Politics: The Dialogue of Psychology with Political Science. *American Political Science Review* 79:293–304.

Smith, L. 1992. The Tyranny of America's Old. *Fortune* 125, no. 1: 68–72.

Social Security Administration. 2000. *Social Security Bulletin, Annual Statistical Supplement*.

Street, D. 1999. Special Interests or Citizens' Rights? "Senior Power," Social Security, and Medicare. In M. Minkler and C. L. Estes, eds., *Critical Gerontology: Perspectives from Political and Moral Economy*, 109–30. Amityville, N.Y.: Baywood.

The Third Rail of Politics. 1982. *Newsweek*, November 24, 24.

Thurow, L. C. 1996. The Birth of a Revolutionary Class. *New York Times Magazine*, May 19, 46–47.

Toner, R. 2000. Basic Differences in Rival Proposals on Drug Coverage. *New York Times*, October 1, A1.

Torrey, B. B. 1982. Guns vs. Canes: the Fiscal Implications of an Aging Population. *American Economics Association Papers and Proceedings* 72:309–13.

A Transcript of the First Televised Debate between Clinton and Dole. 1996. *New York Times*, October 8, A14–17.

U.S. Bureau of the Census. 2000. *Poverty in the United States, 1999.* Current Population Reports: Consumer Income, P60-210. Washington, D.C.: U.S. Government Printing Office.

U.S. General Accounting Office. 1999. *Low-Income Medicare Beneficiaries: Further Outreach and Administrative Simplification Could Increase Enrollment.* Washington, D.C.: U.S. Government Printing Office.

———. 2000a. *Health Care Fraud: Schemes to Defraud Medicare, Medicaid, and Private Health Care Insurers.* Washington, D.C.: U.S. Government Printing Office.

———. 2000b. *Medicare+Choice: Plan Withdrawals Indicate Difficulty of Providing Choice While Achieving Savings.* Washington, D.C.: U.S. Government Printing Office.

U.S. House of Representatives. 1977. *Federal Responsibility to the Elderly: Executive Programs and Legislative Jurisdiction.* Report of the Select Committee on Aging. Washington, D.C.: U.S. Government Printing Office.

Woll, P., and Binstock, R. H. 1991. *America's Political System*, 5th ed. New York: McGraw-Hill.

17

The Financial Problems of the Elderly

A Holistic View

Victor R. Fuchs, Ph.D.

"Grow old along with me! The best is yet to be," wrote Robert Browning in his poem *Rabbi Ben Ezra*. A century later, Robert Butler, a former director of the National Institute of Aging, took a more dismal view of aging, epitomized in the title of his book *Why Survive? Being Old in America* (1975). Why the change in perspective? One possible reason is that an elderly person was a rarity in Browning's time; as the twentieth century drew to a close, however, mortality tables showed that three out of four Americans would reach the biblical "three score and ten." Just being old no longer carries any special distinction.

A Japanese statesman-scholar, Wataru Hiraizumi, recently provided a provocative insight into the effect of an increase in the proportion of elderly persons in a society. Recalling his first few weeks in France in the 1950s, he says, "I suddenly saw the reason for a singular uneasiness. . . . It was the presence of a seemingly inordinate number of old people. . . . They looked vigilant, severe, and vaguely ill-tempered" (2000). He attributed this to the fact that in France at that time more than 11 percent of the population was over 65, whereas in the Japan he had recently left, elderly persons were barely 5 percent of the population.

Probably an even more important reason for the change from Browning to Butler is that improvements in the material condition of America's elderly have been surpassed by rapidly rising expectations. Although today's elderly persons are on average healthier and wealthier than any previous generation in the nation's history, their desires and expectations regarding life in retirement are outpacing the ability of society to fulfill them. Nowhere is this more evident than with respect to health and medical care.

Recent decades have witnessed an unprecedented number of advances in medical technology that, albeit costly, have contributed to longer, better-quality lives for many older Americans. Ten of the most important, as indicated in Fuchs and Sox 2001, are

Balloon angioplasty with stents
Blood-pressure-lowering drugs
Cataract extraction with lens implant
Cholesterol-lowering drugs
Coronary artery bypass graft
Hip and knee replacement
MRI and CT scanning
Mammography
New drugs for depression
New drugs for ulcers and acid reflux

Thanks in part to such innovations (and in part to declines in cigarette smoking), the overall age-adjusted death rate has decreased by 20 percent since 1980. But some major causes of death, such as cancer and diabetes, show little or no decline in mortality. When medical care could do little to extend life for anyone, not much was expected of it. In an era of great progress, however, expectations of further gains accelerate. The more medical care does to keep people alive and healthier, the more is demanded of it.

Moreover, despite the gains in health and wealth, many Americans still experience a troubled old age. In addition to the inevitable loss of family and friends, diminution of status, and existential concerns, many elderly persons face two potentially serious financial problems: lower income and greater expenditures for medical care. Physiological changes are the primary cause of both lower earnings and poorer health. Earnings are also affected adversely by obsolescence of skills and knowledge and by public and private policies that reduce the incentives of older persons to continue working and increase the cost to employers of employing older workers.

These financial problems have been widely discussed in recent years; the chapters in this volume provide additional food for thought. Unfortunately, most policy discussions of the financial problems of elderly persons tend to focus on only one program at a time. Thus, there is a plethora of papers on Social Security, Medicare, Medicaid, employment-based pensions, Medigap insurance, and so on. Sometimes these sharply focused studies are required by legislative or administrative exigencies, but I believe a holistic view is a necessary complement to such fragmented analyses.

A HOLISTIC VIEW

A holistic view focuses simultaneously on the financing of health care and the financing of other goods and services. It also focuses on the expenditures of the elderly that are self-financed as well as on those that are financed by transfers from the young. A holistic view cautions against policy proposals that claim we can patch existing public programs for elderly persons without major changes in policies and behavior. These limited proposals usually include means testing benefits, subsidies, modest increases in taxes, and various administrative maneuvers. When they are examined one program at a time, such proposals may seem reasonable and feasible. The entire package, however, applied to all programs for elderly persons, is likely to create large disincentives for work and saving before retirement and require huge transfers that will ultimately be rejected by taxpayers.

At one time it was reasonable to treat the problem of earnings replacement separately from the problem of paying for health care. Health care expenditures of elderly persons were small relative to expenditures on other goods and services, and a holistic approach was not essential. Now, however, health care expenditures equal or exceed expenditures for all other goods and services for many elderly persons, and given the trends of recent decades, this may be true for the elderly as a group within twenty years.

Artificial separation of the problem of earnings replacement from that of health care payment ignores the fact that there are often trade-offs between the two. Money is money, and for most elderly persons there is never enough to go around. This is self-evident where private funds are concerned. Low-income elderly persons, for example, frequently must choose between prescription drugs and an adequate diet. For middle-income elderly persons, the choice may be between more expensive Medigap insurance and an airplane trip to a grandchild's wedding. Difficult choices are also apparent with respect to public funds. The same tax receipts that could be used to maintain or increase retirement benefits could be used to fund additional health care, and vice versa. Policy analysts who fail to understand that a large increase in Medicare spending will jeopardize the government's ability to fulfill its Social Security commitments ignore the realities of economics and politics.

A holistic approach not only requires analyses that encompass different government programs but also must involve examination of the two-way interactions between changes in the private sector and public programs. For instance, from 1993 to 2000 the share of employers providing health insurance for retirees declined from 40 percent to less than 25 percent (Freudenheim 2000). This change may suggest that government provision of health insurance for retirees should expand, but such expansion could result in further decreases in private coverage.

Another significant trend in the private sector that has major implications for the future financial problems of elderly persons is the shift in private pensions from defined benefit to defined contribution. This change works well for retirees when the stock market is rising briskly, but it looks less attractive when the stock market flattens or goes into decline. Moreover, the 401(k) plans and IRAs that have supplanted the traditional retirement plans typically do not call for automatic annuitization upon retirement. This can be advantageous to retirees who would like access to their money but can be problematic for them and for taxpayers if they lose their retirement savings in bad investments or spend them at too rapid a rate. Furthermore, if annuitization is voluntary, the terms available are likely to suffer from the problem of adverse selection. Hurd and McCarry (2001) have shown that the ability of individuals to predict their longevity is significantly greater than could be expected from chance. For this reason, some compulsory annuitization is probably as necessary as some compulsory enrollment in health insurance.

"FULL INCOME"

To provide a holistic framework for addressing the financial problems of elderly persons, it is useful to think of the "full income" (or its equivalent, "full consumption") of the elderly. I define *full income* as the sum of personal income and health care expenditures not paid from personal income. Two critical questions can be addressed within this framework: (1) How much of the elderly's full income is devoted to health care and how much to other goods and services? (2) How much of the elderly's full income is provided by transfers from the population under age 65 (Social Security retirement payments, Medicare, and similar programs) and how much is provided by elderly persons themselves (earnings, pensions, income from savings, and the like)?

Using data from the Current Population Survey (CPS) (U.S. Department of Commerce and U.S. Department of Labor 1997), the Medicare Current Beneficiary Survey (Health Care Financing Administration 1997), and other sources, with adjustments for underreporting, I estimate that 35 percent of the elderly's full income in 1997 was devoted to health care and 65 percent to other goods and services (see the right-hand column of Table 17.1). I also estimate that 56 percent of full income was provided by transfers from the "young" and 44 percent by elderly persons themselves (see the bottom row of Table 17.1).

Probably the most important information in Table 17.1 is the disaggregation of full income by use *and* source found in the interior of the table. We see that elderly persons are much more dependent on transfers for health care expenditures than for other goods and services. Of the 35 percent of full income that goes for health care, more than three-fourths (27 divided by 35) is provided by the young, as opposed to less than half (29 divided by 65) for other goods and services. This fact combined with the tendency for spending on health care to grow more rapidly than spending on other goods and services will pose major problems for policymakers and elderly persons within two decades.

Table 17.2 shows what the uses and sources of full income would be

Table 17.1. Americans Age 65 or Older, Sources and Uses of "Full Income" in 1997 (percentage distribution)

	Source		
Use	Under Age 65	Age 65 or Older	Total
Health care	27	8	35
Other	29	36	65
Total	56	44	100

Source: Fuchs 2000.

Table 17.2. Projected Uses and Sources of "Full Income" in 2020 under Alternative Assumptions about Gap between Growth of Health and Other

	Gap (percent per annum)			
	0	1	2	3
Use				
Health	35	40	46	52
Other	65	60	54	48
Source				
<65	56	58	60	62
≥65	44	42	40	38

Source: Fuchs 2000.
Note: Assuming that the share of Health and the share of Other provided by <65 remain constant.

in 2020 if the generations under 65 continue to bear the same share of health care and "other" as in 1997. If health care spending does not grow more rapidly than "other" (the first column of Table 17.2), the shares of uses and sources will be identical to those shown in Table 17.1. If health care spending grows 3 percent per annum more rapidly than "other" (the last column in Table 17.2), we see that the health share of full income would jump from 35 to 52 percent and the young would provide 62 percent of full income instead of the 56 percent provided in 1997. These calculations are all per capita; that is, they do not take into account the fact that the ratio of elderly to those under age 65 will be higher in 2020 than it was in 1997. Thus, the figures in Table

17.2 underestimate the potential increased dependency of the elderly on transfers from the young.

Will spending on health for elderly persons grow faster than spending on other goods and services? This question cannot be answered with certainty, but it would be prudent to assume that it will. Over the period 1970–2000, Medicare expenditures per elderly person enrollee grew approximately 2.8 percent per annum faster than GDP per capita (excluding health care expenditures). The growth of the nonhealth economy is an indicator of the rate at which expenditures on "other" could grow. The "gap" of 2.8 percent per annum is attributable primarily to technological advances such as those listed above. Will the pace of technological advance in medicine slow in the next two decades? Not likely. There are currently seven hundred new drugs in development for the diseases of aging, and as the elderly's share of the health care market increases, the share of medical R&D focused on elderly persons is likely to grow.

In theory, advances in medical technology do not necessarily lead to higher expenditures, but in practice that is usually the way it works. The last major exception to this rule occurred a half century ago with the introduction and rapid diffusion of antibiotics. But antibiotics were a very special kind of medical advance. They were given to patients who had life- threatening infections, most of whom who were in otherwise good health. Many beneficiaries were children and young adults who, once the infection was cured, went on to live many years without requiring major medical intervention. By contrast, advances in medical technology that extend life or improve quality of life for older Americans do not offer that same prospect of reducing overall utilization of medical care. Indeed, many expensive interventions, such as open-heart surgery, will only be undertaken on patients who are otherwise in reasonably good health. Moreover, antibiotics were very inexpensive to produce and dispense. By contrast, many of the products currently under development in the biotech and bioengineering laboratories are likely to be expensive to produce and implement.

IMPLICATIONS FOR POLICY

The coming increase in the absolute and relative number of elderly persons will unquestionably increase the burden on the working population and require an increase in taxes. But if the scenario sketched out in Table 17.2 materializes, that is, if health care expenditures for elderly persons grow 2 to 3 percent per annum more rapidly than expenditures on other goods and services, the burden on the young is likely to be unbearable. There seem to be only two possible escapes from this bleak scenario: slow the rate of growth of health care expenditures, or require elderly persons to assume more of the responsibility for paying for their health care.

Slowing the growth of health care expenditures may not be feasible, and even if it is feasible, it may not be desirable. Although advances in technology are the driving force behind the growth of medical expenditures, many of these advances contribute significantly to longer, better-quality lives. Politicians in both parties strongly support increased spending for medical research, and private decision makers in the drug and biotech industries are betting tens of billions of dollars each year that the money to pay for advances in medical technology will be forthcoming. Many economists now assert that the advances of recent decades, albeit expensive, are "good buys" and see no reason why that will not be true of future advances as well.

If health care expenditures for elderly persons continue to grow rapidly, however, and if the ability to finance these expenditures by transfers from the young reaches its limit, the only alternative is for elderly persons to pick up a larger share of the bill. If these payments must come from incomes that grow at only a modest pace, elderly persons will become increasingly "health care poor." Indeed, many are already in that unhappy condition. Although eligible for MRIs, angiograms, bypass surgery, and other high-tech diagnostic and surgical interventions, they do not have the resources to purchase a new mattress, to heat their house to a comfortable temperature in winter, to take a taxi to the doctor, or to access other goods and services that would make life more bearable.

Elderly persons must have additional personal income in order to avoid the scenario in which more and more of them will become "health care poor." They need more income from *savings* (including pensions and investments) and from *earnings,* which means they will have to work more both before and after age 65. Why do millions of Americans reach age 65 so heavily dependent on transfers from the young? One possibility is that their income over the life cycle was so low that they could barely meet everyday expenses, let alone save for retirement. This explanation is undoubtedly correct for some low-income elderly, but analyses of longitudinal data by Venti and Wise (1998) show that inequality in savings for retirement varies greatly even among those with the same earnings prior to retirement. This conclusion holds after adjustments for special factors that affect the ability to save and for differences in investment returns.

An examination of CPS data on sources of income provides additional evidence concerning the question of the relation between saving and income. To obtain the statistics shown in Figure 17.1, everyone 65 and over was sorted into deciles based on their Social Security income, an ordering that is probably similar to one based on lifetime earnings.[1] Within each decile individuals were sorted by savings income (pensions, interest, dividends, and rent) and the 25th, 50th, and 75th percentiles were identified. The results reveal that although savings income tends to be positively correlated with Social Security income, there is great variation *within each decile.* Many elderly persons in the lower deciles have substantial savings income, whereas many in the higher deciles have very little. Consider the striking differences among workers in the middle range of income, that is, Social Security deciles 5 and 6. Those are the quintessential "average workers." At least one-fourth of them have virtually no savings income, but another fourth have savings income of over eight thousand dollars per year. It is clear from these data that when saving is voluntary, many individuals do not save. To provide higher income for future elderly persons and to reduce inequality among them, it will be necessary to introduce some form of compulsory saving.

The other major potential source of increase in income for elderly persons is more paid work. In the late 1990s, mean hours of work per man age 60 was only 1,495 per year, at age 65 only 701 hours, and at age 70 only 338 hours.[2] The comparable figures for women were 926, 423, and 150 hours per year, respectively. Given that most Americans

Savings income

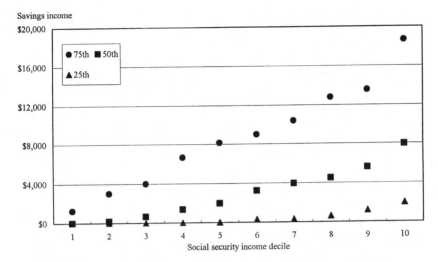

Fig. 17.1. Savings income by Social Security income decile, Americans aged 65 and older, 1997. Symbols represent percentiles. *Source:* Fuchs 1999a.

at these ages are in reasonably good health and suffer from fewer physical limitations than earlier cohorts, there seems to be ample potential for more work.

Since 1975 life expectancy at age 65 has risen appreciably, especially for men. This change, unfortunately, has not been accompanied by any increase in paid work by older men and by only a small increase for women. Thus, the number of years when income must come from sources other than employment has grown, and employment's share of total income was less in 1995 than in 1975. Table 17.3 provides a useful summary of how work has failed to keep pace with increases in life expectancy.

The first row of Table 17.3 presents life expectancy at age 65, a familiar statistic calculated from age-specific mortality rates in the year indicated. It is the mean years of life remaining for the cohort that reached age 65 (in, say, 1995) if it experienced the age-specific mortality that prevailed in 1995. Expected years of work is conceptually similar; it is obtained by combining age-specific rates of work with age-specific survival rates. It shows the years of work that the cohort that reached age 65 (in, say, 1995) would experience if the age-specific work

Table 17.3. Expected at Age 65

Expected	Men			Women		
	1975	1985	1995	1975	1985	1995
Years of life	13.7	14.6	15.6	18.0	18.6	18.9
Years of work (FTE)[a]	2.0	1.7	1.9	0.7	0.7	1.1
Years not at work	11.7	12.9	13.7	17.3	17.9	17.8

Source: Fuchs 1999b.
Note: Based on age-specific mortality and employment rates in the year indicated.
[a]Assuming a full-time work year of 2000 hours.

rate and the mortality that prevailed in 1995 continued through the lifetime of that cohort. The expected years of work are not forecast, anymore than the life expectancies are forecast. The values could be used for forecasting purposes, however, by making assumptions about future trends in age-specific mortality and in age-specific work rates.

Inspection of Table 17.3 reveals that years of life expected at age 65 increased at a rapid pace from 1975 to 1995, more rapidly for men than for women, although the latter still enjoyed a 4.3 year advantage over men in 1995. In contrast to life expectancy, expected years of work remained relatively constant, at about 2 years for men and 1 year for women (full time equivalents). The number of years *not* at work (row 1 minus row 2) rose appreciably for men from 11.7 in 1975 to 13.7 in 1995. Women also show an increase in years *not* at work, from 17.3 to 17.8 years. Health care and consumption of other goods and services in these years not at work must be financed by the accumulated savings of the elderly or by transfers from the young.

To make paid work for older Americans more attractive, there must be a reexamination of all policies that create high implicit marginal tax rates on earnings and employment as well as a review of employment laws, which often make it more costly for employers to hire or retain older workers. In addition to providing more income, there could be additional benefits to elderly persons from making work more feasible and desirable. Work often provides satisfaction, identity, and an opportunity to maintain or develop relationships. Moreover, staying active usually contributes to better health. We should recall the words of another English poet, Alfred Tennyson, who in contemplating Ulysses in retirement has the aging hero say, "How dull it is to pause, to make an end, to rust unburnished, not to shine in use! As though to breathe were life."

ACKNOWLEDGMENTS

I am indebted to the Robert Wood Johnson Foundation and the Kaiser Family Foundation for financial support. The research assistance of Sarah Rosen is also gratefully acknowledged.

NOTES

1. All household income was assumed to be shared equally among the members of the household.

2. These figures were calculated from the 1996–98 Current Population Surveys. They reflect the total annual hours worked for each age-sex group divided by the total number in the group regardless of labor force status.

REFERENCES

Butler, R. N. 1975. *Why Survive? Being Old in America.* New York: Harper and Row.

Freudenheim, M. 2000. *New York Times,* December 31, 38.

Fuchs, V. R. 1999a. Health Care for the Elderly: How Much? Who Will Pay for It? *Health Affairs* 18, no. 1: 11–21.

———. 1999b. Provide, Provide: The Economics of Aging. In A. Rettenmaier and T. R. Savings, eds., *Medicare Reform: Issues and Answers.* Chicago: University of Chicago Press.

———. 2000. Medicare Reform: The Larger Picture. *Journal of Economic Perspectives* (spring): 1–14.

Fuchs, V. R., and H. C. Sox, Jr. 2001. Physicians' Views of the Relative Importance to Patients of Thirty Medical Innovations: A Survey of Leading General Internists. *Health Affairs* 20, no. 5 (September–October).

Health Care Financing Administration (Office of Strategic Planning). 1997. Medicare Current Beneficiary Survey, <http://www.hcfa.gov/surveys/mcbs/Default.htm>.

Hiraizumi, W. 2000. Mass Longevity Transforms Our Society. *Proceedings of the American Philosophical Society* 144, no. 4: 361–83.

Hurd, M. D., and K. McCarry. 2001. The Predictive Validity of Subjective Probabilities of Survival. *Economic Journal,* forthcoming.

U.S. Department of Commerce (Bureau of the Census) and U.S. Department of Labor (Bureau of Labor Statistics). 1997. Current Population Survey, <http://www.bls.census.gov/cps/cpsmain.htm>.

Venti, S. F., and Wise, D. A. 1998. The Cause of Wealth Dispersion at Retirement: Choice or Chance? *American Economic Review* 88, no. 2: 185–91.

Index